Current Topics in Pathology
88

Susan M. Dodd (Ed.)

Tubulointerstitial and Cystic Disease of the Kidney

Contributors
S.M. Dodd   D. Falkenstein   S. Goldfarb
H.-J. Gröne   B. Iványi   T.N. Khan   N. Marcussen
E.G. Neilson   S. Olsen   J.A. Roberts   R. Sinniah
P.D. Wilson   G. Wolf   F.N. Ziyadeh

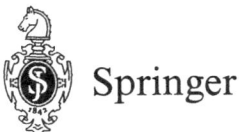

Springer

Susan M. Dodd, Dr.
University of London
The London Hospital Medical College
The Royal London Hospital
Department of Morbid Anatomy
London El 1BB, Great Britain

With 62 Figures and 18 Tables

ISBN-13:978-3-642-79519-0   e-ISBN-13:978-3-642-79517-6
DOI:10.1007/978-3-642-79517-6

Library of Congress Cataloging-in-Publication Data. Tubulointerstitial and cystic disease of the kidney/S.M. Dodd (ed.); contributors, S.M. Dodd... [et al.].   p.   cm. – (Current topics in pathology; 88) Includes bibliographical references and index. ISBN-13:978-3-642-79519-0
1. Kidney, Cystic–Pathophysiology.   2. Kidney tubules–Pathophysiology.   I.
Dodd, S.M. (Susan M.)   II. Series: Current topics in pathology; v. 88. [DNLM: 1. Kidney Glomerulus–pathology.   2. Kidney, Tubules–pathology.   W1 CU821H v. 88 1995/WJ 301T885 1995] RB1.E6 vol. 88 [RC918.C957] 616.07 s–dc20 [616.6′ 107] DNLM/DLC for Library of Congress 95-3278

© Springer-Verlag Berlin Heidelberg 1995
Softcover reprint of the hardcover 1st edition 1995

Typesetting: Thomson Press (India) Ltd., New Delhi

SPIN: 10089894   25/3130/SPS – 5 4 3 2 1 0 – Printed on acid-free paper

List of Contributors

DODD, S.M., Dr.
University of London
The London Hospital Medical College
The Royal London Hospital
Department of Morbid Anatomy
London E1 1BB, Great Britain

FALKENSTEIN, D., Dr.
Division of Nephrology
The Johns Hopkins University School
of Medicine
Ross Building 954
720 Rutland Avenue
Baltimore, MD 21205, USA

GOLDFARB, S., Prof. Dr.
Renal-Electrolyte and Hypertension
Division
700 Clinical Research Building
University of Pennsylvania School
of Medicine
422 Curie Boulevard
Philadelphia, PA 19104-6144, USA

GRÖNE, H.-J., Prof. Dr.
Department of Pathology
Philipps-University of Marburg
Klinikum Lahnberge
Baldinger Str.
35043 Marburg, Germany

IVÁNYI, B., Dr.
Department of Pathology
Albert Szent-Gyorgi University
of Medicine
H-6701 Szeged, Pf. 401
Kossuth L. sgt 40, Hungary

KHAN, T.N., Dr.
Department of Pathology
National University Hospital
National University of Singapore
Lower Kent Ridge Road
Singapore 0511

MARCUSSEN, N., Dr.   University Institute of Pathology
                             Aarhus Kommunehospital
                             Stereological Research Laboratory
                             University of Aarhus
                             Tage-Hansens Gade 2
                             8000 Aarhus C, Denmark

NEILSON, E.G., Prof. Dr.   Renal-Electrolyte and Hypertension
                             Division
                             700 Clinical Research Building
                             University of Pennsylvania School
                             of Medicine
                             422 Curie Boulevard
                             Philadelphia, PA 19104-6144, USA

OLSEN, S., Prof. Dr.   University Institute of Pathology
                             Aarhus Kommunehospital
                             Stereological Research Laboratory
                             University of Aarhus
                             Tage-Hansens Gade 2
                             8000 Aarhus C, Denmark

ROBERTS, J.A.   Department of Urology
                             Tulane Regional Primate Research
                             Center
                             18703 Three Rivers Road
                             Covington, LA 70433, USA

SINNIAH, R., Prof. Dr.   Department of Pathology
                             National University Hospital
                             National University of Singapore
                             Lower Kent Ridge Road
                             Singapore 0511

WILSON, P.D., Dr.   Division of Nephrology
                             The Johns Hopkins University School
                             of Medicine
                             Ross Building 954
                             720 Rutland Avenue
                             Baltimore, MD 21205, USA

WOLF, G., Dr.   Department of Internal Medicine
                             Division of Nephrology
                             University of Frankfurt
                             Frankfurt, Germany

ZIYADEH, F.N., Prof. Dr.   Renal-Electrolyte and Hypertension
Division
700 Clinical Research Building
University of Pennsylvania School
of Medicine
422 Curie Boulevard
Philadelphia, PA 19104-6144, USA

Preface

Over recent years, much renal research has focused on the pathology of the glomerulus, where many primary renal insults occur. However, nearly thirty years have passed since Risdon's study made the apparently anomalous observation that the extent of damage to the tubulointerstitial compartment is the major determinant of renal outcome in a variety of human glomerular diseases.

This volume covers various aspects of tubulointerstitial disease, and starts with an update on cystic disease of the kidney, by Drs. WILSON and FALKENSTEIN, which includes recent experimental data on the altered properties of cystic epithelium.

My own chapter gives an overview of the mechanisms of tubulointerstitial damage in progressive renal disease and includes a discussion of the possible role of cytokines, vasoactive peptides and peptide growth factors found over the last few years to be secreted by renal tubular cells. These comments are expanded in the contribution by Dr. WOLF and Professor NEILSON, who provide a detailed account of the cellular biology of tubulointerstitial growth.

The earliest studies from the 1960s attempted to correlate histomorphometry of the tubulointerstitium with renal outcome. Dr. KHAN and Professor SINNIAH provide us with an update on morphometric methods as applied to the kidney using new techniques. Similar techniques are employed by Dr. IVANYI and Professor OLSEN who give a detailed stereomorphological account of tubulitis both in acute allograft rejection, where its recognition is central to the diagnosis, and in other forms of tubulointerstitial disease.

The apparent disparity between the extent of glomerular damage and progression to chronic renal failure may be related to the presence of atubular glomeruli, where disconnection at the origin of the proximal tubule occurs, and the role of these structures in chronic renal disease is discussed by Dr. MARCUSSEN.

Renal injury is a major cause of morbidity and mortality in patients with diabetes mellitus. Professors ZIYADEH and GOLDFARB describe in detail the characteristic changes that occur in the tubuloepithelial and interstitial compartments of the diabetic kidney.

Dr. GRONE's chapter provides an account of two experimental models of tubular atrophy and cystic hyperplasia and discusses their clinical relevance. The volume is concluded by Dr. ROBERTS with a discussion of the mechanisms of renal damage in reflux nephropathy and of potential prevention of chronic pyelonephritis, the cause of one-fifth of all cases of chronic renal failure.

The topics covered here consider, in some depth, certain aspects of tubulointerstitial disease including recent research which has been facilitated by new techniques and which advance considerably our understanding of various disease processes. It is hoped that they will serve as stimulation for further research in this important area.

SUSAN M. DODD

Contents

The Pathology of Human Renal Cystic Disease

P.D. Wilson and D. Falkenstein

1 Introduction and Classification

Renal cystic disease comprises a wide group of disorders which may be congenital, acquired, sporadic, or genetically determined. All of these disorders have in common the presence of multiple cysts in the kidney, and this may be a primary disease event and lead to organ dysfunction and end-stage renal failure or cyst formation, may be secondary to other tumor or systemic disorders, and may or may not be symptomatic. Several classification schemes for renal cystic diseases have been proposed and modified in the past, and these will probably continue to be modified as more genetic and pathologic information is gathered. One simplified scheme based on current, although necessarily incomplete, published information is suggested in Table 1. For the purposes of classification, the renal cystic diseases have been separated into those of genetic and nongenetic origin and further subdivided into those entities in which renal cyst formation is the primary disease event and those in which cyst formation is a secondary event

Current Topics in Pathology
Volume 88, S.M. Dodd (Ed.)
© Springer-Verlag Berlin Heidelberg 1995

associated with a separate genetic syndrome. It appears that cyst formation in the kidney is a common response to genetic mutation, and an understanding of the molecular basis of these events would be of significant importance in potential retardation of cyst enlargement and eventual gene therapy strategies. The ultimate goal of renal cystic disease research is to isolate and identify the gene responsible for each disease. To date, although significant and rapid progress has been made in the area of cystic disease genetics and the chromosome locations of many of these genes have now been determined, few of the genes themselves have actually been cloned or their encoded protein products characterized.

It might be argued that the most important of the genetic renal cystic diseases—by virtue of its wide clinical impact leading to end-stage renal failure, its extremely high incidence (1:500–1:1000), and complete penetrance—is autosomal dominant polycystic kidney disease (ADPKD). This was formerly known as "adult-onset polycystic kidney disease", but this term is misleading and has been replaced, since, with the advent of improved ultrasonography and CT detection techniques, it is clear that multiple cysts can develop as early as in utero in patients with ADPKD (SEDMAN et al. 1987), although symptoms may take decades to appear. In addition, there have been several reported cases of clear early onset ADPKD in children, leading to renal failure in the first and second decade of life (FICK et al. 1992). ADPKD is the most common lethal genetic disease inherited as an autosomal dominant trait; it affects 500 000 patients in the United States and 6 million worldwide and accounts for 7% of U.S. patients who receive renal replacement therapy by dialysis. Typically, patients present with clinical manifestations in adulthood, including flank and back pain, abdominal enlargement, hematuria, renal stones, recurrent urinary tract infections, a loss of renal concentrating ability, and hypertension. In addition, certain groups (18%) of ADPKD patients have a predisposition to intracranial aneurysms and mitral valve prolapse (25%) (GABOW et al. 1984; HOSSACK et al. 1988; CHAPMAN et al. 1992). Fifty percent of ADPKD patients with renal cysts also exhibit hepatic cysts which arise in the portal tracts and are lined by a single layer of bile duct epithelium. The prevalence of these hepatic cysts in most marked in women patients (EVERSON et al. 1988). In addition, cysts have been found within the pancreas in 5–10% of ADPKD patients and more rarely in seminal vesicles, spleen, and thyroid. Colonic diverticulae are also seen in 25% of these patients (P.A. Gabow, personal communication).

To date, the renal cystic disease that affects approximately 85% of patients with typical ADPKD has been linked to polymorphic markers on the short arm of chromosome 16, confined within a 750-kb pair region of this chromosome between 16p13.3. And recently the gene (PKD-1) has been identified as a 14 kb transcript and partial sequence obtained (REEDERS et al. 1985; GERMINO et al. 1992; EUROPEAN CONSORTIUM 1994). However, lack of homology with known proteins has not shed light on the underlying defect in this disease. However, expression analysis suggest developmental regulation of a membrane protein. In 10–15% of patients with typical ADPKD symptoms the disease is not linked to these markers on chromosomome 16, and they tend to show a slower

Table 1. Classification of renal cystic diseases

Genetic	Inheritance	Chromosome assignment	Gene	Reference
Primary cyst formation				
Autosomal dominant polycystic kidney disease	D	16p13.3	YES	[Reeders et al. 1985; European Consortium 1994]
	D	4q13–q23	NO	[Kimberling et al. 1988, 1993; Peters et al. 1993]
	D	NO	NO	[Daoust et al. 1993]
Autosomal recessive polycystic kidney disease	R	6p21-cen	NO	[Zerres et al. 1994]
Medullary sponge kidney	D	NO	NO	
Nepronophthisis	R	2p	NO	[Antignac et al. 1993]
Medullary cystic kindey disease	D	NO	NO	
Secondary cyst formation				
Tuberous sclerosis	D	9q 34	NO	[Fryer et al. 1987]
		11q 14–23	NO	[Smith 1990]
		12q 22–24	NO	[Fahsold et al. 1991]
		16p 13	YES	[Kandt et al. 1992; Consortium 1993]
von Hippel-Lindau disease	D	3p 25–26	YES	[Seizinger et al. 1991; Latif et al. 1993]
Zellweger's cerebrohepatorenal syndrome	R	NO	NO	
Wilms' tumor (1%)		11p 13	YES	[Call et al. 1990]
Beckwith-Wiedemann syndrome	D	11p 15.5	NO	[Dowdy et al. 1991]
Renal cell carcinoma		3p 14.2	NO	[Gerber et al. 1988]
Meckel's syndrome	R	NO	NO	
Trisomy 21, 13, 18,				
Nongenetic				
Simple cysts				
Acquired cystic disease				
Multicystic dysplasia				
Multilocular cystic disease				

D, Dominant; *R*, recessive

progression to renal failure (KIMBERLING et al. 1988; PARFREY et al. 1990). Recently, this disease has been mapped to chromosome 4q 13–q23, also by linkage analysis with polymorphic markers; this is the first step to narrowing down the search for this gene, which has been given the notation "PKD-2" (KIMBERLING et al. 1993; PETERS et al. 1993). To add to this growing complexity, it appears there may also be yet a third gene causing ADPKD, since a family has been identified whose disease did not segregate with either the chromosome 16 or chromosome 4 polymorphic flanking markers (DAOUST et al. 1993).

Another important genetically determined renal cystic disease is autosomal recessive polycystic kidney disease (ARPKD, formerly known as "infantile polycystic kidney disease". ARPKD is less common than ADPKD, with an estimated frequency of 1 : 40 000, but is a significant cause of death in utero, at birth, or in the early postnatal period, often due to pulmonary insufficiency as a result of failure of lung development, presumably caused in part by encroachment of the enormously enlarged cystic kidneys. Oliguric renal failure may also contribute to early death, but this is usually of secondary importance. Some children with ARPKD manage to survive the postnatal period, but their prognosis is poor due to progressive renal failure and, most commonly, hepatic fibrosis involving the portal tracts. This gene has recently been mapped to chromosome 6p 21–cen. Although several rodent models are available for study that develop renal cysts with an autosomal recessive pattern of inheritance, there is quite a wide spectrum of genetics and pathophysiology in these animal models, including mapping by linkage of murine recessive PKD loci to mouse chromosomes, 9, 12, and 14 in some, none of which are synteneic to human chromosome 6p (NAGAO and TAKAHASHI 1991; TAKAHASHI et al. 1991). This leads to the conclusion that autosomal recessive inheritance of renal cystic disease is a complex process in mice and rats, and none are known to represent the human disease at present. It should also be noted that at this time there are no rodent models of cystic disease known to be inherited as a dominant trait that accurately reflect the pattern of pathology seen in human ADPKD.

Medullary cystic disease, in which, by definition, renal cysts are confined to the medulla, includes medullary sponge kidney which has an incidence of 1 : 5000, is usually sporadic and asymptomatic, but is familial, with a dominant pattern of inheritance in 5% of cases. Medullary sponge kidney does not usually give rise to any significant renal functional impairment per se, but it may be discovered incidentally or as a complication, particularly in patients with urinary tract infections or renal stone formation. No increases in hypertension or alterations in glomerular filtration rate (GFR) or renal plasma flow (RPF) are associated with this disease. However, reduced renal concentrating ability due to vasopressin resistance and impaired urinary acidification due to reduced excretion of titratable acid have been documented in 40% of patients and are consistent with a distal collecting tubule defect. Hypercalciuria and stone formation are particularly common in these patients. No information is available concerning the chromosome location or identity of this disease gene.

The familial nephronophthisis-medullary cystic kidney disease complex has a more significant clinical impact, leading to renal failure in children and adults. These used to be described as two separate disease entities due to their heterogeneity of patterns of inheritance, since in children this is an autosomal recessive trait and in adults a dominant mutation. However, pathologic analysis shows significant overlapping of the features of this disease complex and has led to the conclusion that they should be considered the same disease. Definitive clarification of this question will await future isolation of the gene(s). To date, linkage analysis has shown that the inheritance of juvenile nephronophthisis is linked to a region of human chromosome 2p (ANTIGNAC et al. 1993), and it will be of significant interest, when similar studies are accomplished for adult medullary cystic kidney disease to determine whether this is linked to the same chromosome and locus. Fifty percent of all patients with familial nephro nophthisis-medullary cystic disease inherit this as a receissive trait and these children fail to thrive; they have progressive azotemia, polyuria, and severe renal salt wasting, which typically lead to renal failure in the second decade. It is an important cause of chronic renal disease in children. It has been estimated to account for 15% of end-stage renal failure in children. In the 30% of patients with this disease complex who inherit it as a dominant trait there is also progression to renal failure in adulthood.

Renal cysts can also occur as a sometimes substantial, but secondary component of other hereditary syndromes. These include tuberous sclerosis, an autosomal dominant systemic disease trait of variable penetrance characterized by hamartomatous malformations of the skin, kidney, brain, eye, bone, liver, and lung. Kidney involvement is common (50%) and takes the form of both angiomyolipomas and cysts. Sometimes renal cystic involvement is sufficient to cause renal failure and hypertension. Similarly, renal cystic involvement is common in von Hippel-Lindau disease (cerebroretinal angiomatosis), which is inherited as an autosomal dominant trait and is characterized by angiomatous cysts of the cerebellum, retina, kidney, and pancreas. In addition, an increased incidence of renal carcinoma is seen in association with von Hippel-Lindau disease. It is of interest that tuberous sclerosis appears to be a multigenic dominant disorder, and that one of the disease loci is found on chromosome 16p13, in a region close to the ADPKD (PKD-1) locus. This chromosome 16p gene for tuberous sclerosis was recently isolated and determined to encode the protein "tuberin", which shares homology with a GTPase-activating protein GAP3 (CONSORTIUM 1993). The von Hippel-Lindau gene, also recently isolated, shares a chromosomal location 3p25-26, although quite proximal, with familial renal cell carcinoma found at chromosome 3p14.2 (SEIZINGER et al. 1991). No shared homology with known proteins has been reported to date for this gene (LATIF et al. 1993b).

Other syndromes in which renal cysts occur include Zellweger's cerebrohepatorenal syndrome, Wilms' tumor, Beckwith-Wiedemann syndrome, Meckel's syndrome, and renal cell carcinoma. They also accompany the chromosomal abnormalities trisomy 21, 13, 18, and C. Not only genetic and developmental factors lead to renal cyst formation, however, since simple cysts occur in many kidneys, the numbers of which are known to increase with age. It is clear that certain drugs and dialysis are significant inducers of cyst formation in the kidney and can lead to acquired cystic disease, which also has been suggested to predispose to renal tumor development (HUGHSON et al. 1980).

Therefore, it is clear that renal cyst formation can be a primary or secondary phenomenon and that it can be the result of developmental abnormalities with or without a genetic component as in ARPKD or dysplasia, respectively; a direct result of genetic mutations as in ADPKD, ARPKD, and medullary cystic disease; or the result of factors acquired with age, drugs, or dialysis. Although it is clear that increased genetic information and, ultimately, the isolation and characterization of all the disease genes associated with renal cyst formation will be of paramount importance in the analysis of renal cystic disease, it is also clear that the pathophysiology of each disease process will yield many additional important clues which will allow complete definition of how cysts are formed as a result of developmental, genetic, and non-genetic malformations, and will have an important impact on strategies designed to slow disease progression by cyst expansion. The definition of the epithelial cell phenotype(s) lining renal cysts and of the cellular pathologic processes involved in cyst expansion therefore occupies the rest of this chapter. The majority of experimental information available is related to the genetic malformation ADPKD, since this is a common disease and significant amounts of material are therefore available for study. Recently, interest has also increased in studying other renal cystic diseases, notably 1ARPKD, and it may be anticipated that sufficient information will be obtained to significantly increase our understanding of the pathophysiology of these diseases.

2 Pathology of Autosomal Dominant Polycystic Kidney Disease

Patients with ADPKD usually become symptomatic in adulthood, although childhood onset of clinical symptoms of progressive renal insufficiency has also been reported. ADPKD is characterized by extreme bilateral enlargement of the kidneys due to the presence of multiple cysts, distributed equally throughout the cortex and medulla and resulting in a loss of the reniform structure of the kidney and disappearance of the cortico-medullary boundary. Cysts, which are epithelial lined, spherical, sac-like structures filled with fluid, can vary in size from a few millimeters to several centimeters, and the cyst fluids contained within may vary in color and composition from clear and yellow to turbid and brown, the latter reflecting incidents of hemorrhage into the cyst cavity. The ion and protein content of cyst fluids has been shown to vary from low to high for sodium (<20 to >160 mmol/l), chloride, and potassium, and the presence of epidermal growth factor, erythropoietin, and proteases such as renin has been reported (GARDNER 1969; ECKARDT et al. 1989; DU et al. 1991; TORRES et al. 1992; A.C. Sherwood, personal communication). Kidney enlargement and cyst development usually progress bilaterally and synchronously, although examples of asymmetric renal enlargement have been reported, particularly in the early stages of ADPKD progression. The increase in kidney size and weight has been measured at as much as 12- and 25-fold, respectively (BENNETT et al. 1973; HEPTINSTALL 1992). Microdissection and lectin-staining studies, as well as morphological analysis of ADPKD kidneys in the early stages of cyst enlargement, have established that cysts arise from every segment of the nephron (BAERT 1978; FARAGGIANA et al. 1985), a feature which distinguishes this disease from many other renal cystic diseases, including ARPKD (see Table 2 for summary). This is an important consideration in determining the validity and potential usefulness of experimental animal models, as is inheritance as a dominant trait. To date, no animal models have been characterized that fulfill the criteria of dominant inheritance and slowly progressive renal cystic disease in which all nephron segments are involved. Fortunately, since human ADPKD is a common mutation, and with the advent of tissue culture of microdissected cysts it has never the less been possible to carry out significant studies of the pathophysiology and cellular and molecular biology of ADPKD progression (WILSON et al. 1986, 1991, 1992, 1993a; WILSON and BURROW 1992). In our own laboratory we have examined the pathology of 31 end-stage ADKPD kidneys from nephrectomy specimens taken at the time of surgery, prior to (45%) or after a period of treatment of end-stage renal failure by dialysis. In addition, we have examined 15 early-stage, predialysis and often presymptomatic ADPKD kidneys from victims of automobile accidents or intracerebral aneurysms. All kidneys were prepared at 4° C by in situ perfusion with Eurocollins or UW solution and cross-clamping, identical to the preparation of normal kidneys for use in transplantation, with no period of warm ischemia. Fifty-five normal human kidneys also prepared in this way showed no

Table 2. Pathologic features of venal cystic disease

	ADPKD	ARPKD	Medullary	Nephronophthisis/ medullary cystic
Kidney size	Enlarged	Enlarged	Normal	Shrunken
Reniform shape	No	Yes	Yes	
Region involved	Cortex + medulla	Cortex + medulla	Papilla	Outer medulla
Nephron segment affected	All	CCT, MCT (CNT, TAL)	IMCT	CT, DCT, loops
Cyst-lining epithelium	Flattened Cubold Columnar 1 layer	Cubold 1 layer	Columnar Transitional Metaplastic Squamous	Flattened
Liver cysts	Yes	No	No	No
Liver fibrosis	No	Yes	No	No

CT, collecting tubule; *CCT*, cortical collecting tubule; *MCT*, medullary collecting tubule; *IMCT*, inner medullary collecting tubule; *DCT*, distal convoluted tubule; *CNT*, connecting tubule; *TAL*, thick ascending limb of Henle''s loop

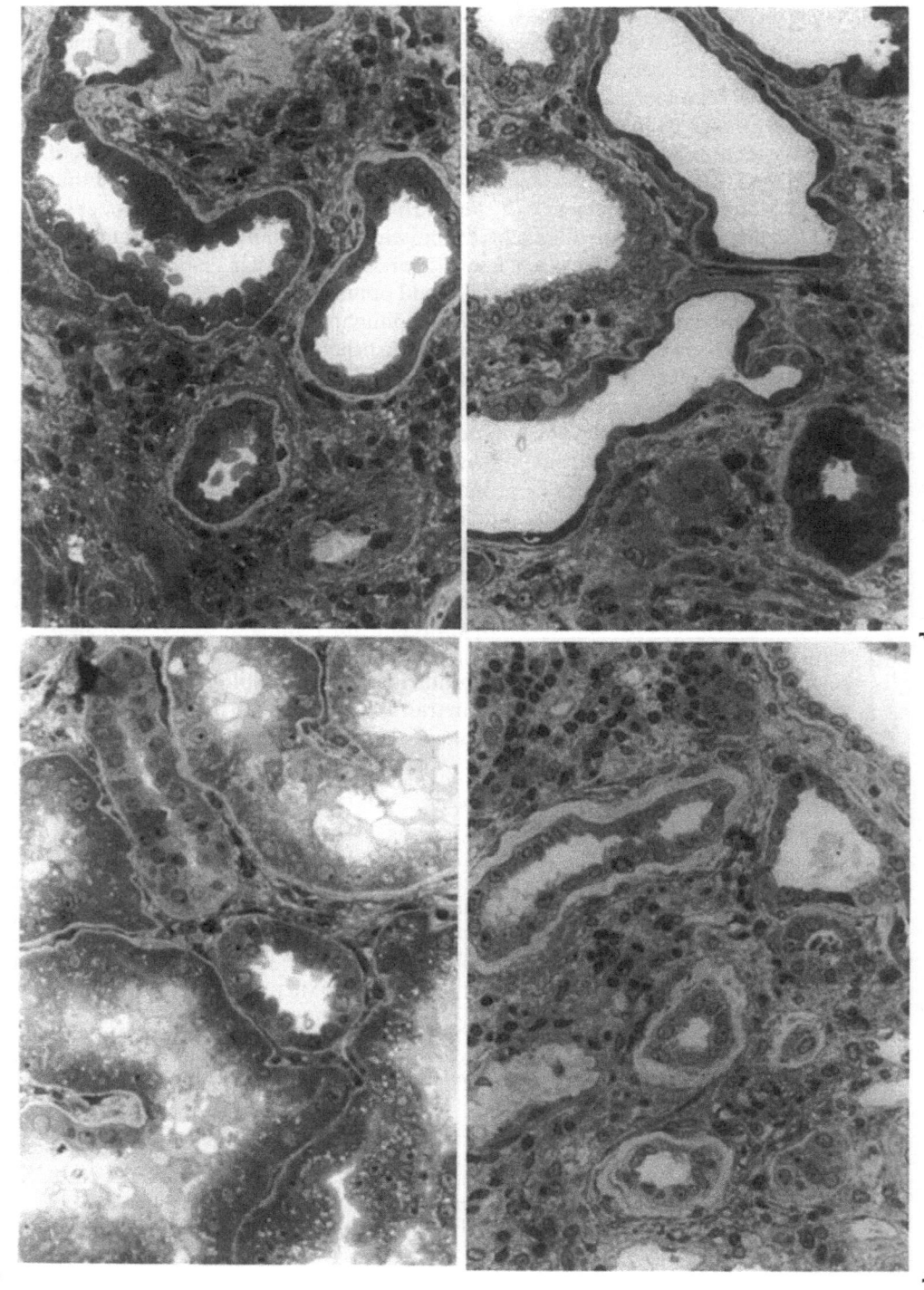

morphological or immunostaining evidence of ischemic injury and were fully viable, as assessed by their successful use for in vitro growth of microdissected tubules. Similarly, the microdissected cysts and tubules from 31 end-stage ADPKD, 15 early-stage ADPKD, and five ARPKD kidneys were fully viable and yielded multiple parallel monolayer cultures.

2.1 Early Stage

In the preazotemic stages of the disease, ADPKD is characterized by the existence of normal renal glomerular and tubule structures interspersed with cysts in varying stages of enlargement (Fig. 1). At these early stages of the disease, it is often possible to discern epithelial phenotypes lining enlarging cysts which resemble proximal tubules, by virtue of their cuboid to columnar nature, clear apical brush border, and rich organelle content (Fig. 1c, d). Other cysts are clearly derived from collecting tubules, as distinguished by a flatter epithelium, few it any apical microvilli lining cyst lumina, and the presence of both dark and light cells, features characteristic of normal human collecting tubule intercalated and principal cells, respectively (Fig. 1d). A thickened basement membrane is a widely described feature of ADPKD cysts (HEPTINSTALL 1992), and even at the earliest stages of expansion, many cysts are lined by epithelia which rest on a clearly thickened basement membrane (Fig. 1b, c, d). It is also of importance to note that the presence of basement membrane thickening is unrelated to nephron segment origin. Although the majority of cysts are lined by a single layer of epithelium, hyperplastic lesions are occasionally seen in which the epithelial cells lining cysts form multilayers (Fig. 1d) or even papillary protrusions. Electron microscopy of multilayered cyst walls shows that these hyperplastic epithelial cells are poorly differentiated and of indeterminate tubule segment origin, and that they rest on a thickened basement membrane (Fig. 2). However, they retain epithelial polarity with apical microvilli and tight junctional specialization areas of cell contact. In trying to gain an understanding of the pathophysiologic mechanisms in ADPKD disease development, it is important to examine those changes associated with the earliest phases of cystic expansion.

◄───

Fig. 1a–d. Light micrographs of preazotemic "early-stage" ADPKD kidneys, 1-μm sections glutaraldehyde fixed, embedded in araldite, and stained with toluidine blue. **a** A relatively normal region of the kidney with proximal tubules and a distal tubule. An abnormal tubule with expanded lumen containing an extrusion body. **b** A region of the same kidney in which several tubules are surrounded by a thickened basement membrane. **c** A region of the same kidney with thickened basement membranes and expansion in the intestitial matrix, which appears cellular and fibrillar (*middle right*). Extrusion bodies are seen in cyst lumens resembling both proximal and dostal tubules. **d** Two cystic tubules of apparent collecting tubule origin with fairly flattened epithelia containing light and dark cells. By contrast, the *upper right* cyst is lined by taller cuboid epithelia with a clear brush border, suggesting a proximal tubule origin. *Lower left*, a hyperplastic cyst in which cells are piled on top of one another

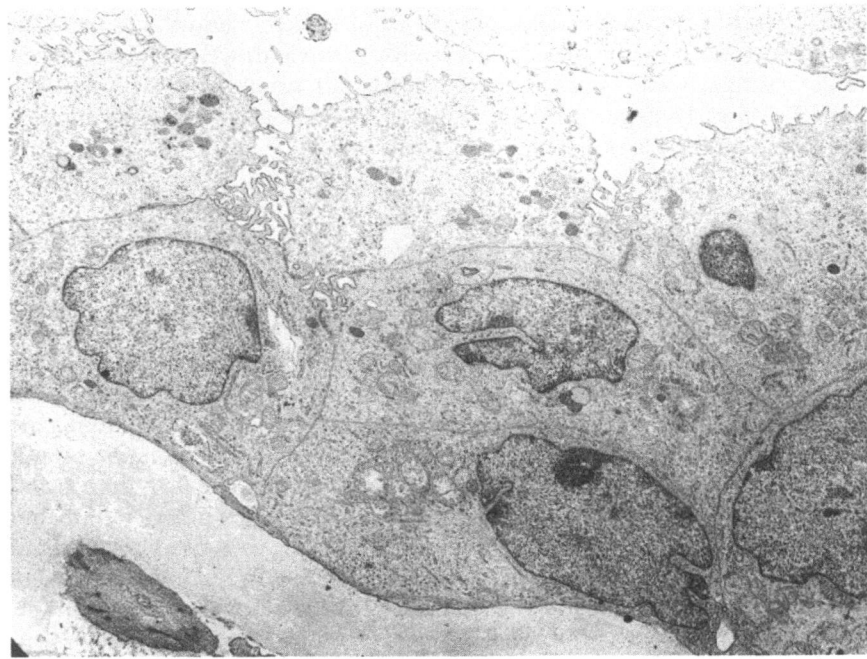

Fig. 2. Electron micrograph of a hyperplastic cyst wall from ADPKD kidney. Note the poorly differentiated cells with apical microvilli, tight junctions, and a thickened basement membrane

The changes seen at these stages are likely to reflect the most important, determining events in cyst formation, an analysis of which might reasonably be assumed to yield pertinent clues to the underlying cause of the disease. In addition to the hyperproliferation and basement membrane abnormalities described above, early changes include the mislocalization of certain key membrane proteins in the polarized epithelia of cysts from the earliest stages of expansion. The most important example of such a change is NaK-ATPase, which is mispolarized to the apical membranes of expanding ADPKD epithelia and contributes to fluid secretion into cyst lumina by virtue of blood-to-lumen sodium ion transport (WILSON et al. 1991; Figs. 16–18). Another common, although less clearly defined feature of early-stage ADPKD kidneys is the frequent occurrence of spherical cell extrusion bodies within the lumina of small cysts, particularly those derived from putative proximal tubules (Fig. 1a, c). At the electron-microscopic level these bodies appear to be membrane-bound, viable regions of cytoplasm containing numerous mitochondria and ribosomes and endoplasmic reticulum (Fig. 3). The significance of these bodies is unknown, but it is interesting to speculate that they may be related to apoptotic bodies, particularly since it has recently been shown that bcl-2-deficient mice have polycystic kidneys (VEIS et al. 1993). Another feature characteristic of early-stage ADPKD kidneys and not seen in end-stage kidneys is that many tubules which

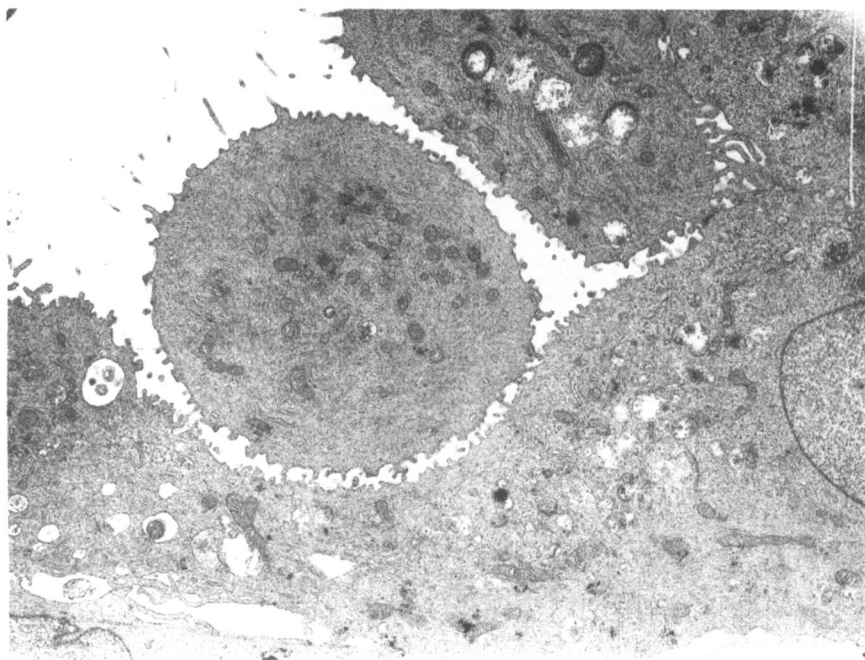

Fig. 3. Electron micrograph of a call extrusion body in the lumen of an expanding cyst. There is a clear plasma membrane with rudimentary microvilli and normal mitochondria, rough endoplasmic reticulum, and free ribosomes

are not cystic and do not have expanded lumina are grossly enlarged in diameter and cell size, suggesting hypertrophy of the epithelium. These epithelia frequently show much stronger immunostaining reactions for many protein products than their normal, non-PKD counterparts, which may be indicative of generalized increases in protein synthesis in precystic ADPKD tubules or may be the result of up-regulation of specific genes.

2.2 End Stage

In ADPKD kidneys from patients with end-stage renal failure, when all normal renal function has ceased, light-microscopic examination of the kidneys shows numerous cysts of varying sizes, again usually lined with a single layer of epithelium, which may range from extremely flattened through cuboid to columnar in appearance (BERNSTEIN 1976; CUPPAGE et al. 1980 and Figs. 4 and 5). These epithelia are less easy to interpret concerning segment of origin, since there is a loss of normal differentiated features (WILSON et al. 1986; MCATEER et al. 1988). At the electron-microscopic level, cyst-lining epithelial cells are struc-

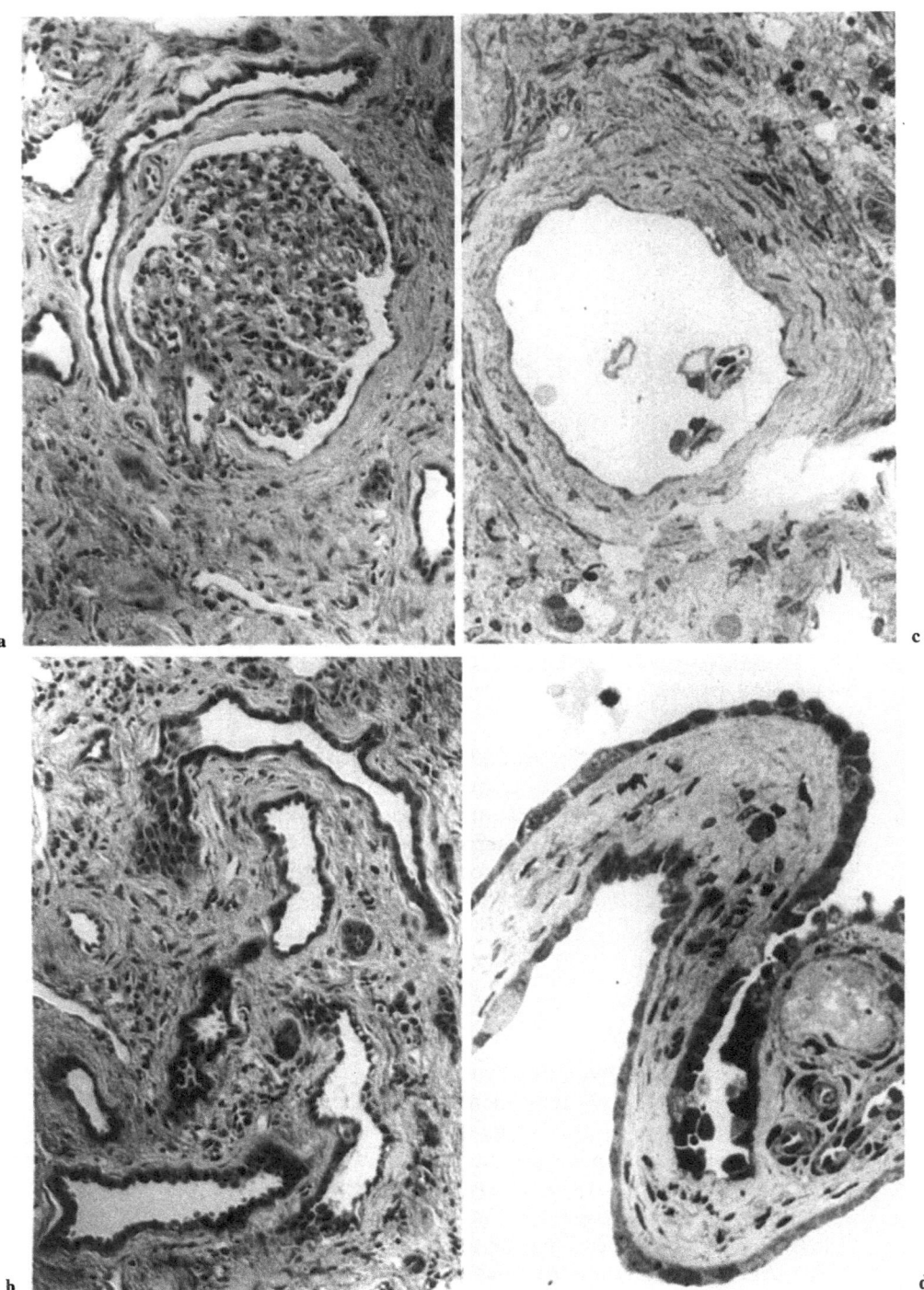

turally polarized since they rest with their basal cell membranes on a basement membrane of varying thickness and their apical surfaces show some specialization in the form of rudimentary microvilli (Fig. 5). All epithelia form tight sheets in which adjacent cells are tightly apposed to one another. In some, wide intercellular spaces are also seen (Fig. 6d). All epithelial cells, however, are interconnected by specialized tight junctions and form morphologically normal desmosomes and zonula adherens (Fig. 6). Intracellular features of ADPKD epithelia typically include an apparent overabundance of cytoskeletal filaments with the morphological features of actin and cytokeratin (Fig. 7a, b), reduced numbers of apical endocytic vesicles (Fig. 8b), and moderate numbers of rather disorganized sets of organelles including mitochondria, lysosomes, and rough endoplasmic reticulum (Fig. 5, 7, and 8). Normal renal structures are rare in end-stage kidneys, although occasional, relatively normal glomeruli are seen (Fig. 4a). Frequently, however, glomerular contents show atrophy and lead to the establishment of glomerular cysts, lined only by an extremely thin layer of flattened epithelial cells of parietal epithelial origin (Fig. 4b). In general, the structure of the tissue is a mixture of epithelial cysts, some with areas of hyperplasia (Fig. 4b) interspersed within an expanded fibrotic interstitium containing stromal cells, extracellular matrix including collagen fibrils, and small, thin-walled blood vessels (Figs. 4, 5, and 9). It has been reported that these blood vessels in ADPKD kidneys contain renin (GRAHAM and LINDOP 1988), which, together with renin synthesized in ADPKD epithelia and secreted into cyst fluids, might contribute to the high incidence of hypertension in these patients (TORRES et al. 1992). The composition of the interstitium in ADPKD is quite characteristic; often it is diffuse and cellular in appearance (Fig. 4), suggesting aberrant proliferation of fibroblasts. In addition, these cells have been shown to synthesize erythropoietin (ECKARDT et al. 1989), which is consistent with the clinical finding that this group of patients are less anemic than non-ADPKD chronic renal failure patients. At the electron-microscopic level fibroblasts are seen interspersed within a loose fibrillar extracellular matrix containing loose collagen bundles (Fig. 5). Inflammatory infiltrates are rarely associated with this type of interstitial fibrosis. The degree of interstitial fibrosis in ADPKD can vary quite substantially. In general, the fibrosis increases with degree of disease development, such that in the early stages of ADPKD cyst expansion increased numbers of stromal cells can be seen with little expansion of the interstitial matrix (Fig. 1); later, in end-stage ADPKD, this progresses to considerable expansion of the

◀───

Fig. 4a–d. Light micrographs of end-stage ADPKD kidneys. **a, b, c** are formaldehyde-fixed, paraffin-embedded 6-μm sections stained with hematoxylin and eosin; **d** shows a 1-μm araldite section of glutaraldehyde-fixed material stained with toluidine blue. **a** Relatively normal glomerulus is surrounded by a fibrotic interstitium containing epithelial-lined cysts of varying sizes. **b** More cysts and fibrotic interstitium. Note the epithelial hyperplasia in one cyst. **c** An apparent glomerular cyst in which the glomerular contents appear to have undergone atrophy, leaving a cyst lined by extremely flattened epithelium derived from the parietal epithelial cells of the glomerulus. **d** Morphological heterogeneity of cyst-lining epithelial cells. The interstitium contains fibrils and thin-walled blood vessels (*lower right*)

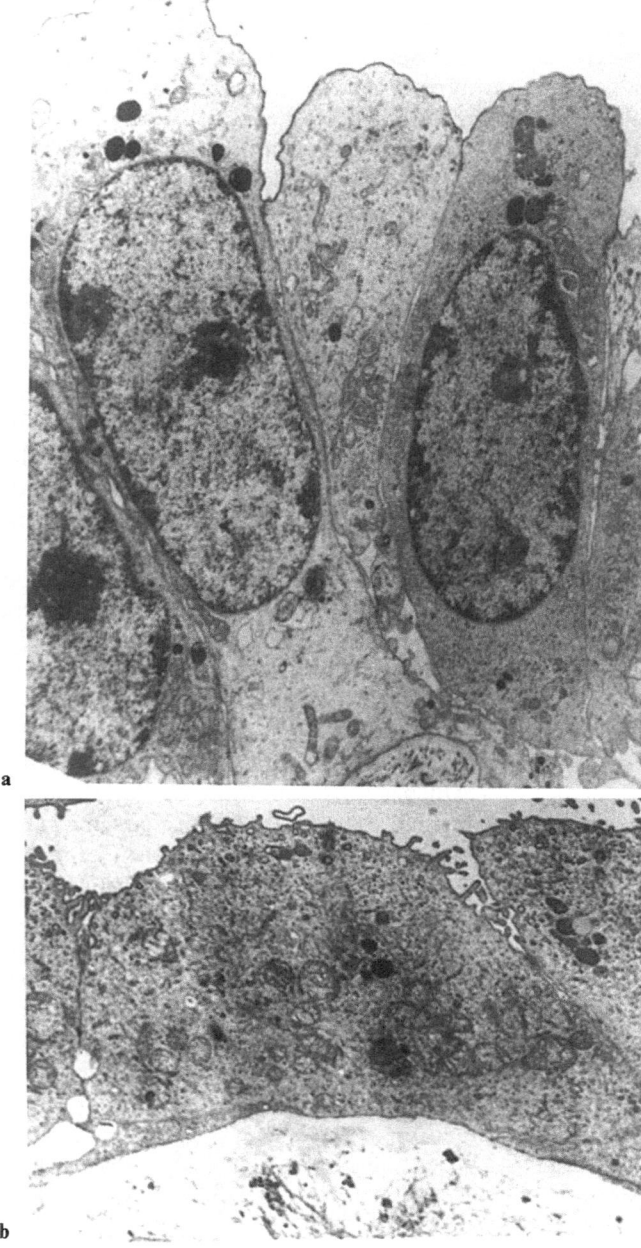

Fig. 5a–d. Electron micrographs of ADPKD cyst epithelial calls, glutaraldehyde-fixed sections. **a** Columnar epithelia with apical intercellular tight junctions but few microvilli or basolateral membrane infoldings. The cytoplasm contains few organelles including mitochondria, lysosomes, and endoplasmic reticulum. **b** Cuboidal epithelium probably of collecting duct principal cell origin. Note the base of a cilium, intercellular tight junctions, rudimentary apical microvilli, and relatively few organelles including mitochondria, lysosomes, and endoplasmic reticulum.

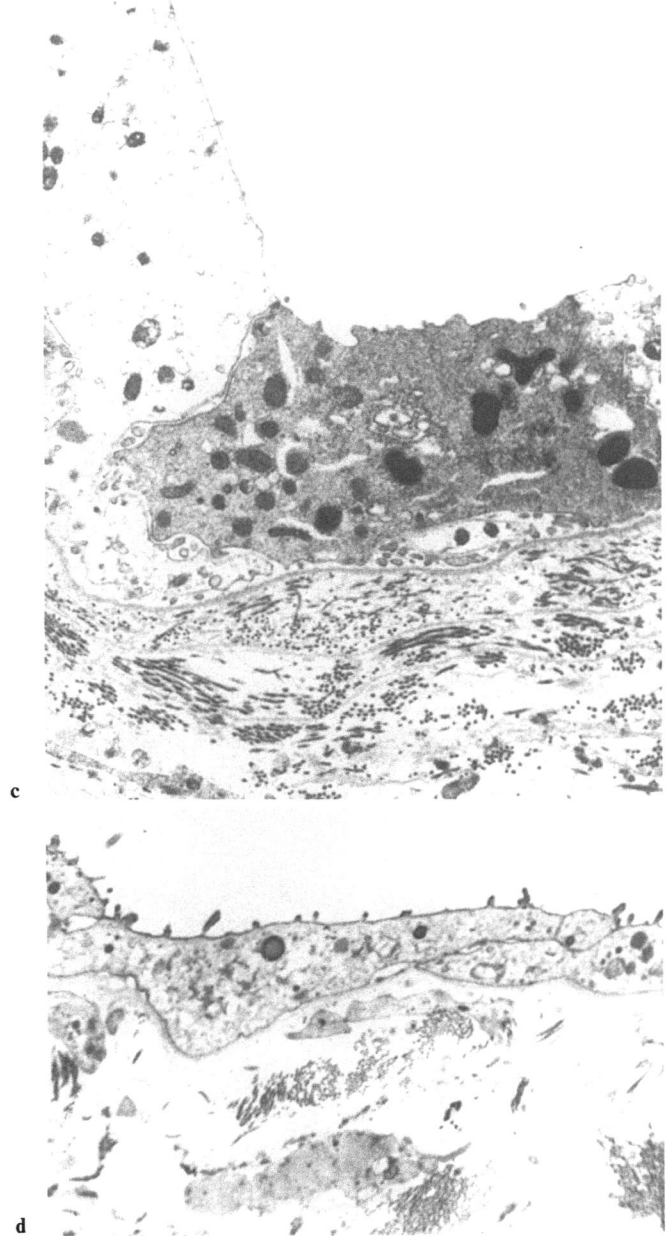

Fig. 5. c A cyst apparently derived from a collecting tubule. The dark cell contains numerous lysosomes, while the light cell is relatively depleted of cellular contents. Note the apical intercellular tight junctions and extensive extracellular matrix. A laminated basement membrane is present with bundles of collagen between the layers. **d** An extremely flattened cyst epithelium with rudimentary apical microvilli and intercellular tight junctions. The extracellular matrix contains fibroblasts, amorphous fibrils, and loose arrays of collagen

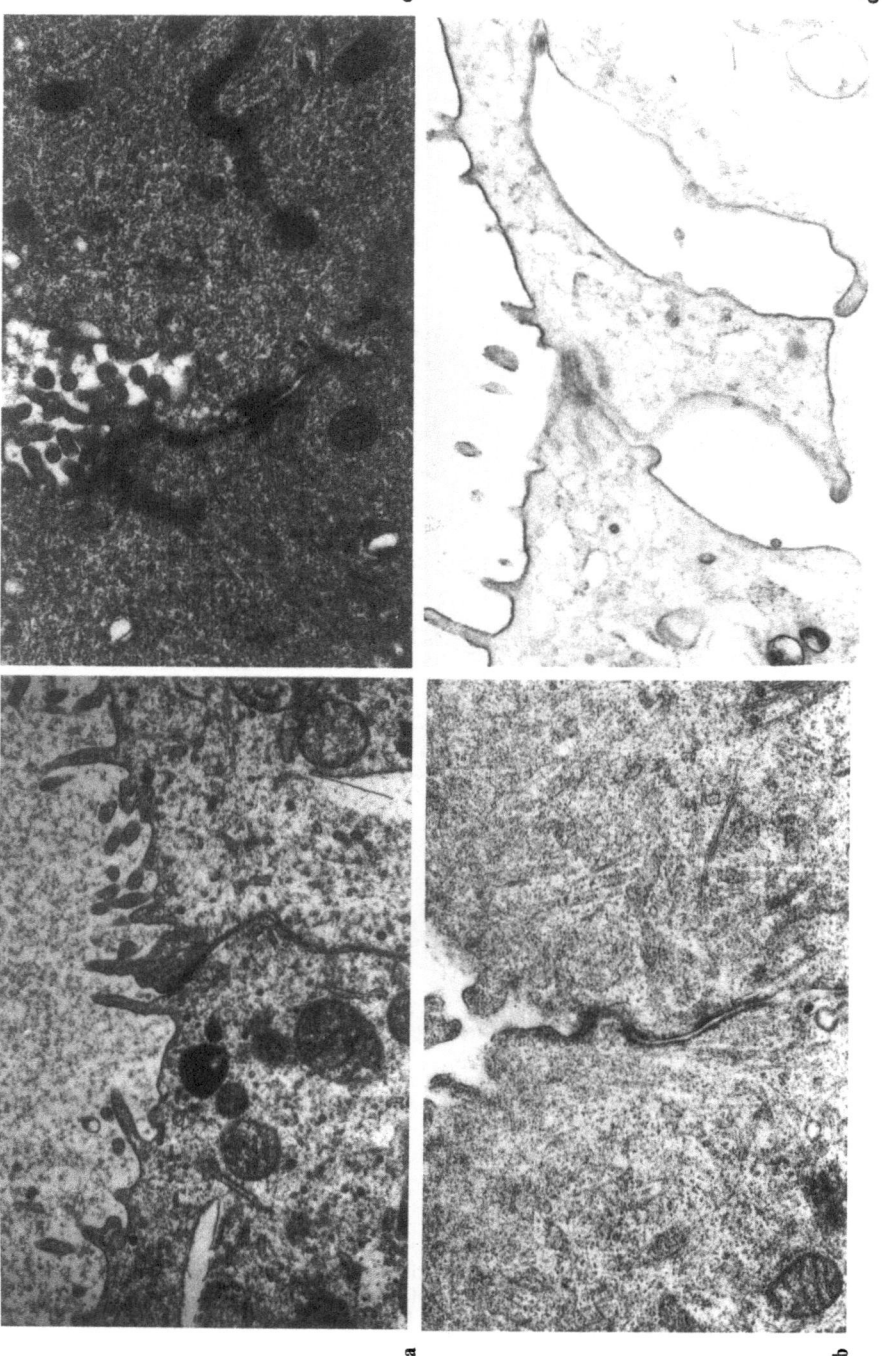

Fig. 6a–d. Electron microscopy of tight junctions in a variety of cystic epithelial cell types. All junctional specializations are located at the apical aspect of the cells and vary in depth and electron density

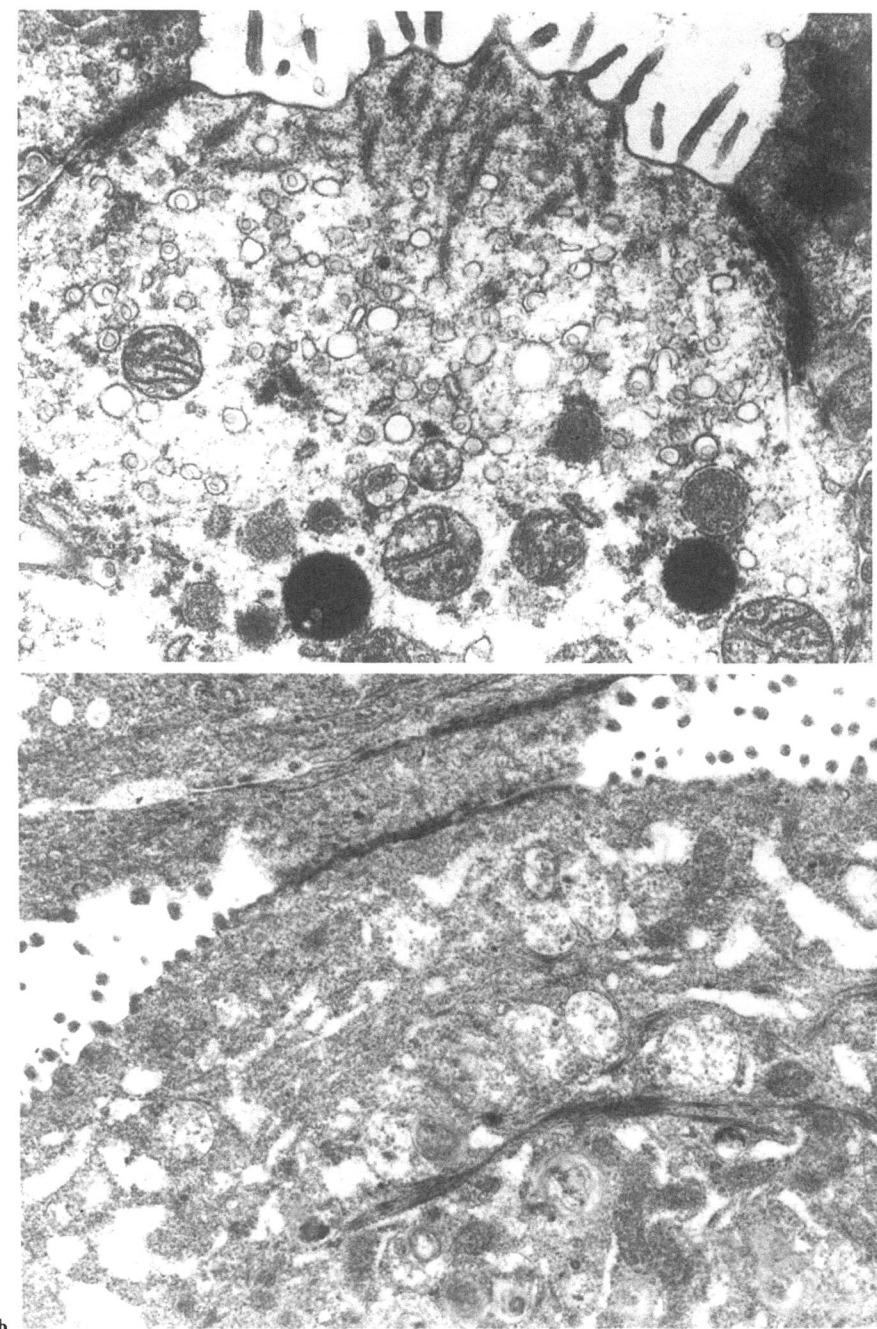

Fig. 7a, b. Electron microscopy of cytoskeletal fibril enrichment in ADPKD epithelia. **a** A cyst epithelial cell with enrichment of microfilaments extending from the base of apical microvilli. Note the deep intercellular tight junctions. **b** Intracellular microfilament bundles in the cytoplasm of a cyst epithelial cell

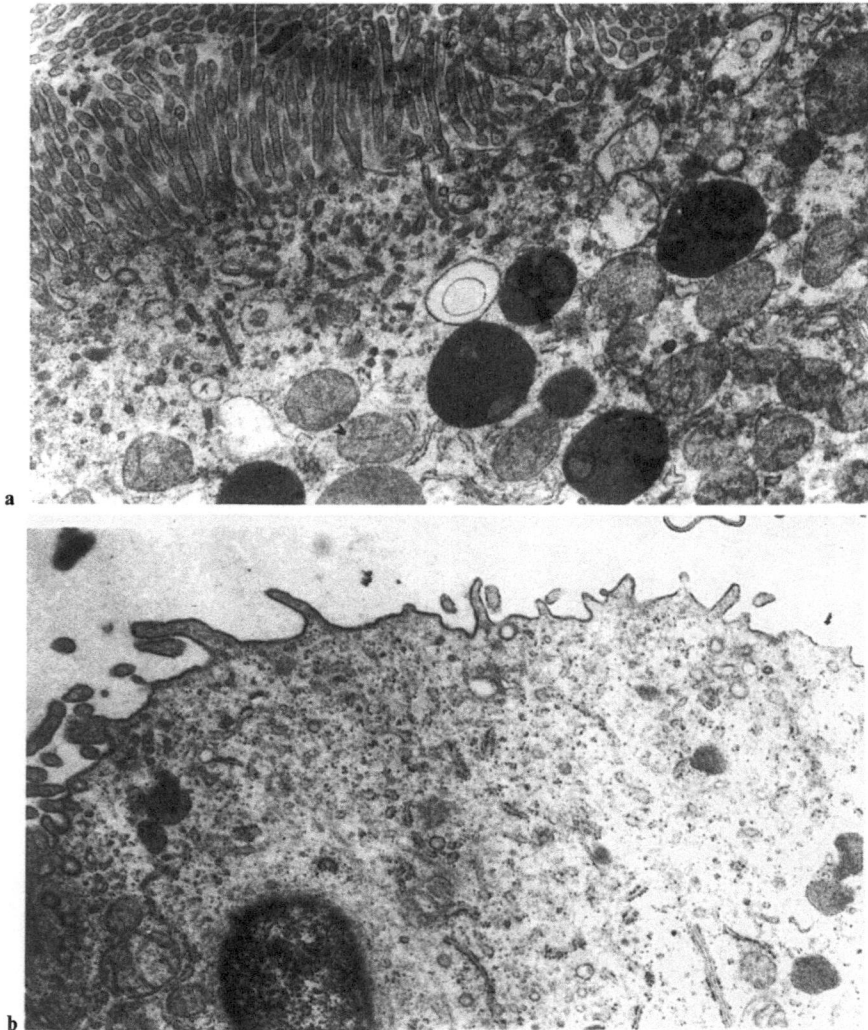

a

b

Fig. 8a, b. Electron microscopy of apical endocytic vesicles. **a** Sub-apical brush border region of a typical proximal tubule from a normal human kidney. Not the extensive network of vesicles and tubulovesicular structures associated with endocytosis. **b** Similar region from an ADPKD cyst epithelial cell. Note the reduction in number of endocytic vesicles

extracellular matrix in the form of diffuse amorphous fibrils and collagen bundles (Fig. 5).

Purely morphological analysis of human ADPKD kidneys has therefore led to seveal areas of study to determine potential mechanisms of disease. It is clear that cyst formation is a continual and dynamic process in the ADPKD patient. It is most likely that patients bearing the ADPKD gene(s) are born with a complement of cysts, which may or may not be of sufficient size to be detected by ultrasonography or other means. It is not known whether all cysts are preformed before birth or whether some normal tubules at birth are later converted to the cystic phenotype. Since it has been estimated that only 2% of tubules become cystic in end-stage ADPKD patients (GRANTHAM et al. 1987), it would be feasible for all cystic events to have occurred during nephrogenesis. The progressive loss of renal function and increase in renal mass due to cystic enlargement (GREGOIRE et al. 1987) is consistent with a declining number of normal functional nephrons. Since it has been clearly demonstrated by extensive freeze-fracture analysis that the majority of ADPKD cysts have no connections with their tubule of origin (EVAN and MCATEER 1990), it has been suggested that cysts close off from their tubule origin early in the expansion process. Together, these findings suggest that the progressive expansion of cystic tubule epithelia and expansion of the interstitium contribute to progressive destruction of normal renal parenchyma. The typical absence of symptoms of renal insufficiency until later decades is consistent with the existence of a large functional reserve in normal kidneys; symptoms become evident only once a critical minimal threshold has been reached. Regarding progression, it has been difficult to

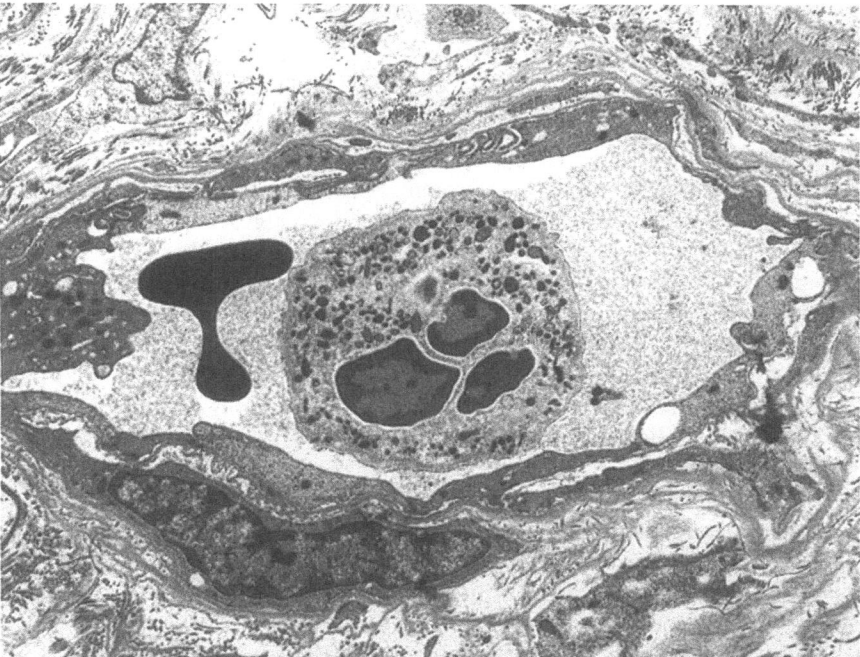

Fig. 9. Electrom microscopy of a thin-walled blood vessel in the interstitium of an end-stage ADPKD kidney. Note the single layer of endothial cells and one pericyte. The lumen contains a red blood cell and a polymorphonuclear leukocyte

explain why, when the gene penetrance in ADPKD is thought to be close to 100% (Dalgaard 1957; Dobin et al. 1993), there is still a wide range of variation in rapidity of progression to renal failure, ranging from the first to the eighth decade with some patients never reaching the end stage. It may be that the variable degree of interstial fibrosis is an associated detrimental factor leading to more rapid destruction of normal renal tubules (Kuo and Wilson 1991; Norman et al. 1992).

3 Pathology of Autosomal Recessive Polycystic Kidney Disease

The characteristics of ARPKD is kidneys of infants resemble those of ADPKD in some respects but differ significantly in others (Table 2). As in ADPKD, both kidneys of infants with ARPKD are greatly enlarged, and cyst formation occurs throughout the cortex and medulla. However, unlike ADPKD, the reinform shape (and infantile lobation) and cortico-medullary distinction of the kidney are retained and all cysts are minute in size (1–2 mm in the cortex, somewhat larger in the medulla) in comparison with ADPKD, where there is much variation in size and they can reach several centimeters. Also, unlike ADPKD, cysts are seen as fusiform dilatations running radially through the cortex and medulla and represent ectatic expansion of collecting tubules, as shown by dissection and lectin-staining studies (Osathanondh and Potter 1964; Faraggiana et al. 1985 and Fig. 10b). Cysts are also sometimes seen to branch, which is consistent with a collecting tubule origin. Occasional connecting tubules and thick ascending limbs are enlarged as well. (Holthofer et al. 1990; Heptinstall 1992). Expansion of collecting tubules is uniform in both kidneys, and inner and outer medullary and cortical collecting tubules are all involved in cystic enlargement. Since the developmental pattern of collecting tubule branching is normal, it is thought that this disease affects predominantly the last generation of collecting tubules. In other respects early renal development appears normal, since the normal numbers of nephrons are formed, glomeruli and proximal convoluted tubules appear normal, and normal profiles of proximal tubules and loops are seen between cystic tubules (Fig. 10a, b). Cysts are usually lined by a single cell layer of cuboid epithelium, although this can be layered in hyperplastic areas (Fig. 10d). In the past, it was thought that the extracellular matrix was not involved in the pathogenesis of cyst enlargement in ARPKD. However, experimental studies are in progress to re-examine this conclusion, as some areas of thickened basement membrane and apparent fibroblast and interstitial matrix expansion can frequently be identified in human ARPKD (Figs. 10c, d and 11a). Electron microscopy confirms a collecting tubule origin for cyst-lining epithelial cells in ARPKD since they exhibit some distinctive features reminiscent of collecting tubule cells, such as the presence of a single apical cilium and short and rudimentary microvilli, consistent with a principal cell of origin (Hjelle et al. 1990; Falkenstein et al. 1993 and Fig. 11b). However, the presence of numerous mitochondria, lysosomal bodies, and glycogen distinguish them from the normal collecting tubules (FALKENSTEIN et al. 1993 and Fig. 11a).

Changes in the liver are also characteristic for ARPKD, since congenital hepatic fibrosis is common, involving the portal tracts, and consists of increases in fibrous connective tissue. There is also some increase in bile ducts with some dilatation and a branching pattern leading to ring formation, which is characteristic during normal differentiation of tubular bile ducts.

Much information regarding ARPKD has been derived from the study of the several animal models that result in the autosomal recessive inheritance of rapidly progressive renal cystic disease. Many studies have focused on the *cpk* mouse and have yielded significant advances in understanding the mechanisms of hyperplasia, differentiation, and epithelial polarity. However, some caution should be applied in complete extrapolation from these animal models to human ARPKD because some significant phenotypic differences exist, including the absence of a hepatic fibrosis component in the *cpk* mouse. Likewise, full pathologic characterization of the several other spontaneous and induced mouse mutations will be needed to allow a true evaluation of their suitability as models for human ARPKD.

4 Pathology of Medullary Cystic Disease

4.1 Medullary Sponge Kidney

Medullary sponge kidney leads to cyst formation in the papillary collecting ducts in all pyramids of both kidneys. Since this is associated with normal developmental patterns of branching and attachment of the collecting ducts and is frequently associated with congenital abnormalities including Marfan's disease, the Beckwith-Wiedemann syndrome, and congenital hemihypertrophy, it is thought to be a developmental anomaly. The kidneys are usually normal in size and calcium deposits are frequently seen in the ectatic or cystic papillary collecting tubules. Cysts are small and lined with columnar, transitional, or metaplastic squamous epithelium, and prominent inflammatory infiltrates are seen near the papillary tips.

4.2 Familial Nephronophthisis-Medullary Cystic Disease Complex

The complex is inherited as a recessive trait by 50% of patients and as a dominant trait by 30%. This disease(s) is characterized by shrunken kidneys in which small cysts of up to 1 cm in diameter are seen in the medulla near the cortico-medullary boundary, distinguishing this disease clearly from medullary sponge kidney. The segments involved in cystic dilation are the loops of Henlé; distal convoluted tubules and the collecting tubules and cysts are lined by a flattened epithelium. In

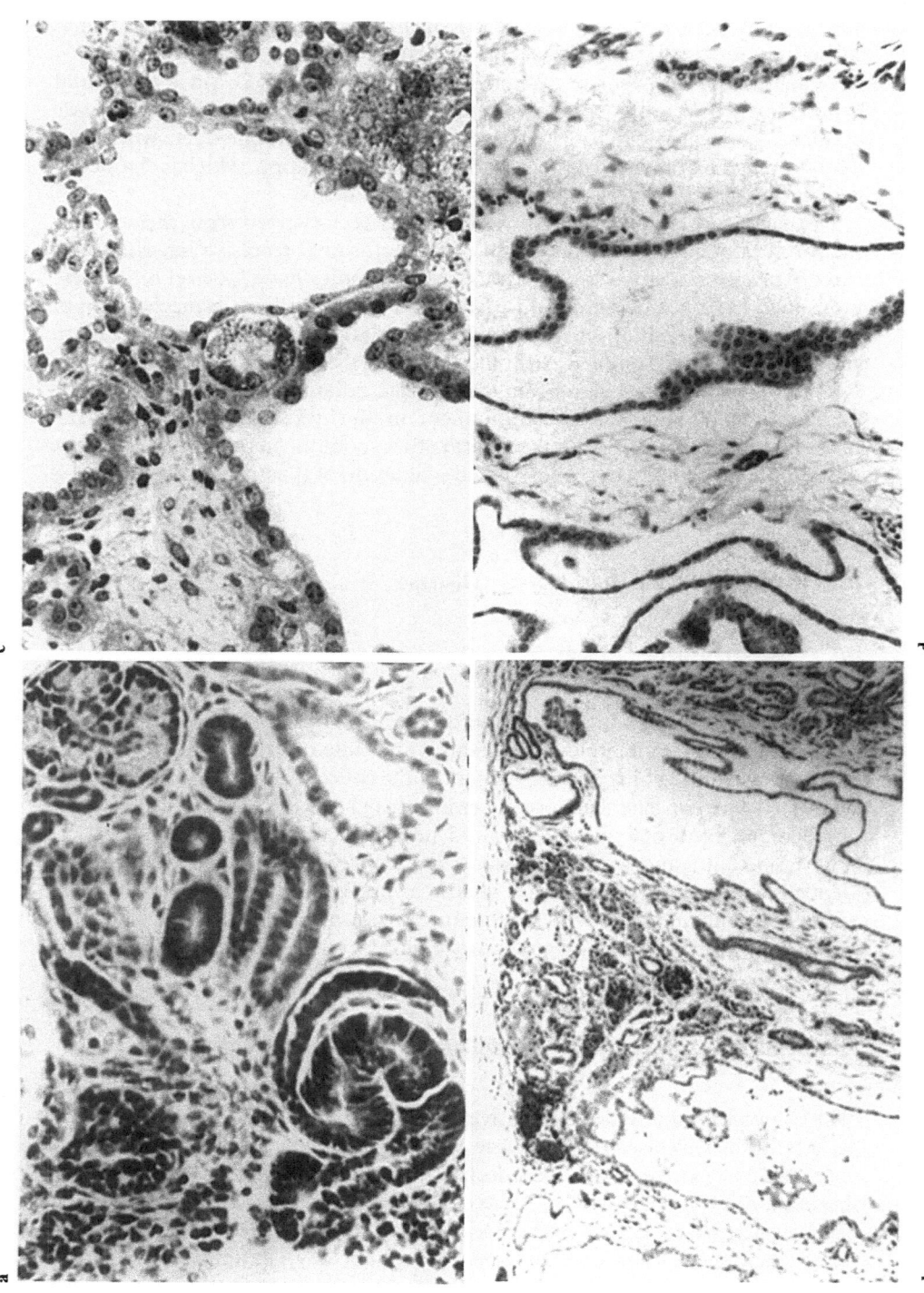

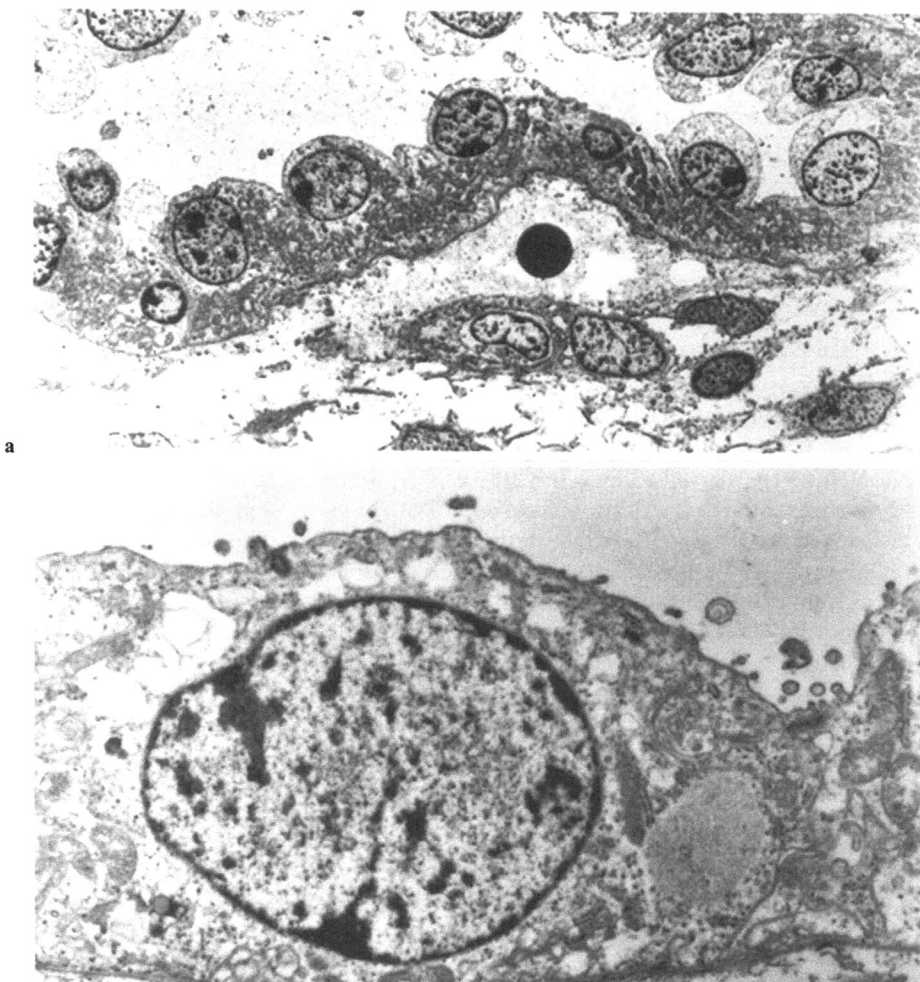

a

b

Fig. 11a, b. Electron micrographs of ARPKD cyst epithelial cells. **a** Note the cuboid epithelium with apically located nuclei, relatively rich in organelles including mitochondria and lysosomes. The interstitium contains several fibroblasts, amorphous fibrils, and little collagen. **b** High-power view of a cystic epithelial cell. Note the apically located intercellular tight junction at the *right* and the base of a cilium at the apical surfac (*left*). The cell is rich in organelles and endoplasmic reticulum and contains intracellular glycogen (*lower right*)

◄━━━

Fig. 10a–d. Light micrographs of ARPKD kidney from 19 weeks gestation; 6-μm sections of paraformaldehyde-fixed material embedded in paraffin and stained with hematoxylin and eosin. **a** High-power view of the extreme cortical region. Undifferentiated metanephric blastemal cells can be seen on the *left*, with a condensate, S-shaped body closely apposed to its inducing collecting tubule and at the *top right*, a fetal glomerulus. The appearance of all these structures is quite normal. Only one expanded collecting tubule can be seen *lower right*. **b** Low-power view of the same ARPKD kidney. Large ectatic expansions can be seen in cortical this, with apparently normal regions of nephrogenic zones between the large cysts. **c** In the medullary region the cyst-lining epithelia are seen to be cuboid. Note the nonexpanded tubule between the cysts and some cellular and fibrillar appearance in the interstitium. **d** Note the region of epithelial hyperplasia in one cyst and the fibrillar nature of the intervening interstitium

addition, many glomeruli are seen to be sclerotic, and tubular atrophy and thickening of basement membranes is widespread. Diffuse interstitial fibrosis is also a feature of this disease, particularly in the areas of tubular atrophy. Chronic nodular inflammatory infiltrates containing Tamm-Horsfall protein are also often seen (HEPTINSTALL 1992).

5 Pathology of Renal Cystic Disease Accompanying Genetic Syndromes

5.1 Tuberous Sclerosis

Tuberous sclerosis is an autosomal dominant trait with variable gene penetrance. Renal involvement is seen in approximately 50% of these patients and may take the form of angiomyolipomas (tumor-like nodules of varying size composed of mature adipose tissue, smooth muscle, and thick walled blood vessels) or cortical and medullary cysts of varying size. These changes are often bilateral. Cyst-lining cells are characteristically large and hyperplastic with acidophilic or clear cytoplasm; they form multilayers, papillary lesions, or sometimes fill the lumen (BERNSTEIN et al. 1987). These characteristics are consistent with a more proliferative lesion than ADPKD or ARPKD. Not surprisingly, therefore, there is an increased incidence of renal cell carcinoma in these patients.

5.2 Von Hippel-Lindau Disease

Von Hippel-Lindau disease is an autosomal dominant trait causing angiomatous cysts of the cerebellum, retinal angiomatosis, and cysts in the pancreas and kidneys. Renal involvement is expressed in approximately 66% of patients and may take the form of cysts and/or renal carcinoma. Cyst epithelia are flattened, sometimes hyperplastic, and may even form small nodules of renal cell carcinoma from within the cyst. In light of the common occurrence of renal cell carcinoma in 25% of these patients, it was of considerable interest that the VHL gene has been mapped to the same chromosome (3p) as some renal cell carcinomas, albeit at a locus (3p 25–26) more proximal to that of familial type renal cell carcinoma at 3p 14.2 (Table 1).

5.3 Multilocular Renal Cysts

Multilocular renal cysts are characteristic of cystic neoplasms and have been described in multilocular cystic nephroma, renal cystadenoma, and solid nephroblastoma (Wilms' tumor). In these conditions, large encapsulated cysts are characteristically lined with cuboid cells which morphologically resemble collecting tubules but show aberrant lectin and antibody staining.

6 Pathology of Nongenetic Cystic Disease

Acquired cystic disease can be induced by hemodialysis and is estimated to affect 40% of these patients. The severity correlates with the duration of the therapy. Typically, these cysts are lined by flattened cuboid epithelium and filled with clear cyst fluid, but hyperplastic and dysplastic epithelia have also been reported. In contrast to ADPKD, continuity between the cysts and tubules of origin is thought to be retained (HEPTINSTALL 1992). Other nongenetic inducers of renal cyst formation include obstruction, drugs, toxins, and increasing age.

7 Cell Culture Studies of ADPKD and ARPKD

In an attempt to increase our understanding of the underlying mechanisms leading to the formation and expansion of renal cysts in these diseases, experimental approaches have been developed. Much information has been obtained by the establishment of cell culture techniques in which cyst-lining epithelia and fibroblasts from genetically determined cystic kidneys can be cultured in pure cell populations and compared rigorously with those of normal human renal fibroblasts and tubule epithelia of defined nephron segment origin (WILSON et al. 1986; FALKENSTEIN et al. 1993; KUO and WILSON 1990). This has been a particularly fruitful approach to the study of genetic cystic disease, since such culture systems allow the discrimination between genetically determined alterations in cells, which are retained through the several passages of which these primary cells are capable, and those due to epigenetic phenomena or nonspecific cell damage such as ischemic injury, since these influences are either lethal and result in nonviability of cells in vitro or are rapidly lost in proliferating systems. The majority of studies of human cells have been carried out in ADPKD, since this is a disease of high prevalence and tissue availability is therefore high (WILSON et al. 1986; MCATEER et al. 1988; MANGOO-KARIM et al. 1989; TORRES et al. 1992). In our laboratory we have studied 31 end-stage and 15 early-stage ADPKD kidneys in this way and have compared them with tubules and fibroblasts derived from 55 normal human kidneys. In addition, although ARPKD is a less common disease, the primary culture technique has also been used to examine epithelial characteristics in ARPKD cystic-kidneys, and in our own laboratory we have been able to generate both epithelial and fibroblast cultures from four ARPKD kidneys (HJELLE et al. 1990; FALKENSTEIN et al. 1993; NORMAN et al. 1993), which are yielding insights into growth, polarity, and transport defects in these cells.

Table 3. Protein alterations in ADPKD epithelia

Changes associated with increased proliferation
EGF receptor apical mislocation
Calpactin I apical mislocation
PCNA aberrant expression
Pax-2 aberrant expression
WT-1 aberrant expression
AKT (RAC-1) aberrant expression

Changes associated with fluid secretion
Na + K + -ATPase apical mislocation
Na + K + 2Cl- basal location
cAMP
CHIP 28

Pathologic studies led to the reasoning that, in order to derive a cyst by expansion of a normal renal tubule, there must be an increase in the number of epithelial cells to account for the expansion of the tubule wall (WELLING and WELLING 1988), and this has been verified experimentally by demonstration of mitotic figures and PCNA (proliferating cell nuclear antigen) staining, indicative of cells in S phase of the cell cycle in ADPKD and ARPKD kidneys in vivo (Table 3). In addition to this abnormal cell proliferation, a second essential criterion for formation of a cyst is that fluid accumulate in the lumen, which implies abnormal ion and fluid transport mechanisms in renal cystic epithelia. This was further implicated when theories of obstruction were disproved by freeze-fracture electron microscopy, showing that ADPKD cysts close off from their tubule of origin early after formation (EVAN and MCATEER 1990). This has led to the current thinking that aberrant secretion is a major mechanism of fluid accumulation in cyst lumina (WILSON and BURROW 1992; GRANTHAM 1993). To fully characterize these fundamental altered properties of ADPKD (and ARPKD) epithelia, therefore, it is clear that cell culture techniques are the methods of choice for examining hyperproliferation and secretion.

8 Hyperproliferation

The first studies in which ADPKD epithelia were placed into primary tissue culture showed that when identical numbers of microdissected ADPKD cyst epithelial cells and normal human proximal tubule, thick ascending limb, or collecting tubule cells were plated onto collagen-coated plastic, the ADPKD cells exhibited a hyperproliferative growth defect (WILSON et al. 1986). Although ADPKD cells do not exhibit faster doubling times than their age-matched normal epithelial cell counterparts, the ADPKD epithelia acquire increased cell numbers by virtue of their ability to go through approximately three times more rounds of division and to survive through more passages than normal cells. In addition, the ADPKD epithelial cells can be maintained in a fully functional state for much longer periods than normal microdissected tubule epithelia (CARONE et al. 1989b; WILSON 1991a, b, c, 1992; WILSON and BURROW 1992). These studies suggested that ADPKD epithelia have a genetically determined predisposition to proliferate and an ability to go through more rounds of division than normal cells. This increased capacity to proliferate would therefore render the cystic tubule susceptible to cell division and inappropriate tubule growth in vivo, so that such cells would be "set up" for cyst formation in the presence of the suitable stimulus. The next question was to determine what mechanisms might be responsible for stimulation of this proliferative potential in vivo in ADPKD kidneys.

Regarding cells in culture and cells during developmental programs, including renal development, it is known that major stimulators of cell division emanate from the influence of the extracellular matrix and from soluble growth factors, both mechanisms working via stimulation of specific cell receptors.

8.1 Basement Membrane and Extracellular Matrix Abnormalities

Morphological studies described major abnormalities in matrix in ADPKD, both in the form of thickened cystic tubular basement membranes, even in the early stages of tubular expansion, and in the expansion and composition of the interstitial stroma (Figs. 1, 2, 4, 5). ADPKD epithelia in vitro have also been shown to synthesize and secrete an abnormal basement membrane in vitro (WILSON et al. 1986, 1992 and Fig. 12). Although normal renal tubule epithelia in vitro synthesize and secrete a thin electron-dense layer resembling a normal basement membrane (Fig. 12a), ADPKD epithelia extrude numerous proteinacious spheroids of ruthenium red-positive material, indicative of sulfated proteoglycan, into the basal extracellular space from intracellular vesicles (Fig. 12b). Vesicles containing these spheroids can also be seen within ADPKD epithelial cells (Fig. 12b, c and d), and when growth in three-dimensional semisolid gels (Matrigel) they reconstituted the typically amorphous matrix fibrillar pattern seen in vivo (Fig. 12d). Further studies in our own and other laboratories have identified a major abnormality in heparan sulfate processing by ADPKD epithelial cells which may have an impact on the proliferative abnormality (CARONE et al. 1989a; JIN et al. 1992; WILSON et al. 1992). In addition, type-IV collagen gene expression has been shown to increase in end-stage ADPKD kidneys, although no major abnormalities in laminin expression were seen at the mRNA or protein levels (WILSON 1991c). The relative importance of basement membrane protein abnormalities in renal cyst formation remains to be determined. This is an appealing concept as a primary alteration in cyst formation in ADPKD and other forms of cystic disease, since changes in compliance or composition in the extracellular milieu would provide a unifying theory to rationalize the findings of cyst formation in several extrarenal tissues (GABOW et al. 1984). Consistent with this notion, basement membrane abnormalities have

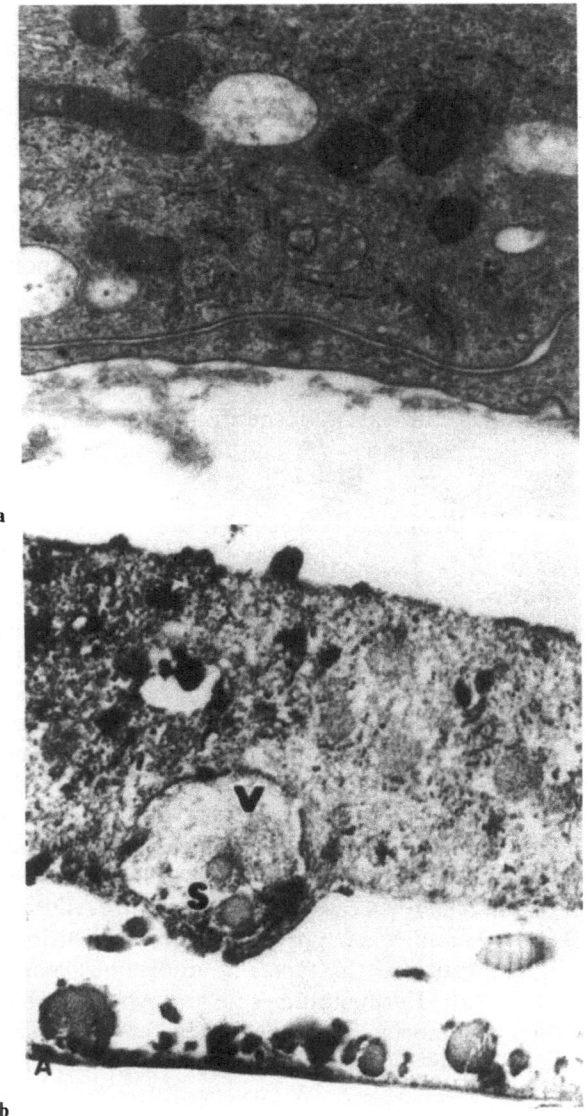

Fig. 12a–d. Electron micrographs of basement membrane region of cultured normal and ADPKD epithelial cells. **a** Basal region of a microdissected culture of normal human proximal tubule epithelia grown to confluence of Teflon and sectioned side-on. The cell has apparently synthesized a morphologically relatively normal basement membrane with a thin electron-lucent area immediately adjacent to the basal aspect of the organelle-rich cell and a thin electron-dense lamina densa. This is characteristic of confluent monolayers of normal human renal epithelia grown in defined media. **b** An ADPKD epithelial cell of the flattened type in culture contains large vesicles (*V*) which can be seen as

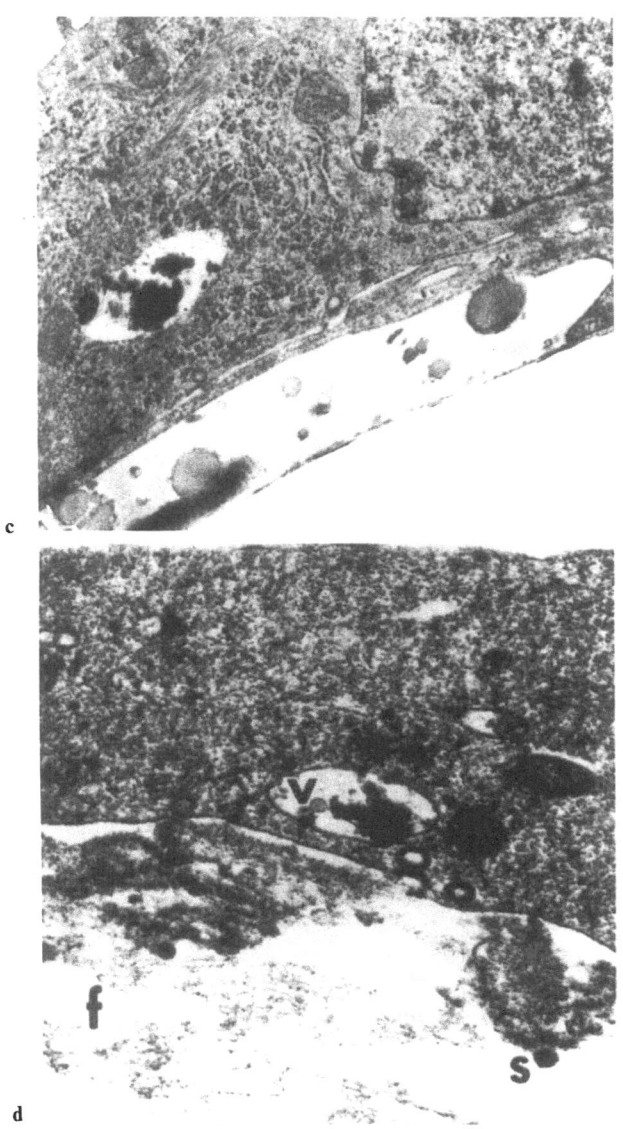

c

d

proteinacious spheroids (*S*); they are apparently extruded from the basal aspect of the cell into the extracellular matrix beneath the cell. Both intracellular and extracellular spheroids have stained for ruthenium red, suggesting their proteoglycan composition. **c** An ADPKD epithelial cell of the cuboidal type contains a large vesicle which can be seen as ruthenium-red-positive spheroids. These are also seen in the extracellular space beneath the cells. **d** Appearance of the extracellular matrix of an ADPKD cell grown in a three-dimensional gel (Matrigel). A few small spheroids can still be seen (*s*), together with large accumulations of fibrils (*f*), which range from amorphous to dense

been reported in nephronophthisis (ZOLLINGER et al. 1980) and murine models of
ARPKD (EBIHARA et al. 1988). However, the occurrence of similar changes in
drug-induced, nongenetic rat models of cystic disease suggests that this may
not be a genetic determinant of polycystic kidney disease (BUTKOWSKI et al. 1985).

8.2 Interstitial Abnormalities

Stromal-epithelial interactions have long been known to play important roles in
epithelial differentiation, development, and tumor formation. A renewed interest
in and appreciation for this phenomenon has been stimulated by the studies of
MONTESANO et al. (1991a, b), who have shown that fibroblasts secrete factor(s)
such as hepatocyte growth factor that influence tubule formation by dog renal
epithelial cells in vitro. Morphological studies show that there is rapid and often
extensive expansion of the interstitium of ADPKD kidneys as they progress to
end-stage renal failure. Our findings also suggest that similar, less extensive
morphological alterations can be seen in ARPKD kidneys, characterized by
increases in interstitial fibroblasts and extracellular proteins. Using the cultured
cell system for comparison of ADPKD and normal, age-matched human
kidneys, we have determined that primary fibroblasts for ADPKD kidneys are
hyperproliferative, go through many more rounds of division and passages than
their normal kidney counterparts, and even exhibit some features akin to
"transformed" cells, in that they will form colonies in soft agar (KUO and WILSON
1991). Despite this even more pronounced hyperproliferative defect than that of
ADPKD epithelial cells, ADPKD fibroblasts are not truly neoplastically transformed since they are not immortal in vitro and have never established permanently growing cell lines spontaneously. These studies suggest that not only the
epithelia, but also the fibroblast component of ADPKD kidneys are hyperproliferative, and co-culture studies are in progress to determine whether these
interstitial cells exert a significant influence on epithelial components and vice
versa. Current studies suggest that alterations in cysteine and metalloproteinase
secretion may also play an important role in the altered epithelial-stromal
interactions associated with cyst formation both in ADPKD and in ARPKD
(HARTZ and WILSON 1994; NORMAN et al. 1993). This is of particular interest in
light of the finding that inhibition of collagenase prevented tubule formation of
a dog kidney epithelial cell line (MDCK) in three-dimensional gels in vitro and
led instead to cyst formation (MONTESANO et al. 1991b).

8.3 Growth Factor Interactions

Our studies of human ADPKD in vitro suggested that these epithelial cells had a
higher proliferative capacity than normal epithelial cells. To determine the relevant

in vivo mechanisms that might be operative in cyst epithelial cell proliferation a series of in vitro studies were carried out to establish the proliferative profile of these cells in response to a number of well-known epithelial cell growth factors. It was established that ADPKD cells were abnormally hyper-responsive to proliferative stimulation by epidermal growth factor (EGF) (WILSON 1991a; WILSON et al. 1993a). Subsequent studies showed that the pre-pro-EGF ligand was synthesized in large amounts by ADPKD cyst epithelial cells, and that it was processed and secreted in mitogenic concentrations into the cyst fluids. In normal renal tubule epithelia, the receptors for EGF are located on the basolateral epithelial cell membranes. Since ADPKD cyst-lining epithelia are essentially tight and have normal occluding intercellular tight junctions, the presence of EGF in the lumen would have a mitogenic effect in vivo only if receptors were present on the apical (luminal) cell membranes of epithelial cells. Immunostaining, radioactive-ligand binding studies, and Western analysis with anti-phosphotyrosine antibodies showed this indeed to be the case, and these receptors were fully functional with respect to their ability to dimerize and autophosphorylate in the presence of ligand (DU and WILSON 1994 and Fig. 13d). These properties of abnormal receptor localization were retained in cell cultures of ADPKD epithelia (Fig. 14c), further suggesting that this is a fundamental change in these cells. In addition to this mispolarization of approximately 60% of EGF receptor protein to the apical cell membranes, an increase in EGF receptor number was demonstrated, which was partially accounted for by transcriptional up-regulation (KLINGEL et al. 1992; WILSON et al. 1993a), but may also be influenced by decreased degradation of receptor-ligand complexes since lysosomal proteinases are significantly reduced in ADPKD (HARTZ and WILSON 1994). These studies suggest a significant role for EGF as a mediator of ADPKD epithelial hyperproliferation by an autocrine mechanism in vivo. In addition, the apical disposition of EGF receptor is marked in human ARPKD cyst epithelia both in vivo and in vitro (FALKENSTEIN et al. 1993 and Fig. 13b, 14b), and these findings correlate with similar findings of apical EGF receptor localization in cystic tubules of *cpk* mice (E. Avner, personal communication). It is also of interest that calpactin II (lipocortin I), a cellular substrate for the EGF receptor, is also localized to the apical membranes of ADPKD but not of normal renal epithelial cells (A.C. Sherwood, personal communication). Other growth factor receptor alterations are seen, although their specific relationships to increased ADPKD epithelial cell proliferation have not yet been examined. These include apical disposition of the hepatocyte growth factor receptor (HGF) and increased expression of a serine/threonine receptor protein, the product of the AKT (RAC-1) oncogene, particularly in hyperplastic foci of cyst-lining epithelia in ADPKD (K. Amsler, personal communication).

In addition to epithelial proliferation, fibroblast proliferation has been examined in vitro. Using a similar mitogenic profiling approach, we found that acidic fibroblast growth factor (aFGF) was a most potent mitogen for ADPKD but not for age-matched normal human renal fibroblasts (KUO and WILSON 1991). In these studies it was also shown that acidic FGF is secreted into the culture medium by ADPKD fibroblasts, suggesting that this growth factor may play a role in the

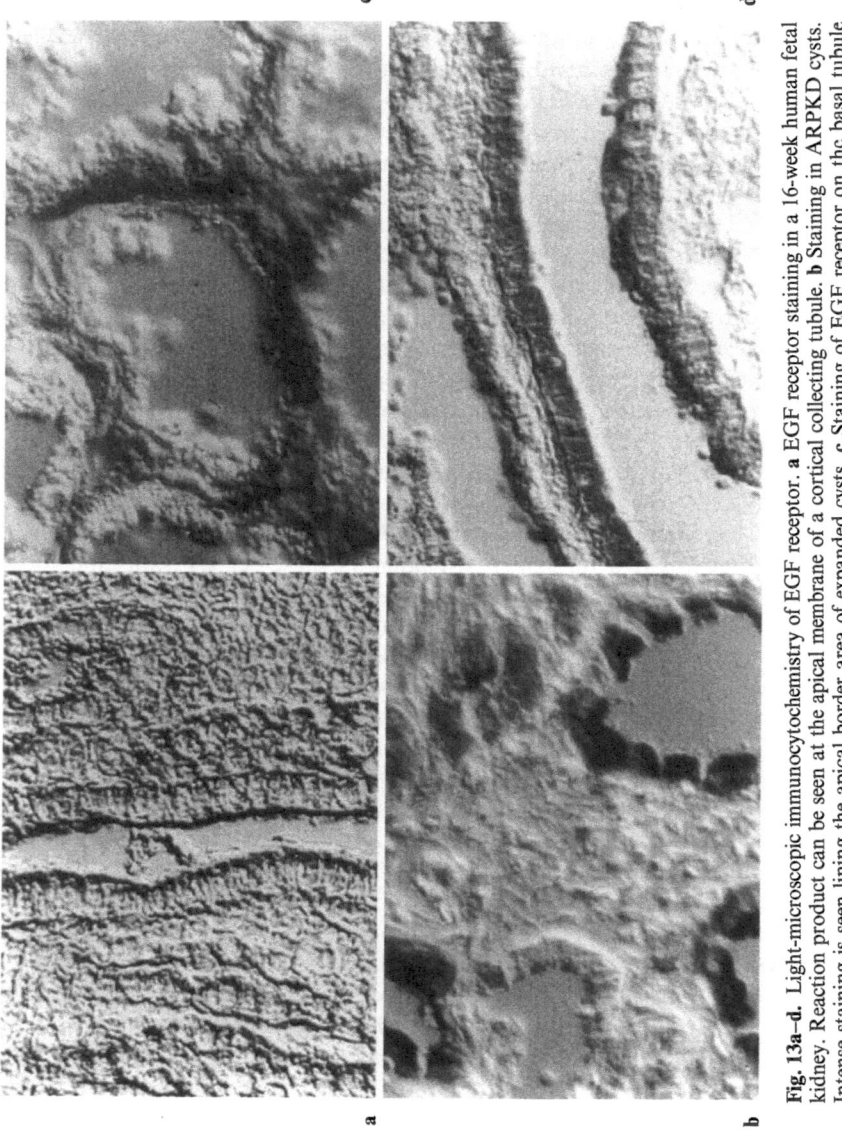

Fig. 13a–d. Light-microscopic immunocytochemistry of EGF receptor. **a** EGF receptor staining in a 16-week human fetal kidney. Reaction product can be seen at the apical membrane of a cortical collecting tubule. **b** Staining in ARPKD cysts. Intense staining is seen lining the apical border area of expanded cysts. **c** Staining of EGF receptor on the basal tubule membranes in normal adult kidneys. **d** Immunostaining for EGF receptor in end-stage ADPKD kidney. Some reaction product is seen on the basal epithelial cell surfaces, but the most intense reaction is at the apical membrane of cystic epithelia

inappropriate expansion of the stromal cell component of the ADPKD inter-stitium. In vitro studies are in progress to determine whether similar mechanisms may operate in ARPKD.

8.4 Transcription Factor Expression

At the most fundamental level, the proliferation of cells in organs in vivo is controlled by the activation of transcription, which is regulated by a myriad of transcription factors. Although some of these nuclear proteins are of general significance to all cell types for cell division, it has become clear that certain transcription factors are associated in a specific manner with cell proliferation in specific organs and at specific stages in development; for instance, Pax-2 and WT-1 are specifically involved in the control of renal cell proliferation during nephrogen-esis (PRITCHARD-JONES et al. 1990; DRESSLER and DOUGLASS 1992). Abnormal transcriptional activation during tumorigenesis is well known, and transgenic mice expressing the oncogenes *c-myc* and T antigen exhibit numerous proliferative and cystic lesions in many organs, including the kidneys (BRINSTER et al. 1984; MACKAY et al. 1987; TRUDEL et al. 1991). However, the lesions in these mice are more profoundly proliferative in nature than is seen in human ADPKD or ARPKD. Indeed, it is of extreme interest and significance that the proliferative lesions in ADPKD and ARPKD are not associated with increased incidence of renal neoplasms and, in several respects, seem to represent a more controlled proliferative response than those associated with neoplastic transformation. It has therefore been of interest to examine the expression of transcription factors normally associated with proliferation during the stage-specific proliferation accompanying renal development, such as WT-1 and Pax-2, which are expressed in normal fetal, ADPKD, and ARPKD kidneys but not in normal adult human kidneys (Tables 3 and 5). These findings are of particular significance in light of the demonstration that mice bearing the Pax-2 transgene also produce cystic kidneys (DRESSLER et al. 1993). This suggests that the re-expression or continued express-ion of renal transcription factors after completion of normal proliferation and differentiation during nephrogenesis might allow the continued, inappropriate proliferation in kidneys and lead to cyst formation.

9 Fluid Transport and Secretion Abnormalities in ADPKD

Since cysts accumulate fluid in their luminal cavities, while normal renal tubules are characterized by their fluid reabsorption properties, it can be reasoned that there are likely to be abnormalities related to fluid and ion transport in cystic kidneys. Since the sodium ion is the major osmotic determinant of fluid movement, and the NaK-ATPase is the active sodium pump responsible for the establishment

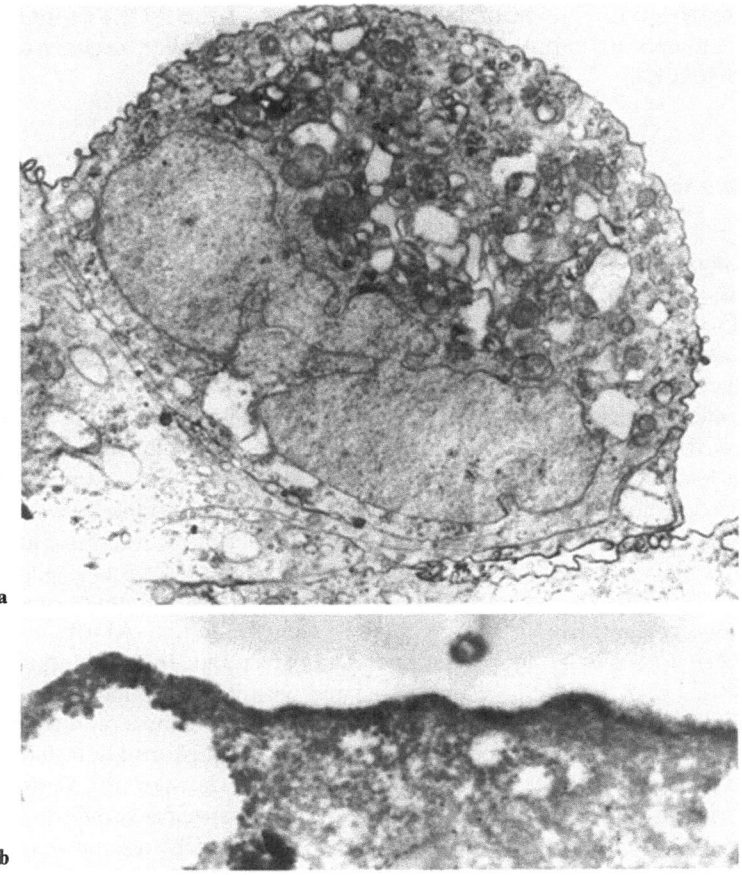

a

b

Fig. 14a–d. Electron-microscopic immunostaining of EGF receptor in filter-grown epithelial calls. Confluent monolayer cultures of cells are fixed in paraformaldehyde for 5 min and undergo pre-embedding immunoreaction with EGF receptor primary antibody, followed by avidin-biotin-peroxidase detection, prior to embedding and sectioning for electron microscopy. **a** Electron-dense reaction on the apical and lateral cell membranes of a human fetal proximal tubule cell in cell vitro. **b** High-power view of electron-dense EGF receptor product on the apical cell surface of an ARPKD epithelial cell in vitro membrane.

of sodium gradients that derive transport in the kidney, it was logical to examine the properties of NaK-ATPase (WILSON et al. 1991). In normal kidneys this enzyme is located exclusively on the basolateral epithelial cell membranes, where it is responsible for pumping sodium out of the cell into the basal cellular (blood) space (Figs. 15 and 16a). Since sodium enters the apical surface of epithelial cells via various transporters as a result of the sodium gradient thus established, the net vectorial transport of sodium is from lumen to blood, i.e., from the apical to the basal side of the epithelial monolayer sheet, and is a consequence of the basolateral location of the NaK-ATPase protein complexes. Both in vivo and in vitro immuno- and enzyme cytochemical localization studies at the light- and electron-

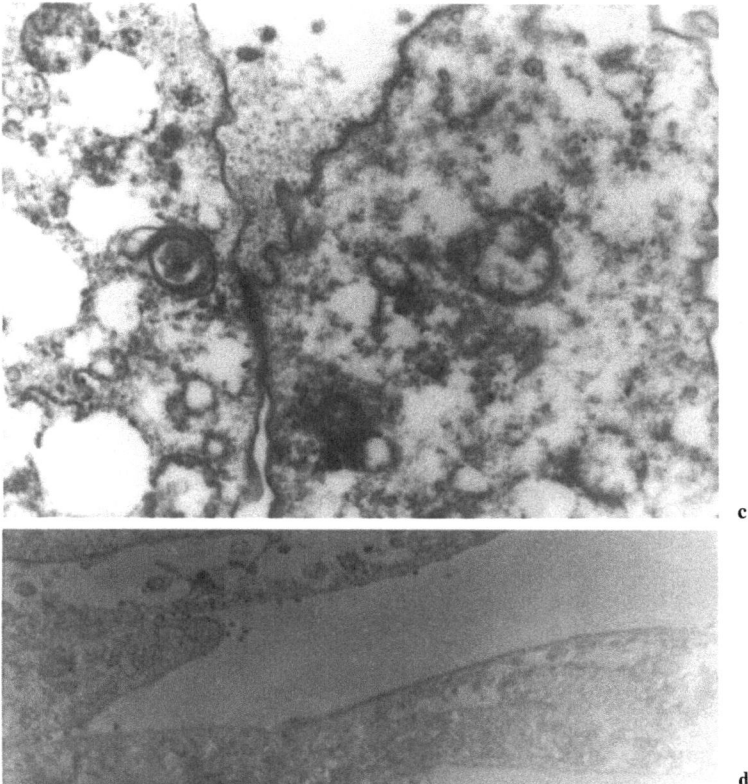

Fig. 14. c Apical localization of EGF receptor in an end-stage ADPKD cultured cell monolayer. Note the tight junction between two cells. **d** An end-stage ADPKD cell processed in a similar fashion, with the exception that no incubation in the presence of a primary EGF receptor antibody was included. Note the lack of reaction product

microscopic levels showed that NaK-ATPase was localized exclusively on the apical, cyst-lining epithelial cell membranes of ADPKD cystic epithelia (WILSON et al. 1991; WILSON and BURROW 1992 and Figs. 16b, c, d, and 17b, c). This was shown to be an early event, since even in minimally expanded microcysts in vivo and in cultures of ADPKD epithelia from early-stage ADPKD kidneys, staining was clearly apical, associated with a brush border (Figs. 16b and 17b). This was in stark contrast to the basolateral membrane staining in normal renal tubule profiles (Fig. 16a). Additional enzymatic, radioligand-binding, and transport studies confirmed that both the normal and mispolarized NaK-ATPase were fully functional (WILSON et al. 1991; WILSON and BURROW 1992). In vitro, net ^{22}Na transport was shown to be from the basal to the apical media compartments of tight ADPKD epithelial monolayers grown on polarized membrane supports (Fig. 18b), and that this transport could be inhibited by ouabain, but only when it was added to the apical cell surface, not when it was added to the basal cell surface (Fig. 18d). This

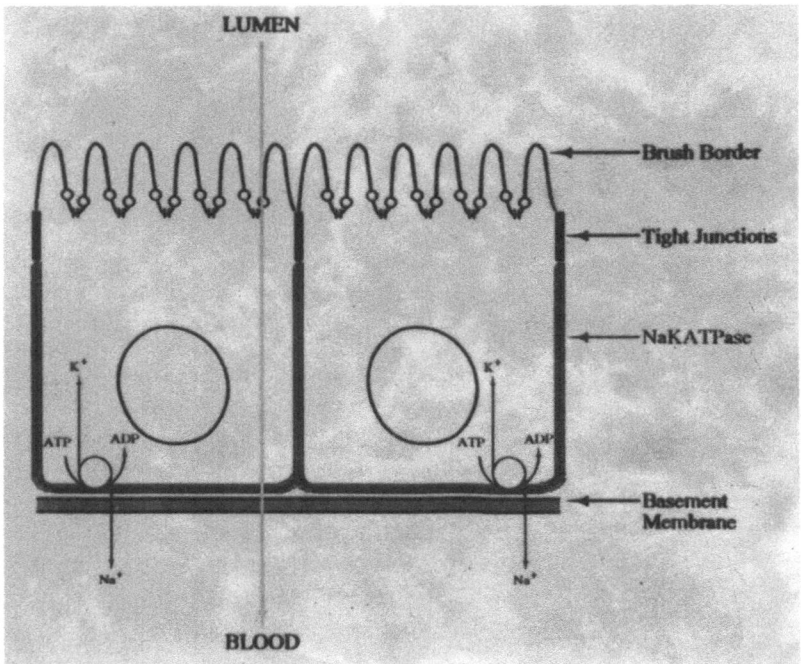

Fig. 15. Mechanisms involved in the vectorial transport of sodium in normal renal tubules

was in direct contrast to the properties of normal renal epithelia grown on membranes in vitro, which transport ^{22}Na only in an apical-to-basal direction (Fig. 18a), a process which can be inhibited only by ouabain when added to the basal compartment (Fig. 18c). These studies showed that NaK-ATPase was dramatically mispolarized in ADPKD epithelial cells both in vivo and in vitro, and that in vitro the functional consequence of the reversal of location was a reversal in the polarity of vectorial transport of sodium from the basal to the apical surfaces of ADPKD epithelial sheets. If this consequence prevails in vivo, it would lead to osmotic fluid secretion into the expanding cystic tubule lumen and to fluid accumulation and progressive expansion.

Further inhibitor studies conducted on polarized ADPKD epithelial cell mono-layers in vitro and functional studies on isolated membrane vesicle transport have been used to further characterize the membrane transporters in these cells. To date, findings include demonstration of an amiloride-sensitive Na-uptake mechanism consistent with an Na^+ channel or Na/H antiporter in the apical cell membranes of cyst-lining epithelia and a bumetanide- and furosemide-sensitive $Na + K + 2Cl$ co-transporter in the basal membranes of cyst epithelial (Wilson et al. 1991). Membrane vesicle studies also suggest that the Na/glucose transporter is function-ally absent from ADPKD and ARPKD kidneys (Hammel and Wilson 1989).

NaK-ATPase is a well-studied enzyme in MDCK and other cell lines, and several mechanisms have been implied as possible regulators for polarized segregation of this membrane protein complex into particular cell membranes

(RODRIGUEZ-BOULAN and NELSON 1989). In normal reabsorptive epithelia, such as those in the normal kidney and intestine, this is restricted to the basolateral membranes, whereas in the retinal epithelium and choroid plexus, where transport is from the basal to an apical surface, NaK-ATPase is located solely on apical membranes. Therefore, it seems that the ADPKD mutation leads to a specific mispolarization of NaK-ATPase to the inappropriate polarized cell membrane, and that this then has dramatic and deleterious consequences for vectorial ion and fluid transport. In MDCK cells, the disposition of the membrane cytoskeletal proteins ankyrin and fodrin (non-red-cell spectrin) have been implicated as regulators of the maintenance of NaK-ATPase polarization (NELSON and HAMMERTON 1989). It is also found that ankyrin and fodrin co-localize at the apical plasma membrane in cyst-lining ADPKD epithelia (WILSON 1991b; WILSON and BURROW 1992). However, in normal kidneys in vivo, ankyrin is associated not only with NaK-ATPase at the basolateral membranes of thick ascending limb tubule epithelia, but also in the apical membranes of proximal tubule cells. Since this association is not seen in normal choroid plexus or retinal epithelial cells, the relative importance of these cytoskeletal proteins in the ADPKD defect remains to be determined. Similarly, the adhesion proteins uvomorulin (E-cadherin) and catenins have been implicated in NaK-ATPase disposition in MDCK cells, but their roles in ADPKD remain to be elucidated (DU and WILSON 1991). The most clear-cut alteration associated with the ADPKD NaK-ATPase abnormality in ADPKD is the aberrant expression of the normally fetal beta-2 isoform in association with the alpha-1 isoform in early- and end-stage ADPKD kidneys (WILSON et al. 1993b). Since NaK-ATPase is a heterodimeric protein complex of alpha and beta isoforms, it is argued that the abnormal presence of the beta-2 isoform instead of the normal adult beta-1 isoform in the complex might direct abnormal cell sorting to the apical instead of basolateral membranes. The precedent for this hypothesis lies in the observation that the presence of beta-2 as the major beta isoform in fetal kidneys is associated with apical localization of NaK-ATPase during normal renal epithelial differentiation during development.

10 Cell Polarity Abnormalities in ADPKD and ARPKD

Since the first demonstration of abnormal polarity of an epithelial membrane protein, the NaK-ATPase, in ADPKD cyst epithelia (WILSON et al. 1991), several other membrane proteins have been found to show abnormalities in polarity (Table 4). These include ankyrin, fodrin, and E-cadherin, which are associated with apical NaK-ATPase and basal Na + K + 2Cl-, all of which have impact on ion and fluid transport abnormalities associated with the fluid secretion in ADPKD cysts. It is of interest that this apical mislocation of NaK-ATPase has also been demonstrated in the *cpk* mouse model for ARPKD (AVNER et al. 1992), although in human ARPKD both apical and basal localization have been seen (FALKENSTEIN et al. 1993; E.D. Avner, personal communication). This may be

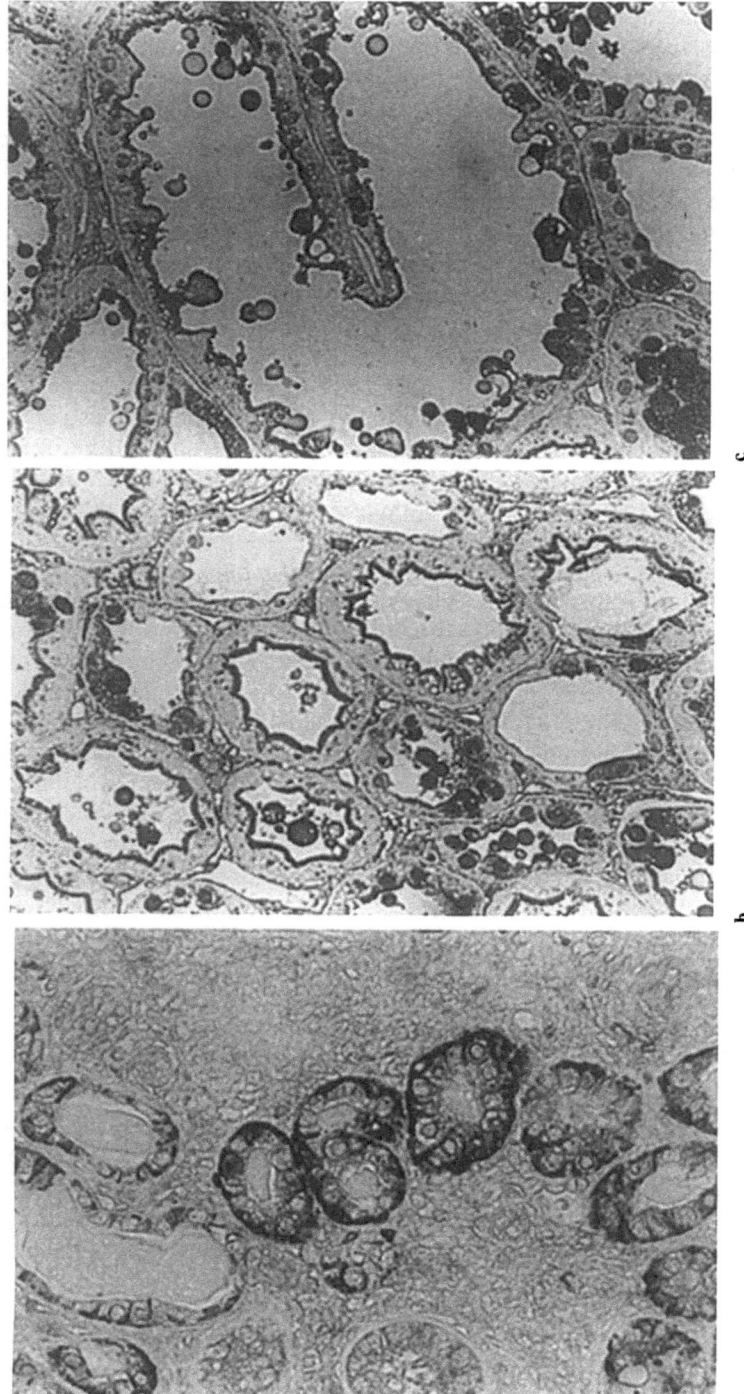

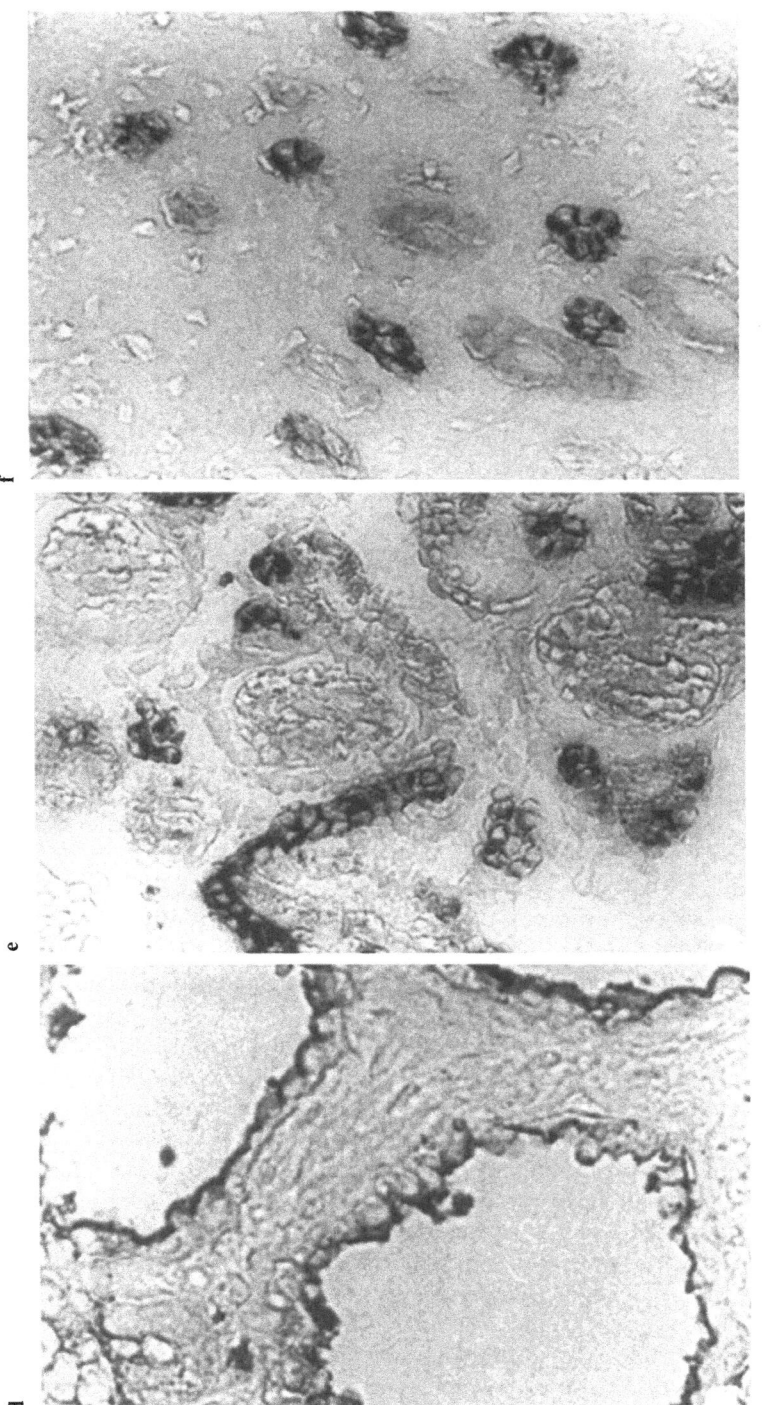

Fig. 16a–f. Light-microscopic immunocytochemistry of NaK-ATPase alpha subunit in human kidneys. **a** Basal and lateral epithelial cell membrane staining of normal human renal tubules. **b** Exclusive apical epithelial cell membrane staining in minimally expanded cystic tubules in an early-stage ADPKD kidney. **c** Exclusive apical epithelial cell membrane staining for NaK-ATPase in a larger cyst in an early-stage ADPKD kidney. **d** Exclusive apical epithelial cell membrane staining for NaK-ATPase in a cysts from an end-stage ADPKD kidney. **e** Apical and lateral epithelial cell membrane staining of a recently formed proximal tubule from a 19-week human fetal kidney. Note that the lumen is closed. **f** Apical and lateral epithelial cell membrane staining of NaKATPase in the medullary collecting tubules of a 19-week human fetal kidney

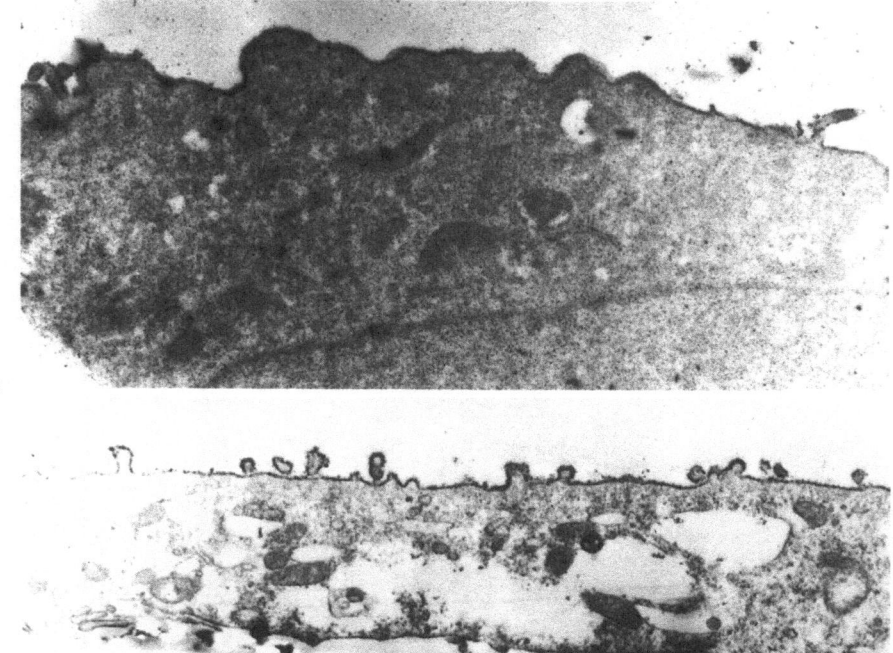

Fig. 17a–c. Electron-microscopic immuno- and enzyme-cytochemistry of NaK-ATPase alpha subunit in confluent monolayer epithelial cell cultures grown on permeable membrane supports. **a** High-power image of electron-dense reaction product on the apical plasma membrane of a human fetal proximal tubule epithelial cell in vitro. **b** Intense reaction product for NaK-ATPase on the apical plasma membrane of an early stage ADPKD epithelial cell in vitro.

a reflection of the small size (1–2 mm) of ARPKD cysts compared with ADPKD cysts, which can reach several centimeters and contain tens to even hundreds of millimiters of cyst fluid, and may implicate the proliferative defect as the predominant cause of cyst formation in ARPKD, while the transport defect may be the predominant feature in ADPKD.

Another membrane protein which exhibits marked, but not complete reversal of polarity in ADPKD and ARPKD is the EGF receptor (WILSON 1991b; WILSON et al. 1993a). As discussed above, this mislocalization to apical membranes of cyst-lining epithelia provides the mechanism whereby EGF can directly induce proliferation in vivo by an autocrine mechanism. This then suggests that alterations in polarity can have (a) significant impact on renal cell function by influencing important changes in ion transport, and also on proliferation by enabling response to ligands. Since the alterations are manifest in both ADPKD and ARPKD, this may invoke a common underlying mechanism resulting in cyst formation in these disease entities.

To determine the extent of membrane protein polarity abnormalities in ADPKD and ARPKD, a more comprehensive survey of polarized membrane

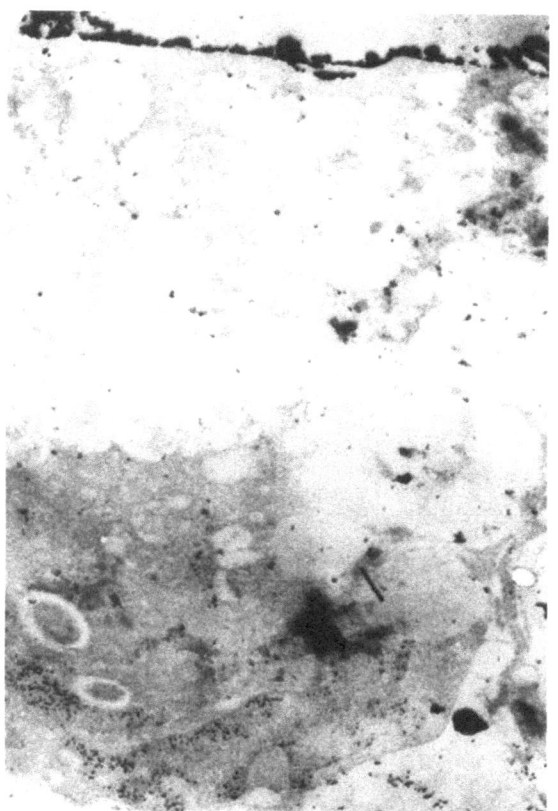

c

Fig. 17. c Intense reaction product for NaK-ATPase activity on the apical membrane of an end-stage ADPKD epithelial cell in confluent culture

protein localization has been carried out in our laboratory. It should be emphasized that many membrane proteins do not change in their polarized distribution in ADPKD or ARPKD epithelia (Table 4). For instance GP330, the P-glycoprotein product of the multi-drug transporter gene glycophosphatidyl-inositol-anchored membrane proteins, alkaline phosphatase, leucine aminopeptidase, and trehalase retain their apical location, while band-3 protein, type-IV collagen, heparan sulfate proteoglycan (HSPG), laminin, and its alpha-6 integrin receptor retain their basal locations. This then excludes the possibility that there is a complete reversal of whole cell polarity and is consistent with the morphological findings showing retention of apical brush borders, basal basement membranes, and apically located intercellular tight junctions. Therefore, specific membrane proteins are affected by an alteration in polarized distribution, and it is to be hoped that precise definition of those groups of proteins so affected point to particular candidate proteins as the underlying cause of cyst formation in ADPKD and ARPKD. The information to date suggests that some protein related to cellular sorting of membrane proteins on

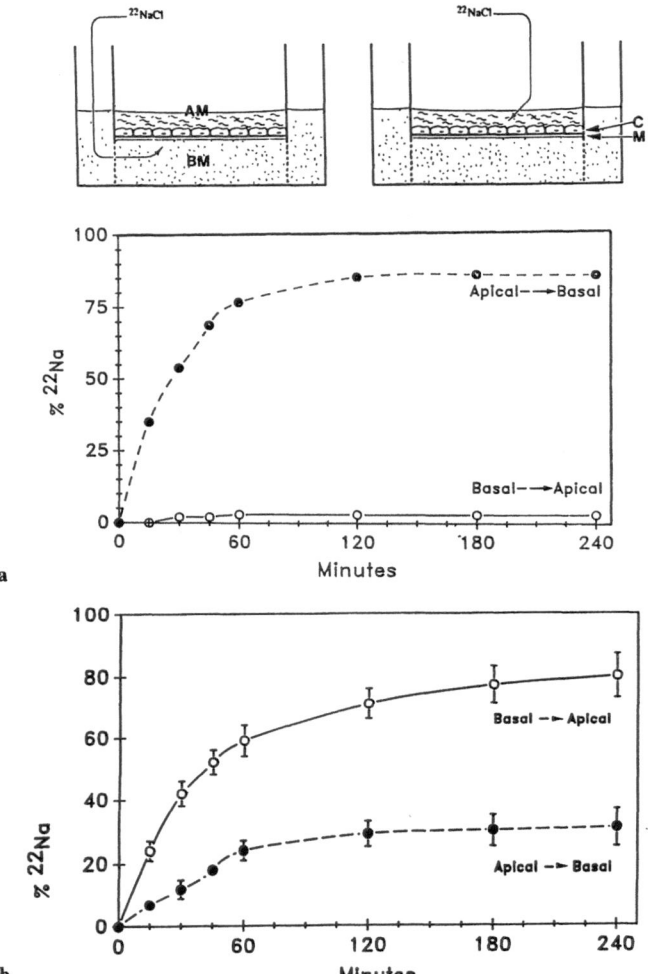

Fig. 18a–d. ^{22}NaCl transport in polarized confluent human renal epithelial monolayer cultures grown on permeable membranes. Renal epithelial cells (*C*) are grown to confluence on a collagen-coated permeable membrane (*M*) and ^{22}NaCl is added to either the apical (*AM*) or basal (*BM*) medium compartment. Transepithelial sodium transport is measured by sampling of the media compartments and counting of radioactivity by liquid scintillation. **a** Results of such studies in confluent monolayers of normal adult human collecting tubule epithelia. Transepithelial transport of sodium was detected only when it was added to the apical compartment, not to the basal compartment. This is consistent with exclusive apical-to-basal vectorial transport of sodium in normal renal epithelia. **b** In parallel studies carried out on tight confluent monolayers of ADPKD epithelia there was significant transepithelial transport of sodium when it was added to the basal surface and some as well when it was added to the apical surface. The net tansport, however, was from the basal to the apical compartment, which is consistent with vectorial transport from the basal (blood) to apical (cyst fluid) surfaces of ADPKD cyst epithelia. **c** Inhibition of normal apical-to-basal ^{22}Na transport was effected by ouabain, but only when it was added to the basal medium compartment, not when it was added to the apical compartment. This is consistent with basal membrane localization of ouabain-sensitive NaK-ATPase in normal human renal epithelia. **d** Inhibilion of ADPKD basal-to-apical transport of ^{22}Na was effected by ouabain when added to the apical medium compartment, but not when it was added to the basal compartment. This is consistent with an apically located, ouabain-sensitive NaK-ATPase in ADPKD cyst epithelia

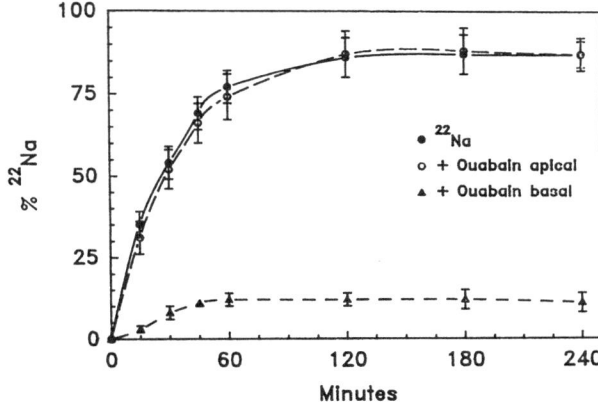

c

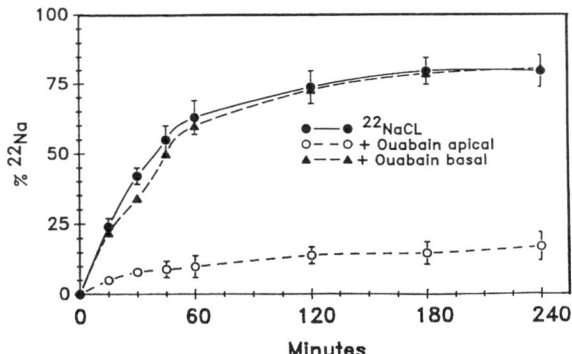

d

Fig. 18. c, d

the secretory pathway may be involved at a fundamental level. Several proteins that act at the trans-Golgi network level to direct vesicular transport of proteins suggest themselves as potential candidates, but clarification will await combination of the genetic, cellular, and molecular approaches being undertaken.

11 Renal Development and Cystic Disease

It is clear that many of the renal cystic lesions described are developmental in origin. They may be due to nongenetic mechanisms as in renal dysplasia or obstruction, or they may be the result of clearly arrested development at a specific stage of the differentiation process leading to nephrogenesis, occurring early, as in

Table 4. Polarized membrane proteins in ADPKD

Polarity	Protein
Basal to apical	Na + K + -ATPase
	Fodrin
	Ankyrin
	Uvomorulin
	EGF receptor
	Calpactin
	c-Met
	CHIP 28
Intracellular to apical	Cathepsin B
	Cathepsin H
	TIMP
	Gelatinase A
Apical to basal	$Na^+K^+2CI^-$
	Cathepsin B (secreted)
Apical no change	Alkaline phosphatase
	GP330
	alpha 95 kD
	MDR P-glycoprotein
	GPI-linked
	Leucine aminopeptidase
	Trehalase
Basal, no change	Band 3
	Transferrin receptor
	Integrin (alpha 6)
	HSPG
	Collagen IV
	Laminin

medullary cystic disease, or in the final stages of ureteric branching, as in ARPKD. This concept is substantiated in the liver pattern in ARPKD, as the angulated branching of bile ducts to form rings is atypical of a stage that precedes differentiation of normal tubular bile ducts.

ADPKD was long considered an adult-onset disease that reflected conversion of normal into abnormal tubules in adulthood. However, recent improvements in ultrasonography and imaging techniques, increased clinical surveillance of ADPKD families, and detailed analysis of preazotemic ADPKD kidneys have led to the realization that ADPKD cysts may form as early as in utero, and the possibility that ADPKD may indeed represent a developmental abnormality has been reinvoked (WILSON and BURROW 1992). To examine the hypothesis that ADPKD refelects arrested development, we have conducted several studies comparing the properties of proteins of normal human fetal kidneys during development with those of ADPKD and ARPKD kidneys in vivo and in vitro (FALKENSTEIN et al. 1993 and Table 5). Most significant, it is clear that during normal renal development there are stages when NaK-ATPase and EGF receptor expression are clearly apical in polarized but not yet fully differentiated renal tubule epithelia (Figs. 13a, 14a, 16e, f, and 17a). This suggests that although renal tubule formation is a rapid and continual process from 6 to 30 weeks of gestation

Table 5. Expression of fetal phenotypic characteristics in ADPKD and ARPKD epithelia

	Fetal	Adult	ADPKD	ARPKD
Apical NaK-ATPase	$+$	$-$	$+$	$+$
	$\alpha_1\beta_2$	$\alpha_1\beta_1$	$\alpha_1\beta_2$	$\alpha_1\beta_2$
Apical EGF receptor	$+$	$-$	$+$	$+$
Pax-2 expressed	$+$	$-$	$+$	$+$
WT-1 expressed	$+$	$-$	$+$	ND
Glycogen	$+$	$-$	$+$	$+$
Microfilaments	$+$	$-$	$+$	
Lamellar bodies	$+$	$-$	$+$	$+$
Albumin	$+$	$-$	$+$	ND

and the conversion from undifferentiated mesenchyme to structurally polarized epithelium takes only 1 week, the fine details of specific membrane protein segregation to final polarized locations may take many weeks, even until after birth. It is apparent that some membrane proteins polarize more quickly than others. For instance, tight junctional specializations occur in the earliest phases of epithelial differentiation at the S-body stage, and proteins including alkaline phosphatase and the MDR protein are also quick to polarize to their final apical membrane locations in S-bodies and early proximal tubules. At the other extreme, however, proteins such as the band-3 transporter are not expressed until after birth, NaK-ATPase and EGF receptor occupy an intermediate position with regard to rate of acquisition of the adult pattern of polarization. The NaK-ATPase complex is highly and differentially expressed early in renal development, but in the earliest stages in newly formed proximal tubules and in medullary collecting tubules it is found on the apical as well as lateral membranes (Figs. 16e and f). The situation is similar for the EGF receptor, with apical localization being distinctive in early proximal tubules and in collecting ducts (Figs. 13a and 14a). This is interest since both of these proteins are found in apical locations in ADPKD and in ARPKD (Figs. 13b,d, 14b,c, 16b,c,d, and 17b,c), which then has dramatic functional consequences for renal tubule expansion into cysts. These correlative findings are therefore consistent with the notion that even ADPKD may represent an arrested developmental state. It could be argued that such tubules with fetal-type protein distribution are the subset responsible for subsequent expansion and gradual destruction of those tubules that have normal or adult patterns of polarization. A more extensive analysis is in progress to validate or refute this assertion which has already yielded some important additional correlations between protein expression during development and ADPKD, including the persistent expression of the transcription factors Pax-2 and WT-1. It remains to be determined whether these correlations of structure and protein expression reflect true arrested development and persistence of protein expression or re-expression of fetal proteins by susceptible adult tubules in ADPKD.

12 Conclusions and Perspectives

From this apparently complicated picture a generalized concept has been hypothesized; i.e., a candidate gene product for the ADPKD gene may be

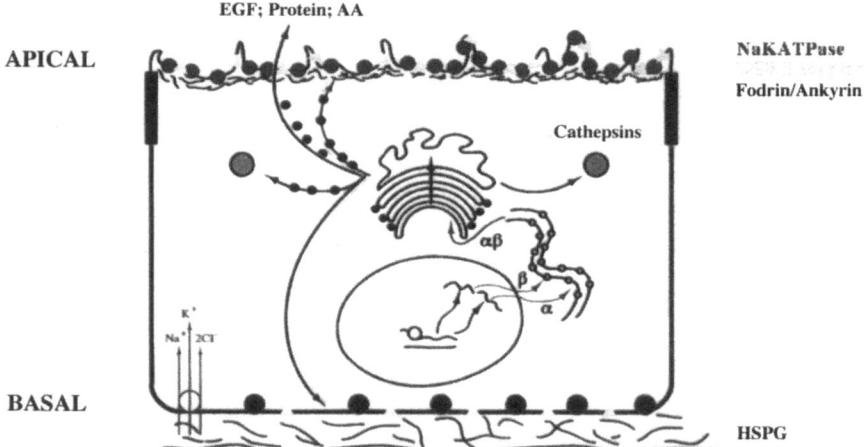

Fig. 19. Phenotype of an ADPKD epithelial cell. Membrane proteins are synthesized on ribosomes, assembled and processed in the endoplasmic reticulum, and further processed by post-translational modification by passage from the cis- to trans- side of the Golgi. In the trans-Golgi network signal mechanisms are involved in the direction of vesicular transport of membrane proteins to their final destinations at polarized plasma membranes. It is hypothesized that in ADPKD there is a defect in this intracellular protein sorting mechanism, and that this may reflect an arrested developmental programming

a protein involved in the ordered sorting of membrane proteins to their polarized segregated membranes, a process that takes place during renal development. This is likely to involve signals that direct proteins to certain subsets of intracellular vesicles for their conveyance to the membrane in question. Precedent exists for these types of proteins, including rab proteins, which are responsible for the transport of proteins from the region of the cell in which they are sorted, the trans-Golgi network, to their final destination at the apical or basolateral cell membrane, or for secretion. A genetic defect which interferes in some fairly minor way with one or more of these sorting signals might be sufficient to cause disturbance of membrane protein polarity without disrupting polarity completely (lethally), thus leading to a "disturbed" phenotype such as the ADPKD cyst epithelial cell (Fig. 19).

As this review of current developments in the field of human renal cystic kidney diseases has shown, the major part of experimental information available concerns alterations associated with human ADPKD, although it should be emphasized that information is also available on murine models of recessive PKD, particularly the *cpk* mouse, which has not been covered in depth here. An attempt has been made to concentrate on human manifestations of renal cystic disease, as it is not clear how far extrapolations can be drawn between the many animal models and disease genes of different chromosome locations with human ARPKD. This situation will become clearer when the chromosome location, and ultimately the gene for ARPKD are identified. In attempting to search for basic mechanisms . underlying cystic disease it is also important not to oversimplify, since there are apparently several ways to induce a cyst. It may be the result of a genetic or nongenetic mechanism and may or may not be associated with more general systemic and frankly neoplastic disorders. Regarding the group of genetic diseases where cyst formation is the primary event, it is important to bear in mind some fundamentals of autosomal inheritance that will have impact on future analysis and ultimately, hopefully on retardation and prevention treatment strategies by "designer drugs" and gene therapy. In those diseases that are the result of recessive mutations, the affected individual is a homozygote bearing two abnormal alleles that lead to a loss of gene function. The treatment for these diseases will necessitate restoration of this lost function, most likely by introduction of the new normal gene. Autosomal dominant mutations such as ADPKD present a more complicated and currently less certain scenario. Since the affected individuals are heterozygotes, the disease is a reflection of the presence of one abnormal allele which might lead to a loss of normal gene function due to a "gene dosage" effect, and therefore be analagous to the situation in recessive disease. Alternatively, however, the abnormal allele may result in the acquisition of an abnormal function, a so-called gain of function mutation. If the second alternative proves to be the case, successful treatment of the disease will necessitate an inhibition of this abnormal function by specifically targeted effectors. In this case, gene therapy may not be the treatment of choice, rather the design of specific drugs would be invoked. In any event, precise definition of the pathophysiologic consequences of the disease phenotype is essential, since only with such an understanding will it be possible to retard progression of the disease in individuals already carrying genes resulting in renal cystic disease.

References

Antignac C, Arduy CH, Beckman JS, Benessy F, Gros, F, Medhioub M, Hildebrandt F, Dufier J, Kleinknecht C, Broyer M, Weissenbach, J, Habib R, Cohen D (1993) A gene for familial juvenile nephrononphthisis (recessive medullary cystic kidney disease) maps to chromosome 2p. Nature Genet 3: 342–345

Avner ED, Sweeney WE, Nelson WJ (1992) Abnormal sodium pump distribution during renal tubulogenesis in cogenital murine polycystic kidney disease. Proc Natl Acad Sci USA 89: 7447–7451

Baert L (1978) Hereditary polycystic kidney disease (adult form): a microdissection study of two cases at an early stage of the disease. Kidney Int 13: 519–525

Bennett AH, Stewart W, Lazarus JM (1973) Bilateral nephrectomy in patients with polycystic renal disease. Surg Gynecol Obstet 137: 918

Bernstein J (1976) A classification of renal cysts. Perspect Nephrol Hypertens 4: 7–30

Bernstein J, Evan AP, Gardner KJ (1987) Epithelial hyperplasia in human polycystic kidney diseases. Its role in pathogenesis and risk of neoplasia. Am J Pathol 129: 92–101

Brinster RL, Chen HY, Messing A (1984) Transgenic mice harboring SV40 T-antigen genes develop characteristic brain tumors. Cell 37: 367–379

Butkowski RJ, Carone FA, Grantham JJ, Hudson BG (1985) Tubular basement membrane changes in 2-amino-4,5-diphenylthiazole-induced polycystic kidney disease. Kidney Int 28: 744

Call KM, Glaser T, Ito CY, Buckler AJ, Pelletier J, Haber DA, Rose EA, Kral A, Yeger H, Lewis WH, Jones C, Housman DE (1990) Isolation and characterization of a zinc-finger polypeptide gene at the human chromosome 11 Wilms' tumor locus. Cell 60: 509–520

Carone FA, Hollenberg PF, Nakamura S, Punyarit P, Glogowski W, Flouret G (1989a) Tubular basement membrane change occurs pari passu with the development of cyst formation. Kidney Int 35: 1034

Carone FA, Nakamura S, Schumacher BS, Punyarit P (1989b) Cyst-derived cells do not exhibit accelerated growth or features of transformed cells in vitro. Kidney Int 35: 1351–1357

Chapman AB, Rubinstein D, Hughes R, Stears JC, Earnest MP, Johnson AM, Gabow PA, Kaehny WD (1992) Intracranial aneurysms in autosomal dominant polycystic kidney disease. N Engl J Med 327: 916–920

Consortium TECITS (1993) Identification and characterization of the tuberous sclerosis gene on chromosome 16. Cell 75: 1305–1315

Consortium (1994) The polycystic kidney disease 1 gene encodes a 14 kb transcript and lies within a duplicated region of chromosome 16. Cell 77: 881–894

Cuppage FE, Huseman RA, Chapman A, Grantham JJ (1980) Ultrastructure and function of cysts from human adult polycystic kidneys. Kidney Int 17: 372–81

Dalgaard OZ (1957) Bilateral polycystic disease of the kidneys: a follow-up study of 284 patients and their families. Acta Med Scand 158: 1

Daoust MC, Bichet D, Somlo S (1993) A French-Canadian family with autosomal dominant polycystic kidney disease unlinked to ADPKD 1 and ADPKD 2. JASN 4: 262

Dobin A, Kimberling WJ, Pettinger W, Bailey WJ, Shugart YY, Gabow P (1993) Segregation analysis of autosomal dominant polycystic kidney disease. Genet Epidemiol 10: 189–200

DIowdy SF, Fasching CL, Araujo D, Lal K, Livanos E, Weissman BE, Stanbridge EJ (1991) Suppression of tumorigenicity in Wilms' tumor by the p15.5-p14 region of chromosome 11. Science 254: 293–295

Dressler GR, Douglass EC (1992) Pax-2 is a DNA-binding protein expressed in embryonic kidney and Wilms tumor. Dev Biol 89: 1179–1183

Dressler GR, Wilkinson JE, Rothenpieler UW, Patterson L, Williams-Simons L, Westphal H (1993) Deregulation of Pax-2 expression in transgenic mice generates severe kidney abnormalities. Nature 362: 65–67

Du J, Norman JT, Wilson PD (1991) EGF as an autocrine/paracrine regulator of aberrant cell proliferation in ADPKD. JASN 3: 251

Du J, Wilson PD (1991) Increased distribution of uvomorulin to apical membrane surface in autosomal dominant polycystic kidney disease. J Cell Biol 115: 67a

Du J, Wilson PD (1994) Abnormal polarity of EGF receptors: a mechanism for autocrine stimulation of cyst epithelial proliferation in human autosomal dominant polycystic kidney disease. Am J Physiol (in press)

Ebihara I, Killen PD, Laurie GW, Huang T, Yamada Y, Martin GR, Brown KS (1988) Altered mRNA expression of basement membrane components in a murine model of polycystic kidney disease. Lab Invest 58: 262–269

Eckardt K, Mollmann M, Neumann R, Brunkhorst R, Burger H, Lonnemann G, Skeusch G, Bucholz B, Frei U, Bauer C, Kurtz A (1989) Erythropoietin in polycystic kidneys. J Clin Invest 84: 1160–1166

Evan AP, McAteer JA (1990) Cyst cells and cyst walls. In: Gardner KD, Bernstein J (eds) The cystic kidney. Kluwer, Boston, pp 21–42

Everson GT, Scherzinger A, Berger LN, Reichen J, Lezotte D, Manco JM, Gabow P (1988) Polycystic liver disease: quantitation of parenchymal and cyst volumes from computed tomography images and clinical correlates of hepatic cysts. Hepatology 8: 1627–1634

Fahsold R, Rott HD, Lorenz P (1991) A third gene locus for tuberous sclerosis is closely linked to the phenylalanine hydroxylase gene locus. Hum Genet 88: 85–90

Falkenstein D, Burrow CR, Gatti L, Hartz PA, Wilson PD (1993) Expression of fetal proteins in human polycystic kidney disease epithelia. JASN 4: 813

Faraggiana T, Bernstein J, Strauss L, Churg J (1985) Use of lectins in the study of histogenesis of renal cysts. Lab Invest 53: 575–579

Fick GM, Johnson AM, Strain JD, Kimberling WJ, Kumar S, Manco-Johnson ML, Duley IT, Gabow PA (1992) Characteristics of very early onset autosomal dominant polycystic kidney disease. JASN 3: 1863–1870

Fryer AE, Chalmers AH, Connor JM, Fraser I, Povey S, Yates AD, Yates JR, Osborne JP (1987) Evidence that the gene for tuberous sclerosis is on chromosome 9. Lancet 1: 659–661

Gabow PA, Ikle DW, Holmes JH (1984) Polycystic kidney disease: prospective analysis of nonazotemic patients and family members. Ann Intern Med 101: 238–247

Gardner KJ (1969) Composition of fluid in twelve cysts of a polycystic kidney. N Engl J Med 281: 985–988

Gerber MJ, Drabkin HA, Firnhaber C, Miller YE, Scoggin CH, Smith DI (1988) Regional localization of chromosome 3-specific DNA fragments by using a hybrid cell deletion mapping panel. Am J Hum Genet 43: 442–451

Germino GG, Weinstatsaslow D, Himmelbauer H, Gillespie G, Somlo S, Wirth B, Barton N, Harris KL, Frischauf AM, Reeders ST (1992) The gene for autosomal dominant polycystic kidney disease lies in a 750-kb cpg-rich region. Genomics 13: 144–151

Graham PC, Lindop GB (1988) The anatomy of the renin-secreting cell in adult polycystic kidney disease. Kidney Int 33: 1084–1090

Grantham JJ (1993) Fluid secretion, cellular proliferation and the pathogenesis of renal epithelial cysts. JASN 3: 1843–1857

Grantham JJ, Geiser JL, Evan AP (1987) Cyst formation and growth in autosomal dominant polycystic kidney disease. Kidney Int 31: 1145–1152

Gregoire JR, Torres VE, Holley KE, Farrow GM (1987) Renal epithelial hyperplastic and neoplastic proliferation in autosomal dominant polycystic kidney disease. Am J Kid Dis 9: 27–38

Hammel RL, Wilson PD (1989) Loss of Na-dependent glucose transport in adult human polycystic kidney disease-derived apical membrane vesicles. Kidney Int 37: 225

Hartz PA, Wilson PD (1994) Functional defects in lysosomal enzymes in autosomal dominant polycystic kidney disease (ADPKD): abnormalities in synthesis, molecular processing, polarity and secretion. Am J Physiol (in press)

Heptinstall RH (1992) Pathology of the kidney. Little Brown, Boston

Hjelle JT, Waters DC, Golinska BT, Steidley KR, Burmeister V, Caughey R, Ketel B, McCarroll DR, Olsson PJ, Prior RB, Miller MA (1990) Autosomal recessive polycystic kidney disease: characterization of human peritoneal and cystic kidney cells in vitro. Am J Kidney Dis 15: 123–136

Holthofer H, Kumpulainen T, Rapola J (1990) Polycystic disease of the kidney. Lab Invest 62: 363–369

Hossack KF, Leddy CL, Johnson AM, Schrier RW, Gabow PA (1988) Echocardiographic findings in autosomal dominant polycystic kidney disease. N Engl J Med 319: 907–912

Hughson MD, Hennigar GR, McManus JF (1980) Atypical cysts, acquired renal cystic disease, and renal cell tumors in end-stage dialysis kidneys. Lab Invest 42: 475–480

Jin H, Carone FA, Nakamura S, Liu ZZ, Kanwar Y (1992) Altered synthesis and intracellular transport of proteoglycans by cyst-derived cells from human polycystic kidneys. JASN 2: 1726–1733

Kandt RS, Haines JL, Smith M, Northrup H, Gardner R, Short MP, Dumars K, Roach ES, Steingold S, Wall S, Blanton SH, Flodman P, Kwiatkowski DJ, Jewell A, Weber JL, Roses AD, Pericakvance MA (1992) Linkage of an important gene locus for tuberous sclerosis to a chromosome-16 marker for polycystic kidney disease. Nature Genetics 2: 37–41

Kimberling WJ, Fain PR, Kenyon JB, Goldgar D, Sujansky E, Gabow PA (1988) Linkage heterogeneity of autosomal dominant polycystic kidney disease. N Engl J Med 319: 913–8

Kimberling WJ, Kuman S, Gabow PA (1993) Identification of chromosome site of autosomal dominant polycystic kidney disease unlinked to chromosome 16. JASN 4: 816

Klingel R, Dippold W, Storkel S, Meyer K, Kohler H (1992) Expression of differentiation antigens and growth-related genes in normal kidney, autosomal dominant polycystic kidney disease and renal cell carcinoma. Am J Kidney Dis 19: 22–30

Kuo N, Wilson PD (1990) Mitogenic effects of growth factors in human renal fibroblasts during normal development, aging and polycystic kidney disease. JASN 1: 723

Kuo N, Wilson PD (1991) A role for acidic fibroblast growth factor in the fibroblast proliferative defect of autosomal dominant polycystic kidney disease. J Cell Biol 115: 418a

Latif F, Tory K, Gnarra J, Yao M, Duh F, Orcutt M, Stackhouse T, Kuzmin I, Modi W, Geil L, Schmidt I, Zhon F, Li H, Wei M, Chen F, Glenn G, Choyke P, Walther M, Weng Y, Duan D, Dean M, Glara D, Richards F, Crossey D, Ferguson-Smith M, Paslier D, Chumakov I, Cohen D, Chinault A, Maher E, Linehan W, Zbar B, Larman M (1993) Identification of the von Hippel–Lindan disease tumor suppressor gene. Science 260: 1317–1320

Mackay K, Striker LJ, Pinkert CA (1987) Glomerulosclerosis and renal cysts in mice transgenic for the early regiuon of SV40. Kidney Int 32: 827–837

Mangoo-Karim R, Uchic M, Grant M, Shumate WA, Calvet JP, Park CH, Grantham JJ (1989) Renal epithelial fluid secretion and cyst growth: the role of cyclic AMP. FASEB J 3: 2629–2632

McAteer JA, Carone FA, Grantham JJ, Kempson SA, Gardner KJ, Evan AP (1988) Explant culture of human polycystic kidney. Lab Invest 59: 126–136

Montesano R, Matsumoto K, Nakamura T, Orci L (1991a) Identification of a fibroblast-derived epithelial morphogen as hepatocyte growth factor. Cell 67: 901–908

Montesano R, Schaller G, Orci L (1991b) Induction of epithelial tubular morphogenesis in vitro by fibroblast-derived soluble factors. Cell 66: 697–711

Nagao S, Takahashi H (1991) Linkage analysis of two murine polycystic kidney disease genes, pcy and cpk. Jikken Dobutsn 40: 557–560

Nelson WJ, Hammerton RW (1989) A membrane-cytoskeletal complex containing Na + K + -ATPase, ankyrin and fodrin in Madin Darby canine kidney (MDCK) cells. Implications for the biogenesis of epithelial cell polarity. J Cell Biol 108: 893–902

Norman JT, Kuo N, Wilson PD (1992) Autocrine stimulation of fibroblast growth in autosomal dominant polycystic kidney disease is mediated by acidic fibroblast growth factor. JASN 3: 300

Norman JT, Gatti L, Wilson PD (1993) Abnormal matrix metalloproteinase regulation in human autosomal dominant polycystic kidney disease. JASN 4: 819

Osathanondh V, Potter EL (1964) Pathogenesis of cystic kidneys: historical survey; survey of results of microdissection. Arch Pathol 77: 459

Parfrey PS, Bear JC, Morgan J, Cramer BC, McManamon PJ, Ganlt MH, Churchill DN, Singh M, Hewitt R, Jomlo S, Readers ST (1990) The diagnosis and prognosis of autosomal dominant polycystic kidney disease. N Engl J Med 323: 1085–1090

Peters DJ, Spruit L, Saris JJ, Ravine D, Sandkjl LA, Fossdal R, Boersma J, van Eijk R, Norby S, Constantinou-Deltas CD, Pierides A, Brissenden, JE, Frants RR, van Ommen GB, Breuning MH (1993) Chromosome 4 localization of a second gene for autosomal dominant polycystic kidney disease. Nature Genetics 5: 359–362

Pritchard-Jones K, Fleming S, Davidson D, Bickmore W, Porteous D, Gosden C, Bard J, Buckler A, Pelletier J, Housman D, van Heyningen V, Hastie N (1990) The candidate Wilms' tumour gene is involved in genitourinary development. Nature 346: 194–197

Reeders ST, Breuning MH, Davies KE, Nicholls RD, Jarman AP, Higgs DR, Pearson PL, Weatherall DJ (1985) A highly polymorphic DNA marker linked to adult polycystic kidney disease on chromosome 16. Nature 317: 542–544

Rodriguez-Boulan E, Nelson WJ (1989) Morphogenesis of the polarized epithelial cell phenotype. Science 245: 718–725

Sedman A, Bell P, Manco JM, Schrier R, Warady BA, Heard EO, Butler SN, Gabow P (1987) Autosomal dominant polycystic kidney disease in childhood: a longitudinal study. Kidney Int 31: 1000–1005

Seizinger BR, Smith DI, Filling-Katz KM, Neamann H, Green JS, Choyke PL, Anderson KM, Freiman RN, Klauck SM, Whaley J, Decker H, Hsai YE, Collins D, Halperin J, Lamiell JM, Dostra B, Waziri MH, Govin MB, Scherer G, Drabkin HA, Aronin N, Schinzel A, Martuza RL, Gusella JT, Haines JL (1991) Genetic flanking markers refine diagnostic criteria and provide insights into the genetics of von Hippel-Lindau disease. Proc Natl Acad Sci USA 88: 2864–2868

Smith M (1990) Mapping of a gene determining tuberous sclarosis to human chromosome 11q14–11q23. Genomics 6: 105–114

Takahashi H, Calvet JP, Dittemore HD, Yoshida K, Grantham JJ, Gattone V (1991) A hereditary model of slowly progressive polycystic kidney disease in the mouse. JASN 1: 980–989

Torres VE, Donovan KA, Scicli G, Holley K, Thibodeau SN, Carretero OA, Inagami T, Mcateer JA, Johnson CM (1992) Synthesis of renin by tubulocystic epithelium in autosomal-dominant polycystic kidney disease. Kidney Int 42: 364–373

Trudel M, D'Agati V, Costantini F (1991) C-myc as an inducer of polycystic kidney disease in transgenic mice. Kidney Int 39: 665–671

Veis DJ, Sorenson S, Shutter JR, Korsmeyer SJ (1993) Bcl-2-deficient mice demonstrate fulminant lymphoid apoptosis, polycystic kidneys and hypopigmented hair. Cell 75: 229–240

Welling LW, Welling D (1988) Theoretical models of cyst formation and growth. Scanning Microsc 2: 1097–1102

Wilson PD (1991a) Aberrant epithelial cell growth in autosomal dominant polycystic kidney disease. Am J Kidney Dis 16: 634–637

Wilson PD (1991b) Cell Biology of human autosomal dominant polycystic kidney disease. Semin Nephrol 11: 607–616

Wilson PD (1991c) Tubulocystic epithelium. Kidney Int 39: 450–463

Wilson PD, Schrier RW, Breckon RD, Gabow PA (1986) A new method for studying human polycystic kidney disease epithelia in culture. Kidney Int 30: 371–378

Wilson PD, Sherwood AC, Palla K, Du J, Watson R, Norman JT (1991) Reversed polarity of Na + -K + -ATPase: mislocation to apical plasma membranes in polycystic kidney disease epithelia. Am J Physiol 260: F420–F430

Wilson PD, Hreniuk D, Gabow PA (1992) Abnormal extracellular matrix and excessive growth of human adult polycystic kidney disease epithelia. J Cell Physiol 150: 360–369

Wilson PD, Burrow CR (1992) Autosomal dominant polycystic kidney disease. Adv Nephrol 21: 125–142

Wilson PD, Du J, Norman JT (1993a) Autocrine, endocrine and paracrine regulation of growth abnormalities in autosomal dominant polycystic kidney disease. Eur J Cell Biol 61: 131–138

Wilson PD, Gatti L, Burrow CR (1993b) Expression of the beta-2 isoform of NaK-ATPase during human renal development and in polycystic kidney disease. Mol Biol Cell 4: 34a

Zerres K, Mucher G, Bachner L, Deschennes G, Eggerman T, Kaariainen H, Knapp M, Lennert T, Misselwitz J, von Muhlendahl KE, Neumann HPH, Pirson Y, Rudnik-Schoneborn S, Steinbicker V, Wirth B, Scharer K (1994) Mapping of the gene for autosomal recessive polycystic kidney disease (ARPKD) to chromosome 6p21–cen. Nature Genetics 7: 429–432

Zollinger HU, Mihatsch MJ, Edefonti A, Gaboardi F, Imbasciati E, Lennert T (1980) Nephronophthisis (medullary cystic disease of the kidney): a study using electron microscopy, immunofluorescence and a review of the morphological findings. Helv Paediatr Acta 35: 509

The Pathogenesis of Tubulointerstitial Disease and Mechanisms of Fibrosis

S. DODD

1 Introduction

Many renal diseases progress inexorably to end-stage renal failure even though the initial renal insult may be transient. Most patients with a glomerular filtration rate below 25 ml per minute will eventually require dialysis or transplantation, regardless of the original cause of reduced function. Time plots of the reciprocal of serum creatinine concentration suggest steady deterioration of nephron function at rates peculiar to each patient but not characteristic of the underlying disease (MITCH et al. 1976; RUTHERFORD et al. 1977).

Whilst in some cases the disease process responsible for the initial renal injury may remain active throughout the decline into renal failure, in many circumstances renal failure progresses even when a well-defined initiating disease process has undergone spontaneous remission or has been controlled therapeutically. BALDWIN (1977) showed progression of renal disease in patients with acute poststreptococcal glomerulonephritis in the absence of continued immunological injury. Similarly, patients with vesicoureteric reflux often develop progressive glomerulopathy in the absence of hypertension or active urinary tract infection, and despite surgical correction of the reflux (TORRES et al. 1980).

Histopathological studies in diverse forms of human renal disease have revealed hypertrophy, most likely due to hyperfiltration, of the nephron units least damaged by the original disease process (GOTTSCHALK 1971). BRENNER et al. (1982) proposed a 'hyperfiltration' hypothesis based on the rat remnant kidney model of nephron ablation and suggested that the increased pressures and flows acting on remnant glomerular capillaries may be responsible for progression of renal failure after an initial insult has reduced nephron mass. They observed progressive glomerulosclerosis in the remnant kidney due to increased transcapillary passage of plasma proteins and their subsequent deposition in the mesangium (VELOSA et al. 1977) and likened this process to the early glomerular sclerosis seen in children born with reduced numbers of functioning nephrons ('oligomeganephronia') or in patients with unilateral renal agenesis (ELEMA 1976; KIPROV et al. 1982).

The clinical relevance of intraglomerular hypertension and chronic glomerular hyperfiltration observed in the rat remnant model and the subsequent histopathological changes have been questioned. NOVICK et al. (1991) found that long-term renal function in man remained stable in most patients with a reduction of renal mass of more than 50%, although the patients were at increased risk of developing proteinuria, glomerulopathy, and progressive renal failure.

Thus, the role of glomerular injury and scarring in the progression of renal disease has been intensively studied, although evidence that changes in the tubulointerstitial compartment are the major determinant of renal outcome has been available for some time.

2 Tubulointerstitial Changes
Correlate with Renal Disease Progression

In 1968, RISDON et al. made an apparently anomalous discovery: it is the degree of tubulointerstitial pathology that correlates most closely with declining renal function, even in primarily glomerular diseases. They attempted to correlate the extent of histological abnormalities in 50 cases of chronic glomerulonephritis with renal function, using a semiquantitative technique and light microscopy, with the following results. There was a statistically highly significant correlation between the extent of the tubular changes and the degree of functional deterioration measured by creatinine clearance, plasma creatinine and the ability of the kidney to concentrate and to acidify the urine. Correlation of the same degree was not seen with glomerular damage.

Two years later, a group of researchers in Washington extended this work, firstly with a method for assaying and classifying histopathological changes in renal disease and secondly by correlating these structural abnormalities with function (SCHAINUK et al. 1970; STRIKER et al. 1970). Their work on the histopathological assessment of renal biopsies attempted to introduce a novel semiquantitative grading scheme into the interpretation of renal morphology which appeared to provide a framework for reproducible recording by different observers in a form suitable for statistical analysis. Having done this, they attempted to apply the method to 70 patients who had renal biopsies, comparing their histopathological data to the patients' glomerular filtration rate (GFR), renal plasma flow, and concentrating and acidifying capacities. Their results showed that a reduction in GFR, renal plasma flow, concentrating ability or ammonia excretion following an acid load showed a substantial relationship to abnormalities of the tubules and interstitium, regardless of the type of renal disease. Only a modest relationship was found between functional abnormalities and glomerular disease, even in conditions primarily affecting the glomeruli.

Bohle and colleagues, in Germany, confirmed these findings with a series of detailed histomorphometric studies that put the issue beyond doubt (BOHLE et al. 1977a, b, c, 1979). They studied large numbers of renal biopsies of specific diseases and were able to show that the appearance of the tubulointerstitial compartment in the initial biopsy was the main histological predictor of whether renal function would be preserved or lost. They found that in extreme cases, relatively normal glomerular appearances could co-exist with a severely impaired GFR, while highly abnormal glomerular appearances may be seen with a normal GFR, with these apparent anomalies explicable by the appearance of the tubulointerstitium (BOHLE et al. 1990). They gave as examples membrano-proliferative glomerulonephritis type I with florid glomerular changes but a normal GFR and, similarly, severe glomerular amyloidosis or diabetic glomerulosclerosis where virtual obliteration of the glomerular tufts had occurred but with sparing of the tubulointerstitium.

However, in some diseases these findings were not confirmed. BENNETT et al. (1982) studied IgA nephropathy and failed to find a correlation between decline in GFR and expansion of the tubulointerstitium. Indeed, many other factors need to be considered in the assessment of renal biopsies for fibrosis. Bohle's group in Germany demonstrated an increase in fibrosis with age (RIEMENSCHNEIDER et al. 1980). If morphometric studies are being undertaken, it should also be remembered that interstitial oedema and inflammatory cell infiltration can widen the interstitium without fibrosis being present (HOOKE et al. 1987).

3 Mechanisms of Tubulointerstitial Injury

For nearly 30 years, therefore, evidence has accumulated that a primary glomerular disease can cause damage to the tubulointerstitium which results in typical features of a chronic inflammatory process, tubular atrophy, interstitial fibrosis and interstitial mononuclear cell infiltration. FINE et al. (1993) proposed a sequence of events to explain these histological features and the gradual loss of filtration accompanying them.

They suggested that the process starts with injury to the glomerulus and ends with loss of glomerular function secondary to events taking place in the tubulointerstitial compartment. They proposed compromise of microvascular blood flow as the initial change leading to ischaemia and atrophy of tubules. Alternatively, the tubules may be damaged by filtration of noxious molecules or by immunological attack from an interstitial inflammatory infiltrate. Subsequent interstitial deposition of extracellular material occurs, which may be from fibroblasts or tubular cells and which is subject to a number of paracrine growth systems. This chapter discusses the various stages in the progression to tubulointerstitial fibrosis.

4 Interstitial Microvascular Injury

BOHLE et al. (1981) demonstrated obliteration of the post-glomerular peritubular capillary network in renal biopsies (performed for a variety of pirmary glomerular diseases) in which an increase in renal interstitial volume was due to interstitial fibrosis. The experiment involved point-counting on semithin sections and went on to show that it is primarily the peritubular capillaries that are destroyed by the formation of interstitial collagen. They concluded that the energy-dependent metabolism of the tubular cells is severely impaired due to the increased length of diffusion and tubular cell ischaemia (VON GISE et al. 1981; FINE and NORMAN 1992). This is compounded by the fact that the pO_2 of much of the kidney is below that of systemic arterial blood, such that any compromise in blood flow will be rapidly reflected by decreased function (BREZIS et al. 1984).

It has also been shown that the renal oxygen requirement is increased by a variety of adaptive processes in the remnant kidney (HARRIS et al. 1988; SCHRIER et al. 1988). If five sixths of the rat nephron population is removed surgically and the remaining kidney removed and perfused in vitro, its oxygen consumption after 4 weeks is equivalent to that present in the intact kidney (HARRIS et al. 1988). SCHRIER et al. (1988) suggested that the increased oxygen consumption in the remnant kidney is associated with enhanced oxygen free radical formation, resulting in tissue injury in the presence of inadequate free radical scavengers. Other researchers showed an increase in renal cortical tissue malondialdehyde, a product of oxygen radicals, in the rat remnant kidney model (NATH et al. 1987).

The mechanisms which lead to a loss of the postglomerular circulation are not precisely known, but it seems likely that systemic hypertension is contributory. Based upon experiments involving direct measurement of glomerular haemodynamics in animal models, it has been established that 'glomerular capillary hypertension' is common to many forms of glomerular disease (ZATZ et al. 1986; ANDERSON et al. 1986). This results from dilatation of the afferent arteriole, combined with systemic hypertension. However, due to dilatation of the efferent arteriole (PELAYO et al. 1990a, b), the raised pressure would be transmitted beyond the glomerulus into the peritubular capillary network. This involves a significant drop in pressure due to the interposition of a resistance vessel, the efferent arteriole. The response of a vessel wall to small alterations in capillary pressure depend on the physical environment of the capillary; for instance, the response of the glomerular capillary surrounded extensively by the urinary space will differ from that of the peritubular capillary which abuts tubular basement membrane directly and then extracellular matrix.

It has been observed that, whilst tubulointerstitial injury is generally prominent in the remnant kidney, this histological feature is absent if the blood pressure is normal. BIDANI et al. (1990) studied a Wistar rat remnant kidney model and found that the majority of animals remained normotensive after five sixths renal ablation with a remarkable preservation of renal structure. The remnant kidneys showed features of hypertrophy but no significant atrophy of tubules, interstitial fibrosis or hyalinised glomeruli. The central role of systemic hypertension in the evolution of renal disease is also confirmed by the observation that renal function can be improved in patients with chronically diseased kidneys by better systemic blood pressure control, specifically in diabetic nephropathy by the use of angiotensin-converting enzyme (ACE) inhibition (BJORCK et al. 1986). Similar results have been obtained in the rat remnant model (PELAYO et al. 1990b). This protective effect of ACE inhibition may be mediated by an improvement in the postglomerular circulation due to afferent arteriolar dilatation (NORMAN et al. 1992a).

Early, at least, in any disease process, the rise in postglomerular resistance due to obliteration of the peritubular capillary bed could result in glomerular enlargement (BOHLE et al. 1981). In animal models, following subtotal nephrectomy, enhanced glomerular haemodynamics due to glomerular capillary distension appear to lead to glomerular hypertrophy (DIAMOND and KARNOVSKY 1987). Using a variety of rat remnant kidney models, YOSHIDA et al. (1989) found a correlation between glomerular hypertrophy and sclerosis. Previous models of unilateral nephrectomy which impose a hypertrophic stimulus on the remnant kidney and glomeruli have been found to accelerate the glomerular sclerosing process in experimental models of glomerulonephritis (TEODORU et al. 1959) and minimal-change disease (GLASSER et al. 1977). It is also well known that in both animal and human forms of diabetes mellitus, marked renal and glomerular hypertrophy precedes the development of diabetic nephropathy (STEFFES et al. 1978; SEYER-HANSEN et al. 1980). Since hypertrophic glomeruli are more likely to sclerose, it may be that the obliteration of the postglomerular capillary network is one way in which glomerular hypertrophy and sclerosis are linked.

However, compromise of microvascular blood flow need not be due only to structural changes. Any sustained increase in peritubular capillary pressure could adversely affect endothelial, interstitial and tubular cell function with the following effects. It has been shown that, in the rat remnant kidney model, tubular expression of platelet-derived growth factor (PDGF) by collecting ducts was increased with poorly controlled hypertension and decreased with good blood pressure control (KNECHT et al. 1991; NORMAN et al. 1992a). PDGF is known to be not only a potent mitogen for interstitial fibroblasts (KNECHT et al. 1991) but also a powerful vasoconstrictor substance (PELAYO et al. 1990a). Similarly, endothelial cells may produce endothelin, a potent vasoconstrictor peptide (YANAGISAWA et al. 1988), in response to a sustained increase in peritubular capillary pressure. LE HIR and colleagues (1989) showed that during conditions of renal hypoxia, adenosine was produced by interstitial fibroblasts which had direct access to the walls of arteries and arterioles, the nerve endings along vessels and tubules and possibly the erythropoietin-producing cell, where it may have its renal haemodynamic regulatory effects as well as effects on the GFR, tubular transport, and the release of renin and erythropoietin. They found that the most conspicuous accumulation of adenosine-producing fibroblasts was in the vicinity of the arteries and arterioles, around which they often constituted a continuous layer. In addition, tubular cells secreted PDGF (KNECHT et al. 1991), angiotensin II (NAVAR et al. 1992) and endothelin (ONG et al. 1993)

All of these mediators may result in vasoconstriction and increased interstitial fibrosis, and thus in obliteration of the peritubular capillary network. As the vascular bed into which glomerular capillary blood flow empties is progressively obliterated, glomerular function declines and renal failure advances in relation to the degree of interstitial fibrosis.

5 Tubular Cell Injury

5.1 Hypermetabolism

HARRIS et al. (1988) first drew attention to the existence of a hypermetabolic state in the remnant kidney and suggested that this was an important factor in the progression to chronic renal failure. The major oxygen-requiring process in the kidney is tubular transport. Hence, in many forms of renal disease with hypertrophied nephrons, renal oxygen consumption is increased. Later in the disease process, tubular atrophy rather than hypertrophy is the rule, and the adaptive processes with greater oxygen requirements no longer exist (FINE 1986). A high protein diet, which increases sodium reabsorption, will further increase oxygen consumption, which in itself is thought to be damaging to the remnant kidney. The two mechanisms by which increased oxygen consumption may be damaging to the kidney are increased ammoniagenesis and increased generation of reactive oxygen species (ROS).

SCHOOLWERTH et al. (1975) showed an enhanced rate of ammoniagenesis and enzyme activity in rats fed high-protein diets after nephron reduction. HAYSLETT (1979) also showed that adaptive changes in ammonia production occur as functional renal mass is reduced, but studies in human and experimental renal disease show that despite an increase in total ammonia production, ammonia excretion, when adjusted for glomerular filtration rate, is increased severalfold (DORHOUT-MEES et al. 1966; SIMPSON 1971; SCHOOLWERTH et al. 1975). Ammonia production per surviving nephron more than doubles in rats with 70% reduction in renal mass (MACLEAN and HAYSLETT 1980).

NATH et al. (1985) attempted to explain these findings and proposed that local toxic and inflammatory effects of ammonia include a biochemical reaction with the thiolester bond of the third component of complement to promote triggering of the alternative complement pathway. This then culminates in the deposition of complement proteins and initiation of complement-mediated cellular infiltration and tissue injury. HANSCH et al. (1991) showed that this inflammatory cellular infiltration would lead to elaboration of inflammatory mediators and increased collagen synthesis by tubular cells. Peritubular fibrosis occurs, as well as on-going obliteration of peritubular capillaries. BROOIMANS and colleagues (1991) observed the existence of a feedback system under these circumstances and showed that proximal tubular epithelial cells in conditioned medium could synthesise C3, and that its production could be increased in a dose-dependent manner by interleukin 2 (IL-2), produced locally by T cells. Of course, high levels of ammonia normally exist in the renal medulla, where similar damage is not observed. CLARK and colleagues (1990) have demonstrated that a hyperosmolar milieu is able to protect against injury by high ammonia concentrations.

Increased oxygen consumption by the kidney may also lead to the generation of reactive oxygen species. Several groups have shown that treatment of animals with scavengers of superoxide anion, hydrogen peroxide, and hydroxyl radical ameliorates the proteinuria and glomerular injury associated with experimental nephritis (REHAN et al. 1984; SHAH 1988, 1989). Until recently, it was assumed that the source of ROS were neutrophils infiltrating the interstitium (REHAN et al. 1984), but it has now been shown that certain cells intrinsic to the kidney are an important source of ROS. Glomerular mesangial cells in culture produce hydrogen peroxide and superoxide anion in response to opsonised zymosan and immune complexes (BAUD et al. 1983), and resident glomerular macrophages are also capable of generating ROS (BOYCE et al. 1989).

Recent work has also demonstrated that primary cultures of rabbit proximal tubule, cortical collecting duct, and papillary collecting duct produced augmented levels of ROS, specifically superoxide anion and hydrogen peroxide, in response to heat-aggregated immunoglobulin and zymosan (ROVIN et al. 1990). Although the magnitude of ROS generation by renal tubular cells appears to be significantly less than that produced by other renal cell types, it appears that ROS secretion by tubules during immune injury of the kidney participates in the development of interstitial disease which accompanies glomerulonephritis.

Damage due to ROS occurs only when the amount of these substances exceeds the capacity of the kidneys' antioxidant scavenging systems (YOSHIOKA et al. 1990). Within aerobic cells, three antioxidant enzymes—superoxide dismutase, glutathione peroxidase and catalase—are major mechanisms to reduce local levels of ROS (FANTONE and WARD 1982; GRISHAM and McCORD 1986), and in their experiment, YOSHIOKA et al. (1990) demonstrated enhancement of intrinsic antioxidant enzyme activity after renal ischaemia-reperfusion injury in the rat and protection of renal function against ROS-induced injuries. Further studies showed that in subtotally nephrectomised rats, the imposition of increased protein intake was sufficient to cause renal damage arising from oxidant stress (NATH et al. 1990). It appears that in the hyperfunctioning surviving nephron, there is increased sodium reabsorption, and hence oxygen consumption, which generates a variety of ROS at several subcellular loci. Increased rates of oxygen consumption require increased transport of reducing equivalents through the mitochondrial electron transport chain. These augmented rates of transport may generate free electrons that overwhelm the resident mitochondrial antioxidant mechanisms, resulting in peroxidation of mitochondrial membrane lipid. A dietary deficiency of antioxidants, i.e. vitamin E and selenium, imposed on weanling rats caused renal growth and tubulointerstitial damage in the intact, nonmanipulated rat kidney with concomitant reduction of overall somatic growth (NATH and SALAHUDEEN 1990). The authors suggested that augmented rates of ammonia production which antedated the phase of renal growth were in part responsible for the renal damage due to these dietary deficiencies. It has been suggested that the accumulation of ROS in the kidney may directly stimulate renal ammoniagenic pathways (NATH and SALAHUDEEN 1990), or that hydrogen peroxide deaminates amino acids via a metal ion-catalysed reaction with the generation of ammonium bicarbonate (STADTMAN and BERLETT 1988; BERLETT et al. 1990). In the same way that ROS up-regulate collagen gene expression in fibroblasts, so they may in tubular cells (HOUGLUM et al. 1991). The resultant peritubular fibrosis leads to nephron destruction and disease progression.

5.2 Toxicity of Filtered Substances

If the level of proteinuria in a particular renal disease is controlled, then progression to renal failure is slowed (REMUZZI and BERTANI 1990). The beneficial effect of angiotensin-converting enzyme inhibitors on the progression of chronic renal disease may in part be due to their role in reducing proteinuria (NORMAN et al. 1992b).

Two separate studies on focal and segmental glomerulosclerosis suggest that reactive mechanisms triggered by increased protein filtration across the glomerular capillary promote a decline in renal function (WEHRMANN et al. 1990; REMUZZI and BERTANI 1990). These mechanisms include activation of mesangial cells by increased passage of macromolecules, which stimulates production of collagen, laminin and fibronectin, glomerular epithelial cell injury and tubulointerstitial damage. Proteinaceous casts cause dilatation and obstruction of tubules with focal rupture of the tubular basement membrane, triggering an interstitial inflammatory cell reaction (BERTANI et al. 1986). An extreme example of this may be seen in an experimental acute interstitial nephritis induced by the injection of bovine albumin into rats; here, increased vimentin intermediate filament expression is seen in proximal tubules due to endocytic protein uptake, which leads to degradation of lysosomes (EDDY 1989). Subsequent release of degradative enzymes leads to interstitial injury, influx of inflammatory cells and fibrosis. A macrophage-specific lipid chemotactic factor has been detected in the urine of proteinuric rats and human beings (SCHREINER et al. 1992), and cultured rat tubular cells produce the same factor when exposed to high concentrations of albumin (KEES-FOLTS et al. 1992). Production of chemotactic factors by the injured tubule then leads to secondary immune injury to the interstitium.

However, despite the data provided by these animal models, it is well known that proteinuria per se cannot be damaging in human renal disease, as no tubulointerstitial damage is seen in minimal-change disease, where torrential nephrotic syndrome is the rule. This may be related to the highly selective nature of the protein filtered, i.e. albumin. In most other forms of glomerular disease there is increased permeability to larger molecules, which may be injurious to the renal tubule.

Tubulointerstitial injury may occur due to a variety of other macromolecules, for instance, monoclonal light chains in myeloma, which impair proximal tubular transport (SANDERS et al. 1988; SOLOMON et al. 1991), or in Heymann nephritis where lyzozymuria occurs due to failure of normal tubular uptake of filtered lyzozyme, causing proximal tubular injury (ZAMLAUSKI-TUCKER et al. 1990). Tubular injury also occurs in hyperlipoproteinaemia (MOORHEAD et al. 1982), nephrotoxic serum nephritis transferrinuria (ALFREY et al. 1989), complementuria (CAMUSSI et al. 1983), puromycin aminonucleoside nephropathy (DIAMOND and ANDERSON 1990) and glomerular bleeding, where haem-induced tubular damage occurs, probably mediated by iron-dependent free radicals (HILL et al. 1989).

5.3 Immunologically Mediated Tubular Cell Injury

It has been noted in studies of renal transplant recipients that initial ischaemic acute tubular necrosis predisposes to a higher rate of graft loss, apparently due to rejection (HALLORAN et al. 1988). Increased immunogenicity due to ischaemic injury has been suggested as the cause (SHOSKES et al. 1990). In this way a primary nonimmune tubular insult may result in immune-mediated injury. SHOSKES et al. (1990) found increased MHC expression in a unilateral ischaemic mouse kidney model with early class-I antigen expression in tubular cells and late class-II antigen expression by tubular and interstitial cells. MHC antigens serve as targets for T-cell recognition (KLEIN et al. 1981) and, experimentally, increased expression of MHC antigens leads to more efficient T-cell recognition and appropriate effector responses (BEKKHOUCHA et al. 1984; KING et al. 1986; BISHOP et al. 1988). An increased MHC expression in various cell types, particularly epithelial cells, as described here, is an almost invariable accompaniment of chronic inflammation. A similar expression was seen when the tubular toxin, mercuric chloride, given in low doses to cause an autoimmune glomerulonephritis, induced class-II expression in interstitial and tubular cells and class-I expression in proximal tubular, glomerular and endothelial cells (MADRENAS et al. 1991). In this experiment MHC expression was blocked by the administration of a monoclonal antibody to interferon-γ (IFN-γ), indicating that this cytokine, elaborated by T cells, plays an essential role in the phenomenon. The induction of class-II expression on renal tubules using IFN-γ was confirmed in two experimental systems, firstly in a mouse model (SKOSKIEWICZ et al. 1985) and then in cultured renal tubular cells, where certain additional characteristics of accessory cells, namely the expression of TNF-α, were seen (WUTHRICH et al. 1990).

In an immunohistochemical study on human renal biopsies, MULLER et al. (1989) found that normal tubular epithelium lacked HLA-DQ and -DP antigens, but carried -DY and, variably, -DR products constitutively. In patients with a variety of forms of proliferative and nonproliferative glomerulonephritis, they found aberrant expression of HLA-DQ and -DP prior to the development of an interstitial infiltrate and significant fibrosis. A similar pattern of class-II expression was seen on renal tubular cells in a mouse lupus model, prior to the onset of glomerular inflammation and proteinuria, with the expression localised to tubules with dense surrounding mononuclear infiltrates (WUTHRICH et al. 1989). The specificity of an immune response is provided by the interaction of specific T-cell receptors with antigen presented by antigen-presenting accessory cells in the presence of class-II molecules. The avidity of this interaction is increased by the expression of other cell surface proteins, such as intercellular adhesion molecule-1 (ICAM-1), a specific ligand of lymphocyte function-associated antigen-1, which was found to be expressed on the apical border of tubular epithelial cells stimulated by IFN-γ. The expression of ICAM-1 was more rapid, required considerably less IFN-γ for induction, and was more resistant to modulation than class-II antigen (JEVNIKAR et al. 1990). Rapid redistribution of surface ICAM-1 to the basolateral membrane was seen following prior sublethal tubular cell injury, facilitating tubular cell-T cell interaction (MOLITORIS et al. 1989). Using a mouse model, HAVERTY et al. (1989) found that autoimmune tubulointerstitial damage was not induced unless proximal tubular class-II MHC antigen expression was increased.

It seems clear that a primary glomerular insult, whether immune or nonimmune, could lead to nonimmune tubular cell injury, which could in turn cause activation or expansion of interstitial immune cells in response to tubular-derived cytokines (SCHMOUDER et al. 1991). A variety of lymphokines would then amplify class-II and ICAM-1 expression (HALTTUNEN 1990), thus enabling tubular cells to function as antigen-presenting cells, with neo-antigens derived from filtered proteins or ischaemic damage (NEILSON 1989). In addition, specific immune cell-derived factors may regulate renal transport processes and haemodynamics (SCHREINER and KOHAN 1990). For instance, IL-1, secreted by macrophages, induces a natriuresis by direct inhibition of collecting duct sodium reabsorption (BEASLEY et al. 1988), and potent vasoconstrictor compounds are released by glomerular macrophages, including leukotriene D_4 (SCHREINER et al.1984) and thromboxane A_2 (SCHARSCHMIDT et al. 1986), which modulate renal blood flow.

Cultured proximal tubular epithelial cells secrete not only type IV, V and VII (basement membrane) collagens but also smaller amounts of interstitial-type collagens, I and III (HAVERTY et al. 1988) The same group subsequently noted a down-regulation of transcription of type IV collagen by a T-cell-secreted tubular antigen-binding protein, with a concomitant increase in type I collagen synthesis due to stimulation of transcription by various cytokines in a mouse model of autoimmune nephritis (HAVERTY et al. 1992). This process correlates with the morphological changes observed histologically in interstitial nephritis, where tubular atrophy occurs, followed by replacement interstitial fibrosis.

6 The Role of the Interstitial Fibroblast in Renal Fibrosis

Cultured human fibroblasts consist of populations of cells of differing morphology, typed as early, intermediate, late mitotic or postmitotic cells (RODEMANN et al. 1989). The life span and mitotic behaviour of the cells are tissue specific, and even within the kidney the growth patterns of cortical and papillary fibroblasts appear to be different (RODEMANN and MULLER 1991). A substantial body of experimental observations has demonstrated that a number of fundamental phenotypic properties of mesenchymal cells can be stably altered. For example, stable alterations in the proliferative capacity and expression of cellular oncogene products have been observed in mesenchymal cells derived from the affected organs of patients with atherosclerosis (YOSHIDA et al. 1988; PARKES et al. 1991), progressive systemic sclerosis (LEROY 1974), idiopathic pulmonary fibrosis (JORDANA et al. 1988) and interstitial renal fibrosis (RODEMANN and MULLER 1990). In the last experiment, the authors established primary cell cultures of fibroblasts from normal kidneys and from those with interstitial fibrosis. The samples were obtained from renal biopsies of potential allografts which were not grafted due to vascular abnormalities. The number of fibroblasts in the cultures of kidneys with interstitial fibrosis was increased some tenfold compared with cultures of fibroblasts from normal kidneys and showed significant alterations in proliferative capacity and generation time when assessed by clonal growth and kinetic experiments. Gel electrophoresis showed that the fibroblasts from fibrotic kidneys expressed two autocrine growth-promoting proteins not normally present in kidney or skin fibroblasts, and that in cross-feeding experiments, these factors could induce hyperproliferation in normal kidney or skin fibroblasts. It remains to be seen whether the stable alteration in phenotype is due to somatic mutation, or whether it represents an autocrine loop comparable to that seen with PDGF and mesangial cells (SCHULTZ et al. 1988) or fibroblast growth factor in autosomal dominant adult polycystic disease (NORMAN et al. 1992b). Enhanced proto-oncogene expression and transforming activity as seen in human atherosclerotic plaques (PARKES et al. 1991) have not yet been demonstrated in the kidney fibroblast.

7 Tubular Cell-Fibroblast Interactions

Tubular epithelial cells have been found to be a rich source of an array of peptide growth factors such as PDGF, insulin-like growth factor (IGF-1), transforming growth factor-β (TGF-β), epidermal growth factor (EGF), granulocyte-monocyte colony-stimulating factor (GM-CSF) (FRANK et al. 1993; SEGAL and FINE 1989; ROCCO et al. 1992), of cytokines such as monocyte chemotactic peptide-1 (MCP-1) (SCHMOUDER et al. 1991), IL-6 (FRANK et al. 1993), IL-8 and TNF-α (WUTHRICH et al. 1990), C3 component of complement (BROOIMANS et al. 1991) and vasoactive peptides, such as endothelin (KOHAN 1991) and angiotensin II (NAVAR et al. 1992). Many of these substances show segment specificity with EGF synthesised only by the thick ascending limb and the distal tubule (SEGAL and FINE 1989). Endothelin is synthesised by several nephron segments but in differing concentrations, with greatest synthesis occurring in the inner medullary collecting ducts (KOHAN 1991).

Although the function of many of these factors in the normal kidney is not known, it may be that tubules damaged for whatever reason secrete them in excess, recruiting inflammatory cells and initiating fibrosis due to mitogenic stimulation of fibroblasts. Experimental studies suggest that there exists a series of paracrine growth systems, at least for PDGF (KNECHT et al. 1991), endothelin (ONG et al. 1994) and IGF (ROGERS et al. 1991) with regionally specific tubular-fibroblast cell interactions, such that growth factors produced locally within the kidney act on an adjacent cell type which is uniquely responsive to it.

At present, it is not known when these substances are synthesised constitutively or how they regulate normal renal function. It may be that changes in tubular cytokine expression in vivo are related to specific tubulointerstitial pathologies, and therefore that the progression of specific diseases may be altered by blocking synthesis or action of individual compounds.

8 Conclusion

From the evidence that has accumulated over the past 30 years, it appears that tubular cell injury is crucial to the process of tubulointerstitial fibrosis. The injured tubular cell becomes dysfunctional, secreting in excess cytokines, growth factors and vasoactive peptides. The process is perpetuated by subsequent interactions between infiltrating lymphocytes and macrophages, fibroblasts and endothelial cells, with tubulointerstitial scarring and secondary loss of glomerular function.

References

Alfrey AC, Foment DH, Hammond WS (1989) Role of iron in tubulointerstitial injury in nephrotoxic serum nephritis. Kidney Int 36: 753–759

Anderson S, Rennke HG, Brenner BM (1986) Therapeutic advantages of converting enzyme inhibitors in arresting progressive renal disease associated with systemic hypertension in the rat. J Clin Invest 77: 1993–2000

Baldwin DS (1977) Poststreptococcal glomerulonephritis: a progressive disease? Am J Med 62: 1–11

Baud L, Hagege J, Sraer J, Rondeau E, Perez J, Ardaillou R (1983) Reactive oxygen production by cultured rat glomerular mesangial cells during phagocytosis is associated with stimulation of lipoxygenase activity. J Exp Med 158: 1836–1852

Beasley D, Dinarello CA, Cannon JG (1988) Interleukin-1 induces natriuresis in conscious rats: role of renal prostaglandins. Kidney Int 33: 1059–1065

Bekkhoucha F, Naquet P, Pierres A, Marchetto S, Pierres M (1984) Efficiency of antigen presentation to T cell clones by (B cell × B cell lymphoma) hybridomas correlates quantitatively with cell surface Ia expression. Eur J Immunol 14: 807–814

Bennett WM, Walker RG, Kincaid-Smith P (1982) Renal cortical interstitial volume in mesangial IgA nephropathy. Lab Invest 47: 330–335

Berlett BS, Chock PB, Yim MB, Stadtman ER (1990) Manganese (II) catalyzes the bicarbonate-dependent oxidation of amino acids by hydrogen peroxide and the amino acid facilitated dismutation of hydrogen peroxide. Proc Natl Acad Sci USA 87: 389–393

Bertani T, Cutillo F, Zoja C, Broggini M, Remuzzi G (1986) Tubulo-interstitial lesions mediate renal damage in adriamycin glomerulopathy. Kidney Int 30: 488–496

Bidani AK, Mitchell KD, Schwartz MM, Navar G, Lewis EJ (1990) Absence of glomerular injury or nephron loss in a normotensive rat remnant kidney model. Kidney Int 38: 28–38

Bishop GA, Waugh JA, Hall BM (1988) Expression of HLA antigens on renal tubular cells in culture: II. Effect of increased HLA antigen expression on tubular cell stimulation of lymphocyte activation and on their vulnerability to cell-mediated lysis. Transplantation 46: 303–310

Bjorck S, Nyberg G, Mulec H, Granerus G, Herlitz H, Aurell M (1986) Beneficial effects of angiotensin converting enzyme inhibition on renal function in patients with diabetic nephropathy. Br Med J 293: 471–474

Bohle A, Christ H, Grund KE, Mackensen A, Neunhoeffer J (1977a) Serum creatinine concentration and renal interstitial volume. Analysis of correlations in endocapillary (acute) glomerulonephritis and in moderately severe mesangioproliferative glomerulonephritis. Virchows Arch [A] 375: 87–96

Bohle A, Glomb D, Grund KE, Mackensen S (1977b) Correlations between relative interstitial volume of the renal cortex and serum creatinine concentration in minimal changes with nephrotic syndrome and in focal sclerosing glomerulonephritis. Virchows Arch [A] 376: 221–232

Bohle A, Grund KE, Mackensen S, Tolon M (1977c) Correlations between renal interstitium and level of serum creatinine: morphometric investigations of biopsies in perimembranous glomerulonephritis. Virchows Arch [A] 373: 15–22

Bohle A, Christ H, Grund KE, Mackensen A (1979) The role of the interstitium of the renal cortex in renal disease. Contrib Nephrol 16: 109–114

Bohle A, von Gise H, Mackense-Haen S, Stark-Jacob B (1981) The obliteration of the postglomerular capillaries and its influence upon the function of both glomeruli and tubuli. Functional interpretation of morphologic findings. Klin Wochenschr 59: 1043–1051

Bohle A, Mackensen-Haen S, von Gise H, Grund KE, Wehrmann M, Batz C, Bogenschutz O, Schmitt H, Nagy J, Muller C, Muller G (1990) The consequences of tubulo-interstitial changes for renal function in glomerulophathies. A morphometric and cytological analysis. Pathol Res Pract 186: 135–144

Boyce NW, Tipping PG, Holdsworth SP (1989) Glomerular macrophages produce reactive oxygen species in experimental glomerulonephritis. Kidney Int 35: 1093–1106

Brenner BM, Meyer TW, Hostetter TH (1982) Dietary protein intake and the progressive nature of kidney disease: the role of hemodynamically mediated glomerular injury in the pathogenesis of progressive glomerular sclerosis in aging, renal ablation, and intrinsic renal disease. N Engl J Med 307: 652–659

Brezis M, Rosen S, Silva P, Epstein PH (1984) Renal ischemia: a new perspective. Kidney Int 26: 375–383

Brooimans RA, Stegmann APA, van Dorp WT, van der Ark AAJ, van der Wounde FJ, van es LA, Daha MR (1991) Interleukin 2 mediated stimulation of complement C3 biosynthesis in human proximal tubular epithelial cells. J Clin Invest 88: 379–384

Camussi G, Tetta C, Mazzucco G, Vercellone A (1983) The brush border of proximal tubules of normal human kidney activates the alternative pathway of the complement system in vitro. Ann NY Acad Sci 420: 321–324

Clark EC, Hostetter TH, Nath KA, Hostetter MK (1990) Renal medullary solutes impair neutrophil function. Clin Res 38: 464 (abstract)

Diamond JR, Anderson S (1990) Irreversible tubulo-interstitial damage associated with chronic aminonucleoside nephrosis. Am J Pathol 137: 1323–1332

Diamond JR, Karnovsky MJ (1987) Alimentary hypercholesterolaemia selectively aggravates glomerular injury. Kidney Int 31: 383 (abstract)

Dorhout-Mees EJ, Machado M, Slatopolsky S, Klahr S, Bricker NS (1966) The functional adaptation of the diseased kidney. 3. Ammonium excretion. J Clin Invest 45: 289–296

Eddy AA (1989) Interstitial nephritis induced by protein-overload proteinuria. Am J Pathol 135: 719–733

Elema JD (1976) Is one kidney sufficient? Kidney Int 9: 380A

Fantone JC, Ward PA (1982) Role of oxygen-derived free radicals and metabolites in leukocyte-dependent inflammatory reactions. Am J Pathol 107: 397–418

Fine LG (1986) The biology of renal hypertrophy. Kidney Int 29: 619–634

Fine LG, Norman JT (1992) Renal growth responses to acute and chronic injury: routes to therapeutic intervention. J Am Soc Nephrol 2: S202–S211

Fine LG, Ong ACM, Norman JT (1993) Mechanisms of tubulo-interstitial injury in progressive renal diseases. Eur J Clin Invest 23: 259–265

Frank J, Engler-Blum G, Rodemann HP, Muller GA (1993) Human renal tubular cells as a cytokine source: PDGF-β, GM-CSF and IL-6 mRNA expression in vitro. Exp Nephrol 1: 26–35

Glasser RJ, Velosa JA, Michael AF (1977) Experimental model of focal sclerosis. I. Relationship to protein excretion in aminonucleoside nephrosis. Lab Invest 36: 519–526

Gottschalk CW (1971) Function of the chronically diseased kidney: the adaptive nephron. Circ Res 28 [Suppl 2]: 1–13

Grisham MB, McCord JM (1986) Chemistry and cytotoxicity of reactive oxygen metabolites. In: Taylor AE, Matalon S, Ward P (eds) Physiology of oxygen radicals. American Physiological Society, Bethesda, pp 1–18

Halloran PF, Aprile MA, Farewell V, Ludwin D, Smith EK, Tsai SY, Bear RA, Cole EH, Fenton SS (1988) Early function as the principal correlate of graft survival: a multivariate analysis of 200 cadaveric renal transplants treated with a protocol incorporating antilymphocyte globulin and cyclosporine. Transplantation 46: 223–228

Halttunen J (1990) Failure of rat kidney nephron components to induce allogeneic lymphocytes to proliferate in mixed lymphocyte kidney cell culture. Transplantation 50: 481–487

Hansch GM, Schonermark M, Wagner C, Schieren G, Jahn G (1991) The terminal complement complex C5b-9: a possible mediator of acute and chronic glomerulonephritis. In: Hatano M (ed) Proceedings of the XIth International Congress of Nephrology, vol II. Springer, Berlin Heidelberg New York, pp 888–897

Harris DCH, Chan L, Schrier RW (1988) Remnant kidney hypermetabolism and progression of chronic renal failure. Am J Physiol 254: F267–F276

Haverty TP, Kelly, CJ, Hines WH, Amenta PS, Watanabe M, Kefalides NA, Harper R, Neilson EG (1988) Chracterization of a tubular epithelial cell line which secretes the autologous target antigen of autoimmune interstitial nephritis. J Cell Biol 107: 1358–1369

Haverty TP, Watanabe M, Neilson EG, Kelly CJ (1989) Protective modulation of class II MHC gene expression in tubular epithelium by target antigen-specific antibodies. Cell-surface-directed down-regulation of transcription can influence susceptibility to murine tubulointerstitial nephritis. J Immunol 143: 1133–1141

Haverty TP, Kelly CJ, Hoyer JR, Alvarez R, Neilson EG (1992) Tubular antigen-binding proteins repress transcription of type IV collagen in the autoimmune target epithelium of experimental interstitial nephritis. J Clin Invest 89: 517–523

Hayslett JP (1979) Functional adaptation to reduction in renal mass. Physiol Rev 59: 137–164

Hill PA, Davies DJ, Kincaid-Smith P, Ryan GB (1989) Ultrastructural changes in renal tubules associated with glomerular bleeding. Kidney Int 36: 992–997

Hooke DH, Gee DC, Atkins RC (1987) Leukocyte analysis using monoclonal antibodies in human glomerulonephritis. Kidney Int 31: 964–972

Houglum K, Brenner DA, Chojkier M (1991) D-α-tocopherol inhibits collagen $\alpha 1$(I) gene expression in cultured human fibroblasts. Modulation of constitutive collagen gene expression by lipid peroxidation. J Clin Invest 87: 2230–2235

Jevnikar AM, Wuthrich RP, Takei F, Xu H-W, Brennan DC, Glimcher LH, Rubin-Kelley VE (1990)

Differing regulation and function of ICAM-1 and class II antigens on renal tubular cells. Kidney Int 38: 417–425

Jordana M, Schulman J, McSharry C, Irving LB, Newhouse MT, Jordana G, Gauldie J (1988) Heterogeneous proliferative characteristics of human adult lung fibroblast lines and clonally derived fibroblasts from control and fibrotic tissue. Am Rev Resp Dis 137: 579–584

Kees-Folts D, Sadow J, Schreiner GF (1992) Individual fatty acids regulate the production of a macrophage chemotactic factor by proximal tubular cells endocytosing albumin. J Am Soc Nephrol 3: 598 (abstract)

King NJC, Mullbacher A, Blanden RV (1986) Relationship between surface H-2 concentration, size of different target cells, and lysis by cytotoxic T cells. Cell Immunol 98: 525–532

Kiprov DD, Colvin RB, McCluskey RT (1982) Focal and segmental glomerulosclerosis and proteinuria associated with unilateral renal agenesis. Lab Invest 46: 275–281

Klein J, Juretic A, Baxevanis CN, Nagy ZA (1981) The traditional and a new version of the mouse H-2 complex. Nature 291: 455–460

Knecht A, Fine LG, Kleinman KS, Rodemann HP, Muller GA, Woo DDL, Norman JT (1991) Fibroblasts of rabbit kidney in culture. II Paracrine stimulation of papillary fibroblasts by PDFG. Am J Physiol 261: F292–F299

Kohan DE (1991) Endothelin synthesis by rabbit renal tubule cells. Am J Physiol 26: F221–F226

Le Hir M, Kaissling B, Gandhi R, Dubach UC (1989) Fibroblasts may represent the main site of production of interstitial adenosine in the kidney. Kidney Int 36: 319–320

Leroy EC (1974) Increased collagen synthesis by scleroderma skin fibroblasts in vitro. A possible defect in the regulation of activation of the scleroderma fibroblast. J Clin Invest 54: 880–889

Maclean AJ, Hayslett JP (1980) Adaptive change in ammonia exretion in renal insufficiency. Kidney Int 17: 595–606

Madrenas J, Parfrey NA, Halloran PF (1990) Interferon gamma-mediated renal MHC expression in mercuric chloride-induced glomerulonephritis. Kidney Int 39: 273–281

Mitch WE, Walser M, Buffington GA, Lemann J Jr (1976) A simple method for estimating progression of chronic renal failure. Lancet ii: 1326–1328

Molitoris BA, Falk SA, Dahl RA (1989) Ischemia-induced loss of epithelial polarity. Role of the tight junction. J Clin Invest 84: 1334–1339

Moorhead JF, El-Nahas M, Chan MK, Varghese Z (1982) Lipid nephrotoxicity in chronic progressive glomerular and tubulo-interstitial disease. Lancet ii: 1309–1311

Muller CA, Markovic-Lipovski J, Risler T, Bohle A, Muller GA (1989) Expression of HLA-DQ, -DR, and -DP antigens in normal kidney and glomerulonephritis. Kidney Int 35: 116–124

Nath KA, Salhudeen AK (1990) Induction of renal growth and injury in the intact kidney by dietary deficiency of antioxidants. J Clin Invest 86: 1179–1192

Nath KA, Hostetter MK, Hostetter TH (1985) Pathophysiology of chronic tubulointerstitial disease in rats: interactions of dietary acid load, ammonia and complement component. J Clin Invest 76: 667–675

Nath KA, Woolley AC, Hostetter TH (1987) O_2 consumption and oxidant stress in the remnant nephron. Clin Res 35: 553A

Nath KA, Croatt AJ, Hostetter TH (1990) Oxygen consumption and oxidant stress in surviving nephrons. Am J Physiol 258: F1354–1362

Navar LG, Gauthier-Lewis L, Hymel A, Broam B, Mitchell KD (1992) Assessment of intraluminal, kidney and plasma levels of angiotensin I and II in anaesthetized rats. J Am Soc Nephrol 3: 442 (abstract)

Neilson EG (1989) Pathogenesis and therapy of interstitial nephritis. Kidney Int 35: 1257–1270

Norman JT, Gallego C, Bridgman DA, Fogo A, Fine LG (1992a) Enalapril ameliorates interstitial fibrosis in the remnant kidney of the rat. J Am Soc Nephrol 3: 746 (abstract)

Norman JT, Kuo NT, Wilson PD (1992b) Autocrine stimulation of fibroblast growth in autosomal dominant polycystic kidney disease is mediated by acidic fibroblast growth factor. J Am Soc Nephrol 3: 300 (abstract)

Novick AC, Gephardt G, Guz B, Steinmuller D, Tubbs RR (1991) Long-term follow-up after partial removal of a solitary kidney. N Engl J Med 325: 1058–1062

Ong ACM, Jowett TP, Scoble JE, O'Shea JA, Varghese Z, Moorhead JF (1993) The effect of cyclosporin A on endothelin synthesis by cultured human renal cortical epithelial cells. Nephrol Dial Transplant 8: 748–753

Ong ACM, Jowett TP, Firth JD, Burton S, Kitamura M, Fine LG (1994) Human tubular-derived endothelin in the paracrine regulation of renal interstitial fibroblast function. Exp Nephrol (in press)

Parkes JL, Cardell RR, Hubbard FC Jr, Hubbard D, Meltzer A, Penn A (1991) Cultured human atherosclerotic plaque smooth muscle cells retain transforming potential and display enhanced expression of the *myc* protooncogene. Am J Pathol 138: 765–775

Pelayo JC, Noble PW, Riches DWH (1990a) Expression of platelet-derived growth factor A and B mRNA in acute unilateral ureteral obstruction. J Am Soc Nephrol 1: 743 (abstract)

Pelayo JC, Quon AH, Shanley PF (1990b) Angiotensin II control of the renal microcirculation in rats with reduced renal mass. Am J Physiol 258: F414–F422

Rehan A, Johnson KJ, Wiggins RC, Kunkel RC, Ward PA (1984) Evidence for the role of oxygen radicals in acute nephrotoxic nephritis. Lab Invest 51: 396–403

Remuzzi G, Bertani T (1990) Is glomerulosclerosis a consequence of altered glomerular permeability to macromolecules? Kidney Int 38: 384–394

Remuzzi A, Puntorieri S, Battaglia C, Bertani T, Remuzzi G (1990) Angiotensin converting enzyme inhibition ameliorates glomerular filtration of macromolecules and water and lessens glomerular injury in the rat. J Clin Invest 85: 541–549

Reimenschneider T, Mackensen-Haen S, Christ H, Bohle A (1980) Correlation between endogenous creatinine clearance and relative interstitial volume of the renal cortex in patients with diffuse membranous glomerulonephritis having a normal serum creatinine concentration. Lab Invest 43: 145–149

Risdon RA, Sloper JC, De Wardener HE (1968) Relationship between renal function and histological changes found in renal biopsy specimens from patients with persistent glomerular nephritis. Lancet ii: 363–366

Rocco MV, Chen Y, Goldfarb S, Ziyadeh FN (1992) Elevated glucose stimulates TGF-β expression and bioactivity in proximal tubule. Kidney Int 41: 107–114

Rodemann HP, Muller GA (1990) Abnormal growth and clonal proliferation of fibroblasts derived from kidneys with interstitial fibrosis. Proc Soc Exp Biol Med 195: 57–63

Rodemann HP, Muller GA (1991) Characterization of human renal fibroblasts in health and disease: II. In vitro growth and differentiation of fibroblasts derived from kidneys with interstitial fibrosis. Am J Kidney Dis 17: 684–686

Rodemann HP, Bayreuther K, Francz PI, Dittman K, Albiez M (1989) Selective enrichment and biochemical characterization of seven human skin fibroblast cell types in vitro. Exp Cell Res 180: 84–93

Rogers SA, Miller SB, Hammerman MR (1991) IGF1 gene expression in isolated rat renal collecting duct is stimulated by epidermal growth factor. J Clin Invest 87: 347–351

Rovin BH, Wurst E, Kohan DE (1990) Production of reactive oxygen species by tubular epithelial cells in culture. Kidney Int 37: 1509–1514

Rutherford WE, Blondin J, Miller JP, Greenwalt AS, Vavra JD (1977) Chronic progressive renal disease: rate of change of serum creatinine. Kidney Int 11: 62–70

Sanders PW, Herrera GA, Chen A, Booker BB, Galla JH (1988) Differential nephrotoxicity of low molecular weight proteins including Bence Jones proteins in the perfused rat nephron in vivo. J Clin Invest 82: 2086–2096

Schainuck LI, Striker GE, Cutler RE, Benditt EP (1970) Structural-functional correlations in renal disease. Part II: The correlations. Hum Pathol 1: 631–640

Scharschmidt LA, Douglas J, Dunn M (1986) Angiotensin II and eicosanoids in the control of glomerular size in the rat and human. Am J Physiol 250: F348–F356

Schmouder RL, Streiter RM, Wiggins RC, Kunkel SL (1991) Disparate IL-8 and MCP-1 expression in human renal cortical epithelial cells stimulated with interferon-γ. J Am Soc Nephrol 3: 787 (abstract)

Schoolwerth AC, Sandler RS, Hoffman PM, Klahr S (1975) Effects of nephron reduction an dietary protein content on renal ammoniagenesis in the rat. Kidney Int 7: 397–404

Schreiner GF, Kohan DE (1990) Regulation of renal transport process and haemodynamics by macrophages and lymphocytes. Am J Physiol 258: F761–F767

Schreiner GF, Rovin B, Lefkowith J (1984) The anti-inflammatory effects of essential fatty acid deficiency in experimental glomerulonephritis. J Immunol 143: 3192–3199

Schreiner GF, Kees-Folts D, Delmez J (1992) Characterization of a macrophage-specific lipid chemotactic factor in the urine and peritoneal dialysate of nephrotic patients with declining renal function. J Am Soc Nephrol 3: 419 (abstract)

Schrier RW, Harris DCH, Chan L, Shapiro JI, Caramelo C (1988) Tubular hypermetabolism as a factor in the progression of chronic renal failure. Am J Kid Dis 12: 243–249

Schultz PJ, Corleto PE, Silver BJ, Abboud HE (1988) Mesangial cells express PDGF mRNAs and proliferate in response to PDGF. Am J Physiol 255: F674–F684

Segal R, Fine LG (1989) Polypeptide growth factors and the kidney. Kidney Int 36: S2–S10

Seyer-Hansen K, Hansen J, Gundersen HJG (1980) Renal hypertrophy in experimental diabetes. diabetologia 18: 501–505

Shah SV (1988) Evidence suggesting a role for hydroxyl radical in passive Heymann nephritis. Am J Physiol 254: F337–F344

Shah SV (1989) Role of reactive oxygen metabolites in experimental glomerular disease. Kidney Int 35: 1093–1106

Shoskes DA, Parfrey NA, Halloran PF (1990) Increased major histocompatibility complex antigen expression in unilateral ischemic acute tubular necrosis in the mouse. Transplantation 49, 201–207

Simpson DP (1971) Control of hydrogen ion homeostasis and renal acidosis. Medicine (Baltimore) 50: 503–541

Skoskiewicz MJ, Colvin RB, Schneeberger EE, Russell PS (1985) Widespread and selective induction of major histocompatibility complex-determined antigens in vivo by γ interferon. J Exp Med 162: 1645–1664

Solomon A, Weiss DT, Kattine AA (1991) Nephrotoxic potential of Bence Jones proteins. N Engl J Med 324: 1845–1851

Stadtman ER, Berlett BS (1988) Fenton chemistry revisited: amino acid oxidation. In: Simie MC, Taylor KA, Ward JF (eds) Oxygen radicals in biology and medicine. Plenum, New York, pp 131–136

Steffes MW, Brown DM, Mauer SM (1978) Diabetic glomerulopathy following unilateral nephrectomy in the rat. Diabetes 27: 35–41

Striker GE, Schainuck LI, Cutler RE, Benditt EP (1970) Structural-functional correlations in renal disease. Part I: A method for assaying and classifying histopathologic changes in renal disease. Hum Pathol 1: 615–630

Teodoru CV, Saifer A, Frankel H (1959) Conditioning factors influencing evolution of experimental glomerulonephritis in rabbits. Am J Physiol 196: 457–460

Torres VE, Velosa JA, Holley KE, Kelalis PP, Stickler GB, Kurtz SB (1980) The progression of vesicoureteral reflux. Ann Intern Med 92: 776–784

Velosa JA, Glasser RJ, Nevins TE, Michael AF (1977) Experimental model of focal sclerosis. II. Correlation with immunopathologic changes, macromolecular kinetics, and polyanion loss. Lab Invest 36: 527–534

von Gise H, von Gise V, Stark B, Bohle A (1981) Nephrotic syndrome and renal insufficiency in association with amyloidosis: a correlation between structure and function. Klin Wochenschr 59: 75–82

Wehrmann M, Bohle A, Helol H, Schumm G, Kendziorra H, Pressler H (1990) Long-term prognosis of focal sclerosing glomerulonephrosis. An analysis of 250 cases with particular regard to tubulo-interstitial changes. Clin Nephrol 33: 115–122

Wuthrich RP, Yui MA, Mazoujian G, Nabavi N, Glimcher LH, Kelley VE (1989) Enhanced MHC class II expression in renal proximal tubules precedes loss of renal function in MRC/lpr mice with lupus nephritis. Am J Pathol 134: 45–51

Wuthrich RA, Glimcher LH, Yui MA, Nevnikar AM, Dumas SE, Kelley VE (1990) MHC class II, anitigen presentation and tumor necrosis factor in renal tubular epithelial cells. Kidney Int 37: 783–792

Yanagisawa M, Kurihara H, Kimura S, Tomobe Y, Kobayashi M, Mitsui Y, Yazaki K, Goto Y, Masaki T (1988) A novel potent vasoconstrictor peptide produced by vascular endothelial cells. Nature 332: 411–415

Yoshida Y, Mitsumata M, Yamane T, Tomikawa M, Nishida K (1988) Morphology and increased growth rate of atherosclerotic intimal smooth muscle cells. Arch Pathol Lab Med 112: 987–996

Yoshida Y, Fogo A, Ichikawa I (1989) Glomerular haemodynamic changes vs. hypertrophy in experimental glomerular sclerosis. Kidney Int 35: 654–660

Yoshioka T, Bills T, Moore-Jarrett T, Greene HL, Burr IM, Ichikawa I (1990) Role of intrinsic antioxidant enzymes in renal oxidant injury. Kidney Int 38: 282–288

Zamlauski-Tucker MJ, van Liew JB, Goldinger J, Noble B (1990) Persistent proximal tubule dysfunction late in Heyman nephritis. Kidney Int 37: 1536–1542

Zatz R, Dunn BR, Meyer TW, Anderson S, Rennke HG, Brenner BM (1986) Prevention of diabetic glomerulopathy by pharmacological amelioration of glomerular capillary hypertension. J Clin Invest 77: 1925–1930

Cellular Biology of Tubulointerstitial Growth

G. Wolf and E.G. Neilson

1 Introduction and Historical Perspective

The capacity of the kidney to grow has been known for more than 2000 years. Aristotle (384–322 B.C.) was probably the first to describe that animals born with one kidney can develop normally, and that the single kidney is enlarged compared with the kidneys of normal two-kidney control animals (Wolf 1993). In the early nineteenth century, the French physician Pierre-Francois-Olivier Rayer (1793–1867) reported enlargement of the renal cortex in diabetes mellitus and observed that the size of the remnant kidney in patients in whom one kidney is missing approaches that of the two kidneys of healthy individuals (Rayer 1837). Rayer also undertook microscopic studies and found that "if the kidney is partially disorganized, the healthy parts become hypertrophied, resulting in a curious mixture of atrophic and hypertrophic parts" (Ritz et al. 1989). Gustav Simon (1824–1876), a professor of surgery at the University of Heidelberg in Germany, performed the first unilateral nephrectomy in human subjects. The question of whether compensatory renal growth is solely an increase in protein and size (hypertrophy) or rather is caused by proliferation has puzzled students of renal growth for a long time. The famous Viennese pathologist Carl Rokitansky (1804–1878) believed that the increase in renal size after nephrectomy is true hypertrophy of all tissue constituents, whereas Simon thought that an increase in cell number was responsible for compensatory renal growth (Wolf 1993). However, most of these confusing early opinions can be attributed to the different ages of the animals used and the degree of renal ablation.

Current Topics in Pathology
Volume 88, S.M. Dodd (Ed.)
© Springer-Verlag Berlin Heidelberg 1995

Another controversial question persisting to the present is the unclear nature of the factors which stimulate and regulate the growth of remnant renal tissue. For example, Carl Wilhelm Nothnagel from Jena postulated as early as in 1886 that an increase in "nutrient" substances stimulates renal growth. Thus, Nothnagel can be considered the founding father of all subsequent studies defining the importance of growth factors, cytokines, and hormones in the complex regulation of renal growth. In contrast, Sacerdotti introduced, in 1896, the concept that the enlargement of the remaining kidney after uninephrectomy was a necessary response to the need to excrete greater amounts of waste (WOLF 1993). This more mechanical view was later referred to as the "work theory," which considers that a necessary increase in renal function is required as a trigger for kidney growth after ablation. The "work theory" has exerted great influence in the past decade, establishing the concept that increases in glomerular hemodynamics after permanent loss of renal tissues subsequently stimulate the enlargement of remnant nephrons (BRENNER 1985).

This chapter will highlight recent findings thought to be important in the regulation of tubulointerstitial growth at the molecular biological level. Although many cellular mechanisms have been elucidated in cells of nonrenal origin, there is a more recent general agreement that a conceptual framework of common molecular events is responsible for the growth regulation in virtually all cell types (NURSE 1990; MURRAY 1989).

The present paper covers neither the renal hemodynamic alterations associated with adaptive responses after nephrectomy—the "macromolecular" aspects of renal growth, nor the detailed descriptions of models of tubulointerstitial hypertrophy and hyperplasia. This information has been summarized elsewhere (WESSON 1989; WOLF and NEILSON 1991). Some animal models of renal hypertrophy and hyperplasia are described, however, in Table 1.

Table 1. Some in vivo models of tubular hypertrophy and hyperplasia

---

Hypertrophy
  Uninephrectomy in adult animals
  Unilateral obstruction (contralateral kidney)
  High-protein diet
  Insulin-dependent diabetes mellitus
  Ammonium chloride feeding
  Testosterone administration to female animals
  Thyroxine administration

Combined hypertrophy and hyperplastic responses
  Renal ablation in neonatal animals
  Tubular salt overload
  Potassium depletion

Hyperplasia
  Folate nephropathy
  Chemical nephrotoxicity (mercuric chloride, lead
    acetate)
  Renal ischemia with reperfusion

---

2 Importance of the Tubulointerstitial Environment

The tubulointerstitial environment is organized from several distinct cell types which are in close proximity, permitting the interactive engagement of multiple auto-, para-, and endocrine cytokine networks (LEMLEY and KRIZ 1991). The cellular residents of the tubulointerstitium include the various types of tubular epithelium, highly specialized in morphology and function along the nephron, a class of interstitial cells (types I and II in the cortex, types I–III in the medulla), interstitial fibroblasts, vascular endothelium, nerve cells, lymphatics, macrophages, and lymphocytes (TISHER and MADSEN 1988). This cellular registry is supplemented by a vast extracellular matrix containing interstitial collagenous fibres (types-I, -III and -VI collagen), proteoglycans, glycoproteins, and interstitial fluid.

An increasing number of studies suggest that changes in the tubulointerstitial environment are a major determinant in the progression of renal disease even when there is primary glomerular injury (reviewed in NATH 1992). Disturbance of the normal tubulointerstitial architecture is also a common finding in the chronically injured kidney, independent of the anatomical origin or type of primary disease. One invariant denominator of chronic tubulointerstitial disease is the development of interstitial fibrosis (NEILSON 1989). The molecular mechanisms inciting fibrogenesis are incompletely understood and are reviewed elsewhere in this volume. A variety of cytokines, growth factors, and hormones which also influence the growth of tubular cells and fibroblasts are involved in the synthesis and deposition of extracellular matrix components (KUNCIO et al. 1991). Interestingly, several in vitro studies revealed that factors influencing the growth of tubulointerstitial cells also exert fundamental effects on the biosynthesis of various collagens linking growth regulation to interstitial fibrogenesis (WOLF and NEILSON 1991).

3 Hyperplasia Versus Hypertrophy

Quiescent tubular cells can undergo either hyperplasia or hypertrophy, two totally different growth responses (FINE 1986). Cells committed to proliferation double their DNA content and divide during mitosis. In contrast, hypertrophic cells increase their size, protein, and RNA content, but do not duplicate their set of chromosomes. These growth responses are exclusive: a cell can be committed to either mitosis or hypertrophy (WOLF and NEILSON 1991). However, different cell types along the nephron may exhibit a different growth response to the same factor; even adjacent cells of the identical histological type might respond differently, depending on the activation state of the cells, receptor expression for growth factors, influence of growth suppressors, and the genetic program of individual cells.

The regeneration of functional tubular epithelium after acute tubular necrosis is a classical example of a proliferative growth response restoring correct cell numbers to preformed nephrons (TOBACK 1992). In contrast, compensatory renal enlargement following chronic loss of nephrons in the adult kidney after uninephrectomy results in hypertrophy of tubular cells (FINE 1986). However, greater degrees of renal ablation or younger animals shift the compensatory growth response to partial proliferation of remnant tubular cells (WOLF and NEILSON 1991). Compensatory renal growth responses which involve mainly tubular cells, because they constitute the bulk of the renal mass, may, although initially restoring functional renal tissue, ultimately result in maladaptation of renal function. Hypertrophic tubular cells exert a state of hypermetabolism with an increase in oxygen consumption per remaining nephron. It has been proposed that this increase in oxygen consumption leads to cellular damage via the production of oxygen-reactive species or free radicals (CULPEPPER and SCHOOLWERTH 1992; SCHRIER et al. 1988). Adaptive increments in tubular ammoniagenesis associated with compensatory hypertrophy also yield elevated levels of ammonia, which activates C3/C5 convertase (NATH et al. 1985). This leads to tubular deposition of complement factor C5b-9, resulting in inflammation (NATH et al. 1985). These mechanisms may finally produce tubular atrophy and interstitial scarring.

4 Cell Cycle Regulation

Regulation of the cell cycle is the pivotal element controlling whether resting, quiescent cells are committed to mitosis or not (CROSS et al. 1989). Major progress in the molecular biology of the cell cycle over the past few years has added to a detailed picture of how proliferation is controlled. Although knowledge of the cell cycle biology originated from studies with the fission yeast *Schizosaccharomyces pombe* and the budding yeast *Saccharomyces cerevisiae*, as well as with *Xenopus* oocytes, there is general agreement that similar mechanisms are operative in all cell types (GAUTIER et al. 1989; MALLER 1990). Orderly cell division depends on the progression of cells through a cycle of successive phases (LEWIN 1990; CROSS et al. 1989). Quiescent, nondividing cells, enter the cell cycle from the G_0-phase, pass through G_1, initiate their DNA synthesis in the S-phase, and, after progressing through G_2, enter mitosis. Mitosis, with its ordered steps of prometaphase, metaphase, anaphase, and telophase, may be considered cycle itself, interfaced between the G_2- and G_1-phases of the cell cycle (McINTOSH and KOONCE 1989). The organized events during circular progression of the cell cycle require checkpoints at which the successful completion of earlier phases of the cell cycle is controlled. For example, cells can enter mitosis only if the DNA replication in the S-phase has been accomplished. Two general checkpoints have been identified, one in the G_0/G_1 transition governing entry into S-phase, and the other in the G_2-phase, governing entry into the phases of mitosis (HOFBAUER and DENHARDT 1991; PARDEE 1989).

Complex oscillation patterns of expression of various cyclins, changes in phosphorylation patterns of key proteins and activation of distinct phosphatases control the kinetics of the cell cycle. It was known for some time that a poorly characterized factor called maturation promoting factor (MPF), originally isolated from frog oocytes undergoing meiosis, is a major regulator of mitosis (BROEK et al. 1991; GAUTIER et al. 1988). The activity of MPF fluctuates during the cell cycle: the active factor is detectable during mitosis but not during the interphase (GOULD and NURSE 1989). The catalytic subunit of MPF is a 34 000 M_r phosphoprotein with kinase activity called pp34. This phosphoprotein is identical to the product of the cdc2$^+$ gene, originally identified as a gene crucial to mitosis in yeast (CLARKE and KARSENTI 1991; NURSE 1990). The cdc2$^+$ gene is required not only at the onset of mitosis, but also at the so-called start control point of the G_1/S transition; pp34 itself functions as a protein kinase (MALLER 1990). The protein is phosphorylated on both threonine and tyrosine during late interphase (MORIA et al. 1989). The level of pp34 remains constant during the cell cycle and complexes with cyclins, the other constituents of MPF (DRAETTA et al. 1989; PINES and HUNTER 1989). In contrast to pp34, cyclins must accumulate during interphase (DRAETTA et al. 1989). The complex of cyclin and pp34 still lacks activity and is called pre-MPF. This complex is then activated by dephosphorylation of pp34 and phosphorylation of cyclin. The 107-kD phosphoprotein product of the wee 1$^+$ gene prevents the activation of MPF and is a negative regulator of entry into mitosis (PARKER et al. 1992; RUSSELL and NURSE 1987); p107 is also a kinase with the unusual properties of phosphorylating serine/threonine, as well as tyrosine residues (PARKER et al. 1992). The product of the cdc25$^+$ gene, a 67-kD protein, counteracts the mitotic inhibition caused by wee1$^+$ (RUSSELL and NURSE 1986). Although cdc25$^+$ has no sequence homology to known phosphatases, there is overwhelming evidence that cdc25$^+$ directly catalyzes the dephosphorylation of pp34 (GALAKTIONOV and BEACH 1991). Interestingly, the phosphatase activity of cdc25$^+$ seems to be highly substrate specific, and no efficient dephosphorylation of any protein other than pp34 complexed to cyclin has been detected so far. Active pp34 phosphorylates several target substrates, resulting in biochemical changes necessary for mitosis; pp34 kinase phosphorylates laminins B1 and B2 at serine 16 residue as well as with vimentin (OTTAVIANO and GERACE 1985; WARD and KIRSCHNER 1990; CHOU et al. 1990). This phosphorylation plays a major role in the nuclear disassembly, which is an important prerequisite of mitosis. On the other hand, pp34 activity has traditionally been measured as histone H1 kinase, and phosphorylation of this histone may contribute to chromosome condensation by changing nucleosome assembly (ARION et al. 1988).

A more direct role of pp34 in active transcriptional regulation has been suggested by the identification of the carboxyl terminal domain of RNA polymerase as substrate (CISEK and GORDEN 1989). Moreover, recent studies demonstrate that the cyclinA-pp34 complex is associated with the E2F transcription factor, and this complex accumulates during S-phase (DEVOTO et al. 1992). This observation suggests that cyclin A-pp34 possesses sequence-specific DNA-binding activity and may phosphorylate other DNA-bound substrates, offering the possibility of direct transcriptional control of selected target genes (DEVOTO et al. 1992). The cyclin partner of pp34 in the MRF complex can be classified into A and B types which are only weakly related to each other (MALLER 1990). Either A or B cyclins complex with pp34. Cyclin B levels accumulate during the G_2-phase (DRAETTA et al. 1989). The transition from metaphase to anaphase in mitosis leads to the degradation of cyclins, making this the crucial event in exiting mitosis and entering the G_1-phase (NURSE 1990). Cyclins are degraded by ubiquitin-dependent proteolysis (GLOTZER et al. 1991). Recent studies revealed that the cyclin A-pp34 complex is active earlier in the cell cycle than the cyclin B-pp34 complex (REED 1991). It has been proposed that the binding of pp34 to cyclin A controls the G_2/S transition in the cell cycle (REED 1991). In accordance with this hypothesis is the observation that microinjection of antisense cyclin A cDNA or anti-cyclin A antibodies into fibroblasts during G_1-phase led to inhibition of entry into the S-phase and DNA synthesis (GIRARD et al. 1991). Other control elements such as the product of cdc 10^+ gene, which is part of a trans-acting binding factor named DSC1 interacting with the hexamer element ACGCGT, present in the promoters of several target genes, are important for entry into the S-phase (LOWNDES et al. 1992). There is compelling recent evidence that additional cyclins named D and E exist (KOFF et al. 1992). Human cyclin E associates with a cell cycle-regulated protein kinase, the activity of which peaks during G_1, before the appearance of cyclin A. The major cyclin E-associated kinase was identified as a member of the cdc 2^+ family called cdk 2 (cyclin-dependent kinase 2). It is apparent that the assembly of the cyclin E-cdk complex is important for the progression through G_1 (KOFF et al. 1992). Although many details have been worked out regarding the control of this complicated phosphorylation cascade, it is most likely that other important kinases and/or phosphatases will also be identified in this orchestrated progression toward mitosis (CYERT and THORNER 1989).

5 Growth Factors for Tubular Cells

Several investigators have assessed growth-stimulatory effects of cytokines and polypeptide growth factors on different tubular cell lines (for review see KUJUBU and FINE 1989; TOBACK et al. 1990). The biochemical properties of renal growth factors have been extensively reviewed and are summarized in Table 2. In general, serum, epidermal growth factor (EGF; HAVERTY et al. 1988), transforming growth factor α (TGFα; HUMES et al. 1991), hepatocyte growth factor (HGF; IGAWA et al. 1991; ISHIBASHI et al. 1992), fibroblast growth factor (FGF), insulin, insulin-like growth factor-1 (IGF-1; BLAZER-YOST et al. 1992), calcium oxalate monophosphate (LIESKE et al. 1992), and adenosine diphosphate (ADP; KARTHA

Table 2. In vitro effects of cytokines and growth factors
on cultured tubular cells

Proliferation
  Serum
  Epidermal growth factor
  Transforming growth factor α
  Hepatocyte growth factor
  Fibroblast growth factor
  Insulin-like growth factor I
  Insulin
  ADP
  Culture medium with low sodium
  Calcium oxalate monophosphate

Hypertrophy
  Angiotensin II
  NH_4Cl
  High glucose in the medium
  Transforming growth factor β

---

et al. 1987) have been shown in vitro to be mitogenic for tubular cells (Table 2). In contrast, angiotensin II (ANG II; WOLF and NEILSON 1990a), transforming growth factor β (TGF-β; FINE et al. 1985), NH_4Cl (GOLCHINI et al. 1989), and high glucose (ROCCO et al. 1992) induce cellular hypertrophy in cultured tubular cells.

In a series of experiments we have studied the hypertrophogenic actions of ANG II as a single-factor model on a murine proximal tubular cell line (WOLF and NEILSON 1990a; WOLF et al. 1991a, c). Stimulation of quiescent tubular cells with $10^{-8}M$ ANG II for 48–72 h led to an incrase in cellular size, total RNA and protein content, and protein synthesis, but failed to induce mitosis (WOLF and NEILSON 1990a). These effects were mediated by DuP 753-sensible, G-protein-coupled AT_1 receptors, and depended on a decrease in intracellular cAMP (WOLF et al. 1991c). Furthermore, tubular enlargement was associated with an increase in transcription and synthesis of collagen type IV (WOLF et al. 1991a). Activation of immediate early genes is not sufficient to explain ANG II-induced hypertrophy, since a similar pattern of genes is induced by the mitogenic factor EGF (WOLF et al. 1991d). We have isolated a set of ANG II-induced genes by differential hybridization which appears to be associated with hypertrophy (WOLF and NEILSON 1990b, 1993). A further analysis of these genes will help to understand the complex mechanisms of cellular enlargement.

The involvement of single growth factors on renal proliferation or hypertrophy in vivo is more difficult to assess. Acute ischemia reduces renal prepro-EGF mRNA and increases the number of EGF receptors (NORMAN et al. 1990). Subcutaneous administration of EGF enhanced tubular proliferation and functional recovery after acute tubular necrosis (HUMES et al. 1989). EGF precursor is synthesized in the thick ascending limbs of Henle's loop and in more distal tubules (BREYER et al. 1991, MILLER et al. 1992). At 24 h after uninephrectomy, there was an increase in luminal immunostainable EGF in the remnant kidney.

In contrast, staining of EGF was present more diffusely throughout distal tubular cells at 5 and 14 days after uninephrectomy, involving luminal and contraluminal membranes (MILLER et al. 1992). Mice made deficient of circulating EGF by sialoadenectomy failed to undergo compensatory renal growth following unilateral nephrectomy (UCHIDA et al. 1988). Although it appears that EGF may play a role in proliferative regeneration of functioning tubular epithelium after acute necrosis, its function as an initiator of tubular hypertrophy seems unlikely, since hypertrophy occurs prior to any change in renal EGF content (MILLER et al. 1992). Nevertheless, EGF may be involved as a growth promoter in subsequent events of compensatory hypertrophy, perhaps through the stimulation of IGF-1 synthesis.

Several groups have studied the expression of IGF-1 in different models of renal growth (EL NAHAS et al. 1990; FAGIN and MELMED 1987; FLYVBERG et al. 1992; LAJARA et al. 1989; MARSHALL et al. 1991; MULRONEY et al. 1991; STILES et al. 1985). IGF-1 receptors which can undergo autophosphorylation after activation have been localized on the basolateral membrane of the proximal tubule (HAMMERMAN and ROGERS 1987). In addition, several IGF-binding proteins have been characterized (CONOVER et al. 1989). EGF also stimulates IGF-1 expression in renal collecting ducts (ROGERS et al. 1991). In a model of unilateral obstruction, hypertrophic growth of the contralateral kidney was preceded by a rise in extractable IGF-1 protein (MARSHALL et al. 1991). Increases in IGF-1 immunoreactivity in regenerating tubules after ischemia have been reported (DAUGHADAY and ROTWEIN 1989). Earlier studies suggested an increase in IGF-1 mRNA 24 h and IGF-1 protein 4 days after uninephrectomy in the remnant kidney (STILES et al. 1985). This phenomenon occurred independent of changes in growth hormone (GH) secretion. EL NAHAS and co-workers (1990) reported that IGF-1 protein increases and compensatory enlargement of the contralateral kidney occurred after uninephrectomy in GH-deficient dwarf rats, suggesting that GH is not necessary. In contrast, a different study found an increase in the intensity of immunostaining for IGF-1, but no changes in mRNA post nephrectomy (LAJARA et al. 1989). These results indicate that possible translational mechanisms underlie the induction of IGF-1 synthesis during compensatory hypertrophy. Along this line, the initial hypertrophy in experimental diabetes is associated with renal accumulation of IGF-1 protein, but not of mRNA (FLYVBERG et al. 1990). Transcripts for the IGF-1 receptor and receptor binding of the peptide are increased in the kidneys of rats 14 days after streptozotocin-induced diabetes. IGF-1 peptide, but not transcripts, is increased in initial renal hypertrophy in potassium-depleted rats (FLYVBERG et al. 1992). Recent evidence suggests an age-related difference in IGF-1 and IGF-1 receptor steady-state mRNA levels: they were three- to four fold increased in remnant kidneys of immature rats (22–24 days of age), but not in adult rat kidneys (4 months of age) after unilateral renal ablation (MULRONEY et al. 1992a,b). Considering all these findings, there is some evidence that IGF-1 may play a role in hypertrophy. However, it is not clear whether the expression of IGF-1 peptide, in the absence of concomitant changes in mRNA levels, may represent some common epiphenomenon associated with different models of renal hypertrophy rather than being causally connected to the molecular mechanisms of renal enlargement. Furthermore, since IGF-1 is clearly mitogenic for cultured tubular cells (BLAZER-YOST et al. 1992), its role in cellular hypertrophy remains speculative.

Recent interest has focused on HGF, a heterodimer composed of 69-kD and 34-kD subunits, originally identified as a potent mitogen for mature hepatocytes (GRAZIANI et al. 1991). HGF strongly induces mitogenesis in cultured tubular cells of the LLC-PK$_1$ and OK cell lines (ISHIBASHI et al. 1992). These cells also express the receptor for HGF, which is the protein product of the *c-met* oncogene. In contrast, only mesangial cells have transcripts for HGF (where HGF has no effect on proliferation), but not tubular cells (ISHIBASHI et al. 1992). These findings suggest that HGF is produced in mesangial cells and may work on tubular epithelial cells to stimulate proliferation in a paracrine manner. In the remnant kidney, HGF mRNA increased markedly, reaching a maximum 6 h after uninephrectomy in male Wistar rats. In situ hybridization suggests that these transcripts were produced by renal endothelial cells (NAGAIKE et al. 1992). The HGF receptor was greatly reduced 24 h after unilateral nephrectomy, suggesting internalization of the receptor after binding of HGF (NAGAIKE et al. 1991). Thus, HGF may be involved in some way in the growth response after uninephrectomy. However, the strong mitogenic action of HGF on tubules in vitro and the contradictory findings of tubular hypertrophy after uninephrectomy certainly do not make HGF likely to be the single factor causing compensatory hypertrophy.

Many investigators have attempted to isolate, purify, and characterize renal growth factors from plasma of uninephrectomized rats, the so-called renotropins (AVERBUKH et al. 1992; MALT 1983; MANZANO et al. 1989; KANETAKE and YAMAMOTO 1981; HARRIS et al. 1983; LOGAN and BENSON 1990, 1992). Nobody has so far succeeded in purifying such a factor, and the molecular weights of candidate renotropins, estimated by different investigators (12–55 kD), are as variable as the biological effects of these factors. Some, for example, induce production of inositol trisphosphates (BANFIC and KUKOLJA 1988; BANFIC 1990); other factors appear to stimulate prostaglandin synthesis in renal cells from the rabbit (LOGAN and BENSON 1990). Noticeably, all these studies investigated the effect of the proposed serum renotropin on proliferation, an inappropriate assay to measure factors which are supposed to induce compensatory renal hypertrophy (LOGAN and BENSON 1992). In conclusion, there is some evidence that specific renotropins might exist. It is, however, more likely that they represent a heterogeneous group of moieties which may be similar to the polypeptides described above. It appears that not just one humoral factor is responsible for tubular hypertrophy and hyperplasia; rather, the interplay of several growth modulators, in concert with events regulating the cell cycle, determines the net growth responses (hypertrophy or hyperplasia) of tubular cells.

6 Signal Transduction Pathways

As a fairly simple generalization, a growth factor binds to its appropriate receptor and the signal is transduced by G-proteins and/or protein kinases, depending on the type of receptor (CANTLEY et al. 1991; KARIN 1992; MILLER 1991). Subsequent events include the generation of cyclic nucleotides like cAMP and cGMP, or the stimulation of phospholipase C, which hydrolyzes phosphatidyl inositol biphosphate to inositol trisphosphate (IP_3) and diacylglycerol (DAG; PFEILSCHIFTER 1989b). These second mesengers induce release of Ca^{++} from intracellular stores. In addition, growth factors may modulate the activity of transmembrane Ca^{++} channels, resulting in an increased influx of this ion (IRVINE 1992). There is also clear evidence that inositol tetracisphosphate (IP_4) can control Ca^{++} entry (IRVINE 1991). All these second messengers, in turn, can influence the activity of successive protein kinases, such as cAMP-dependent kinases and calmodulin-associated kinases (TAYLOR 1989). The signals are then further transmitted to the nucleus where trans-acting factors influence the activity of key regulators of the cell cycle or the activation of immediate early genes, as described below. Although the different signal transduction pathways have traditionally been considered separate entities, more recent work indicates that considerable networking occurs between all these systems (PFEILSCHIFTER 1989a). For example, activation of protein kinase C (PKC) with phorbol ester increase cAMP in the presence of cholera toxin (ROZENGURT et al. 1987). Domin and Rozengurt demonstrated in 3T3 fibroblasts that persistent occupancy of the V_1 receptor, a guanine-nucleotide-binding protein-coupled receptor, by vasopressin attenuated responsiveness to a polypeptide growth factor (in this case platelet-derived growth factor, PDGF) that initiates responses through a tyrosine kinase (DOMIN and ROZENGURT 1992). Down-regulation of PKC results in an enhanced induction of the urokinase-type plasminogen activator gene expression by cAMP-mediated signals in LLC-PK$_1$ cells, a permanent porcine tubular cell line (ZIEGLER et al. 1991). Moreover, diverse proteins like an isoenzyme of phospholipase C (PLC-g), oncogenes like *c-src* and *c-vav*, the GTPase-activating protein (GAP), and a phosphatase all express a common protein motif consisting of approximately 100 amino acids, the SH2 domain (MACARA 1989; MARGOLIS 1992). These proteins interact via their SH2 domains with autophosphorylated receptors for polypeptide growth factors like EGF after ligand binding. Many ligands induce autophosphorylation of their receptors on tyrosine residues (MARGOLIS 1992). In a secondary step, serine and threonine residues in many target proteins are phosphorylated. Mitogen-activated protein (MAP) kinases are 42- and 44-kD serine-threonine kinases that are activated by tyrosine and threonine phosphorylation in cells treated with mitogens (PELECH and SANGHERA 1992). A MAP-kinase kinase has been identified which phosphorylates MAP kinase, indicating a hierarchic cascade of phosphorylation (ADAMS and PARKER 1992). MAP kinase itself phosphorylates and activates the transcription factor p62TCF which constitutes with the serum-response element, a tertiary complex binding to the *c-fos* promotor (PULVERER et al. 1991; details see below). This pathway provides one example of how signals are transduced from the cell surface to the nucleus, and how this information is translated to changes in transcription of distinct genes. The roles of different signal transduction pathways in tubulointerstitial hypertrophy and hyperplasia have previously been reviewed in detail (WOLF and NEILSON 1991). PKC activity of proximal tubular brush-border membranes is significantly increased after unilateral nephrectomy (BANFIC 1990). A significant increase in the concentration of DAG in remnant kidney cortical tissues as early as 5 min after uninephrectomy has been reported as well (SALIHAGIC et al. 1988). Ischemia and reperfusion resulted in stable increases of phospholipase A2 in the rat kidney (NAKAMURA et al. 1991). A rise in the concentration of cGMP in the contralateral kidney within 2 min after unilateral nephrectomy was found by SCHLONDORFF and WEBER (1978). In contrast, adenylate cyclase activity was significantly lower in cortical membranes from kidneys with compensatory hypertrophy compared with controls (MILANES et al. 1989). These changes in the activation state of signal transduction pathways in the growing kidney probably mirror the stimulation by multiple growth factors and cytokines.

7 Proto-oncogenes and Immediate Early Genes

Proto-oncogenes play a major role in the control of proliferation and hypertrophy in all tissues including renal cells (WOLF et al. 1991b; HERSCHMAN 1991; STRYER and BOURNE 1986; BISHOP 1983). Proto-oncogenes can be functionally classified into different groups. Certain proto-oncogenes encode for growth factors (MULLER et al. 1990), for example the c-sis product, which is the β-chain of platelet-derived growth factor (PDGF; CHIU et al. 1984), and the k-fgf proto-oncogene are related to the FGF (SMITH et al. 1988). A different group of proto-oncogenes are related to receptors for growth factors. Examples of this group are c-erb B, which encodes for a truncated version of the receptor for EGF, and the protein product of c-ros, which shares more than 70% homology with the tyrosine domain of the insulin receptor (ULLRICH and SCHLESINGER 1990; FREEMAN and DONOGHUE 1991). The c-met proto-oncogene encodes for the receptor for HGF, which associates with phosphatidylinositol 3-kinase (GRAZIANI et al. 1991). A third group of proto-oncogenes encode proteins related to G-proteins (c-ras, c-rho proto-oncogenes; MILLER 1991; MILBURN et al. 1990)

Finally, the last group of proto-oncogenes encode for proteins acting in the nucleus as regulators of transcriptional activity (BOETTINGER 1989; HERSCHMAN 1991). They represent primary sets of genes induced after stimulation by various growth factors or mechanical stimulation and have been called immediate early or primary response genes because of their induction kinetics (TRAVALI et al. 1990). We will focus in this chapter solely on this group of genes, since they represent a common mechanism of growth regulation and indicate how various growth factors can induce a group of early genes which regulate the activity of other downstream structural genes (HOFBAUER and DENHARDT 1991). Several primary response genes have been identified using differential hybridization of cells stimulated with serum, various growth factors, cytokines, and phorbol ester (ALMENDRAL et al. 1988; CHAVRIER et al. 1988). Sequences induced by these factors include *c-fos*, *fosB*, *c-jun*, *junB*, *fra-1*, *fra-2*, *Egr-1*, *Egr-2*, *N10*, *TIS11*, *cMG₁*, *c-myc*, *max*, *TIS10*, and *TIS21*. The function of many of these immediate early genes remains uncharacterized. However, a more detailed understanding emerges for the employment of *c-fos*, *c-jun*, *Egr-1*, and *c-myc* in transcriptional regulation. We will therefore focus on these primary response genes.

The induction, regulation, and function of *c-fos* can serve as a paradigm for other primary response genes (GILMAN et al. 1986). This proto-oncogene is a member of a whole family of related genes including *fosB*, *fra-1*, and *fra-2*. Serum and other growth factors induce transcription of *c-fos* in the presence of cycloheximide, indicating that ligand-mediated post-translational actions are sufficient to stimulate its transcriptional activity (SASSONE-CORSI and VERMA 1987). Deletion experiments in the *c-fos* promoter identified a region between nucleotides −322 and −276 as responsible for the ligand-induced transcription of *c-fos* (GILMAN et al. 1986). This element has been named the serum-response element (SRE). Subsequently, the corresponding 508-amino acid protein binding to SRE, the serum response factor (SRF), has been cloned. Growth factor-induced phosphorylation of SRF, perhaps by casein kinase II, appears to be important in the transcriptional activation of *c-fos*. Although many growth factors induce *c-fos* activity through SRE, it is not known whether several competing SRFs exist. Moreover, a second, less potent, serum-response element (SRE-2) has been characterized in the *c-fos* promoter. Induction of *c-fos* by cAMP requires the cAMP-response element (CRFB) at nucleotide −60 as well as an AP-1-like element at −296 (SASSONE-CORSI et al. 1988a). A *cis*-acting element responsible for calcium induction of *c-fos* is identical with CRE. Additional data suggest that cAMP-mediated transcription of *c-fos* involves phosphorylation of a protein binding to CRE by protein kinase A, whereas calcium phosphorylates this peptide by a calmodulin-dependent protein kinase. *C-fos* protein has an auto-negative feedback on its own promoter (SASSONE-CORSI et al. 1988b). *C-fos* mRNA is rapidly degraded. Repeated copies of AUUUA elements in the 3′ untranslated part of the *c-fos* mRNA are responsible for the rapid destabilization (HIPSKIND and NORDHEIM 1991). Apparently the 3′ AU-rich region is necessary for the removal of the poly(A) tail, resulting in a labile, easily degradable RNA. Thus, the concentration of steady-state *c-fos* mRNA may also be determined by post-transcriptional regulation of message stability. Immunoprecipitation of *c-fos* protein revealed a complex of *c-fos* associated with another protein, subsequently identified as the product of the *c-jun* gene (GENTZ et al. 1989; RANSONE and VERMA 1989; TURNER and TJIAN 1989). *C-jun* is the cellular counterpart to the avian sarcoma virus 17 oncogene *v-jun* and displays approximately 80% homology (VOGT and TJIAN 1988). In contrast to the high basal activity of *v-jun*, *c-jun* expression is tightly regulated

(RYSEK et al. 1988). Induction of *c-jun* transcription by phorbol ester is mediated by binding of AP-1 to a high-affinity AP-1 binding site in the *c-jun* promoter region, suggesting positive autoregulation of this immediate early gene (ANGEL et al. 1988). There exist other *c-jun* related genes (*junB, junD*). The *c-jun* protein forms a heterodimer with the protein product of *c-fos*. This heterodimer association occurs through a leucine zipper domain which is different from the DNA-binding site (GENTZ et al. 1989). The *c-jun–c-fos* complex binds to the sequence TGACTCA, the AP-1 site which can be found in the regulatory region of many genes (FRANZA et al. 1988; NAKABEPPU and NATHANS 1989). Dimerization of both proteins through the leucine zipper is necessary for DNA binding to the AP-1 region. The *c-jun–c-fos* heterodimer binds DNA more tightly and activates transcription more potent than the *c-jun* homodimer (TURNER and TJIAN 1989; CHIU et al. 1988). *C-fos* alone fails to form homodimers. A transcriptional activation domain (A1) and an adjacent negative regulatory domain (delta) have been identified in *c-jun* (BAICHWALD and TJIAN 1990). A cell-type-specific inhibitor binding to the A1 and delta regions of the *c-jun* protein has been characterized (BAICHWALD et al. 1991). This specific inhibitor does not bind sufficiently to *c-jun–c-fos* heterodimers. Recently, a signal-transduction pathway that results in an increase in transcriptional activity of *c-jun* and AP-1 by disrupting the *c-jun*-inhibitor interaction has been proposed (GILLE et al. 1992). Various members of the *c-jun/c-fos* family may be associated with each other through the common leucine zipper motif. Since expression of every member of these families is probably independently regulated, and their protein products compete to form dimers through leucine zippers with subsequent binding to AP-1 regions involving cell-type-specific inhibitors, it is obvious that such a multidimensional network modulates gene expression at different levels.

The immediate early gene *c-myc* encodes a short-lived 64-kD nuclear phosphoprotein which is induced early in the G_0/G_1 transition (ASSELIN et al. 1989). *N-myc* and *L-myc* are additional elements of the *c-myc* family (KATO and DANG 1992). Transcription of *c-myc* initiates from two promoters named P1 and P2, which are independently regulated (LÜSCHER and EISENMAN 1990). The *c-myc* protein negatively regulates its own expression at the level of transcription initiation (LGUCHI-ARIGA et al. 1988). Multiply mechanisms regulate *c-myc* gene expression, and different growth factors work through several modes: by influencing initiation of transcription and by abrogation of intragenic pausing, as well as by post-transcriptional stabilization of the mRNA (STUDZINSKI et al. 1986; KAKKIS et al. 1989; NEPVEU et al. 1987). Although it has been known for some time that the *c-myc* protein contains helix-loop-helix and leucine zipper regions in its carboxyl-terminal 85 amino acids, evidence for direct DNA binding or heterodimer formation was inconclusive. However, lately BLACKWOOD and EISENMAN (1991) used a labeled fusion protein containing the carboxyl-terminus region of *c-myc* to screen an expression library in λGT11 constructed from random-primed lymphoblast cell RNA. They came up with a new protein, *max*, which contains adjacent helix-loop-helix and leucine zipper regions (BLACKWOOD and EISENMAN 1991). *Max* forms heterodimers with all three proteins of the *c-myc* family, and these heterodimers bind to the sequence CACGTG (COLE 1991). Interestingly, *max* does not dimerize with other proteins having leucine zipper motifs. This explicit binding to *myc* proteins is likely due to the precise spacing of the helix-loop-helix and leucine zipper domains in *max* and *myc*. A 2.1-kb RNA for *max* is expressed in many tissues at concentrations comparable to those of *c-myc* (BLACKWOOD and EISENMAN 1991). Interestingly as well, an endogenous RNA transcript with homology to the antisense strand of *c-myc* has been identified, offering the possibility of an additional control mechanism (CELANO et al. 1992). Both activation and repression of target genes were observed, depending on the promoter, when *c-myc* was tested in trans-activation experiments. Expression of neural cell adhesion molecule (N-CAM) and major histocompatibility antigen (MHC) class I is suppressed by *c-myc*, whereas the hsp70 promoter plasminogen activator inhibitor-1 (PAI-1) gene is activated (KATO and DANG 1992). However, expression of *c-myc* is typically associated with proliferation, but not with cellular hypertrophy.

The *Egr-1* cDNA (also known as TIS-8, Krox-24, or Zif268) was identified by SUKHATME and co-workers using differential screening of a serum-stimulated fibroblast library (SUKHATME et al. 1987, 1988). Other members of the *Egr-1* family exist (e.g., *Egr-2*, *Egr-3*, *Egr-4*). The human *Egr-1* gene maps to the long arm of chromosome 5 and has two exons and one intron (TSAI-MORRIS et al. 1988). The transcript size of Egr-1 is 3.7 kb. The protein of 533 amino acids reveals in the carboxyl-terminal end a zinc finger structure of the Cys2-His2 class which interacts with specific DNA sequences (SUKHATME 1990). *Egr-1* protein binds with high affinity to the sequence CGCCCCGC. Protein kinase C (PKC)-dependent and -independent signal transduction pathways can induce *Egr-1*. The promoter region of *Egr-1* contains several CREB, SRE, and Sp1 and AP-1 binding sites, suggesting complex regulation by diverse factors (SUKHATME 1990).

C-fos, *c-jun*, *c-myc*, and *Egr-1* are readily induced in cultured tubular cells by mitogenic growth factors such as serum or EGF. Expression of *c-fos* and *Egr-1* has been also reported after ischemia and reperfusion of the kidney (BONVENTRE et al. 1991; OUELLETTE et al. 1990, ROSENBERG and PALLER 1991; SAFIRSTEIN et al. 1990). The increase in *c-fos* and *Egr-1* mRNAs occurs within the first hour of reflow, well before the peak in DNA synthesis is reached. Reperfusion is required for *Egr-1* protein synthesis (OUELLETTE et al. 1990). The *Egr-1* protein was localized to the nuclei of the thick ascending limbs and principal cells of the collecting ducts (BONVENTRE et al. 1991). In a model of regeneration of tubules after folic acid-induced necrosis *c-myc* levels accumulated to very high levels 4–6 h after treatment (ASSELIN and MARCU 1989; COWLEY et al. 1989). The amount of effective transcription throughout the *c-myc* gene remains unchanged after folic acid-induced proliferation, indicating strong post-transcriptional regulatory events (ASSELIN and MARCU 1989). ADP, which is a potent mitogen for the monkey kidney epithelial cells of the BSC-1 line, also induces expression of *c-myc* within 1 h of incubation (KARTHA et al. 1987). Significant increases in *c-myc*, *c-fos*, and *c-Ki-ras* expression were detected in whole kidneys from *cpk* mice, a murine model of autosomal recessive polycystic kidney disease (COWLEY et al. 1991). Nuclear run-on experiments revealed that the *c-fos* and *c-myc* genes are transcriped at higher rates in cystic kidneys (HARDING et al. 1992). *C-myc* mRNA was detected in elongated tubules by in situ hybridization (HARDING et al. 1992). Interestingly, cultures of *cpk* kidneys as well as of kidneys harvested from folic acid-treated animals showed that the level of *c-fos* induction following stimulation with serum was much higher than that in normal renal cells (RANKIN et al. 1992). Mice positive for the *c-myc* transgene driven by an SV 40 enhancer also develop polycystic kidney disease (TRUDEL et al. 1989).

Renal expression of proto-oncogenes is not limited to proliferation of cells. We have demonstrated in a culture model of tubular hypertrophy that angiotensin II induces, under defined culture conditions, the expression of *c-fos*, *c-myc*, and *c-N-ra ras* (Table 3; WOLF and NEILSON 1990a). Moreover, Rosenberg and Hostetter have demonstrated a significant increase in the renal expression of *c-fos* and *Egr-1* after infusion of angiotensin II into the renal artery in vivo that was independent of the arterial blood pressure (ROSENBERG and HOSTETTER 1990). Although some earlier studies investigating immediate early gene expression in compensatory renal hypertrophy after nephrectomy revealed some inconclusive results (NORMAN et al. 1988), recent studies have clearly demonstrated that such genes are also elevated in situations with renal hypertrophy (OUELLETTE et al. 1990; NAKAMURA et al. 1992; SAWCZUK et al. 1988). One hour after uninephrectomy, *c-jun*, *c-fos*, and *c-myc* mRNA levels were significantly increased in the cortex of the remnant kidney (NAKAMURA et al. 1992; SAWCZUK et al. 1990). *C-jun* and *c-fos* expression decreased rapidly to the control levels, whereas *c-myc* showed a more sustained level, decreasing to basal levels after 7 days. Increases in *Egr-1* mRNa levels also occur after uninephrectomy (OUELLETE et al. 1990). The genes *c-H-ras* and *c-K-ras* were induced in the remant kidney after uninephrectomy of mice (BAILEY et al. 1990; NOMATA et al. 1990). Oncogene expression was also detected in contralateral kidneys 15 min after acute unilateral obstruction, which leads to a compensatory hypertrophy of the contralateral kidney (SAWCZUK et al. 1989). Collectively, these results suggest that immediate early genes play a key role in tubular growth. However, their similar induction patterns, by mitogenesis and cellular hypertrophy suggest that the expression is an early common pathway influenced by many factors, and most likely characterizes the generic shift from the G_0- to the G_1-phase of the cell cycle.

Table 3. Oncogenes expressed during tubular hypertrophy and/or hyperplasia

Immediate early genes
  c-jun
  c-fos
  EgR-1
  c-myc

Oncogenes related to G-proteins
  c-Ha-ras
  c-K-ras
  c-N-ras

8 Negative Regulators of Cell Proliferation

The discovery that malignancy can be suppressed when malignant cells are fused with non-malignant ones by Harris and co-workers almost 25 years ago was a high point in the envolution of the concept that cellular growth can also be negatively regulated (Harris et al. 1969). Enormous progress in the molecular biology of tumor-suppressor genes or anti-oncogenes in recent years has provided a detailed picture of how these genes are associated with the regulative elements of the cell cycle. Despite the fact that several tumor-suppressor genes may exist (Lakshmanarao et al. 1991), only the function of the protein products of p53, retinoblastoma gene (Rb), Wilm's tumor gene (WAGR), and growth-arrest-specific (gas) genes have been more thoroughly characterized. Protein p53 was originally identified in a complex with the large T antigen of SV 40 virus by co-precipitation (Levine et al. 1991). Overexpression of p53 mutants immortalize cells, whereas wild-type p53 inhibits transformation and proliferation of cells (Ullrich et al. 1992). Protein p53 is expressed at very low levels in almost all cell types. Expression of wild-type p53 inhibits growth factor-induced G_1- to S-phase progression (Yin et al. 1992) and may directly repress transcription. Transient co-transfection experiments revealed that p53 represses may promoters including *c-fos*, actin, and MDM2, A 10-bp binding site for p53 has been identified, and binding of the protein may occur as a tetramer on two 10-bp binding sites separated by up to 13 bp of random sequence. Since p53 down-regulates the expression of genes which do not contain p53-binding sites, it is likely that other, yet unknown, genes are regulated by p53 which, in turn, suppress the activity of subsequent genes (Mercer et al. 1991). Thus, p53 may regulate transcription of a set of genes which are necessary for the passage from late G_1- to -S phase of the cell cycle. Loss of both alleles of wild-type p53 leads to the ability of cells to amplify at a high frequency caused by changes in cell cycle progression. In addition, a 90-kD cellular phosphoprotein, the protein product of the *mdm-2* oncogene, which binds to the p53 protein has recently been isolated (Momand et al. 1992). Interestingly, when a cosmid expressing *mdm-2* was co-transfected with p53, the transactivation of the p53-responsive element was inhibited, suggesting that *mdm-2* exerts its oncogenic potential by inhibiting the growth suppressive effect of p53 (Momand et al. 1992).

   The product of the retinoblastoma susceptibility gene (Rb) is a 110- to 114-kD phosphoprotein whose phosphorylation depends on the phase of the cell cycle (Buchkovich et al. 1989; Lee et al. 1987a). Rb is unphosphorylated in G_0/G_1 cells, becomes progressively phosphorylated at the G_1/S boundary, and is exclusively phosphorylated during S and G_2 (Mittnach and Weinberg 1991; DeCaprio et al. 1989). This phosphorylation occurs in at least three steps. Only underphosphorylated Rb binds efficiently to the nucleus. Phosphorylation inactivates Rb, and the underphosphorylated form suppresses cell proliferation and promotes cellular differentiation (Lee et al. 1987b). It has been proposed that pp34 kinase is responsible for this phosphorylation (Dou et al. 1992; Lin et al. 1991). Interestingly, transforming growth factor β (TGF-β), which is a known growth-inhibitory cytokine, retains Rb in the underphosphorylated, growth-suppressive state (LAIHO et al. 1990). On the other hand, recent evidence suggests that Rb activates transcription of the TGF-β_2 gene through transcription factor ATF-2 (KIM et al. 1992). Unphosphorylated Rb, but not phosphorylated Rb, associates with the transcrption-activating factor E2F protein (SHIRODKAR et al. 1992). E2F promoter elements are important for transcriptional activation of genes which play a pivotal role during the orderly progression through the cell cycle. The Rb-E2F complex, which forms during G_1 silences transcriptional activity when bound to the E2F target site, providing a clue to how changes in Rb phosphorylation directly influence transcription of regulatory genes (WEINTRAUB et al. 1992; SHIRODKAR et al. 1992; BANDARA et al. 1991).

Recent studies have also classified a series of genes (so-called *gas* genes) which are only expressed only on mRNAs and proteins which are expressed only in quiescent, growth-arrested cells (SCHNEIDER et al. 1988; PHILIPSON and SORRENTINO 1991; MARSHALL 1991). *Gas 1* is an integral membrane protein with two putative transmembrane domains flanking an extracellular region (DEL SAL et al. 1992). Sequence analysis showed no significant homology with other known proteins. The expression of *gas 1* mRNA and protein is significantly increased in growth-arrested cells compared with growing cells in medium containing serum. When such serum-starved NIH 3T3 cells are induced to reenter the cell cycle, *gas 1* expression is promptly down-regulated. *Gas 1* overexpression from a constitutive promoter in serum-stimulated NIH 3T3 cells induced a block in cell cycle progression without affecting the immediate early expression of *c-fos* and *c-jun* (MANFIOLETTI et al. 1990; DEL SAL et al. 1992). In contrast, *gas 1* overexpression had no effect on SV 40-transformed fibroblasts. Another gene of the *gas* family, *gas 5*, is ubiquitously expressed in murine tissues during development and differentiation (COCCIA et al. 1992). Nuclear run-off experiments revealed that the accumulation of *gas 5* mRNA in density-arrested cells is controlled at the post-transcriptional level, whereas in differentiating cells the expression is regulated by gene transcription (COCCIA et al. 1992).

The tumor-suppressor gene for Wilm's tumor, WT1, is expressed at high levels in glomeruli. It appears that WT1 plays a crucial role in proliferation and differentiation of nephroblasts and gonadal tissue. The WT1 protein is 45–49 kD in size and contains a carboxyl terminus which consists of four Cys-His zinc-finger domains, indicating that it functions as a transcription factor. Moreover, two alternative splice sites have been identified in the WT1 gene, resulting in the expression of four distinct mRNA transcripts (BICKMORE et al. 1992). These alternative spliced RNAs encode for proteins with different DNA binding specificity (HABER et al. 1991). The binding sequence for the WT1 protein is similar to the site recognized by the *Egr-1* gene product, implying that WT1 may antagonize the growth-stimulatory trans-activating effects of the *Egr-1* protein (RAUSCHER et al. 1990). Recent experiments using transient transfection assays revealed that the WT1 protein functioned as a repressor of transcription when bound to the *Egr-1* site (MADDEN et al. 1991). This repressive function was mapped to the NH_2-terminus of WT1. However, simple competition between

Egr-1 and WT1 at a single DNA-binding site seems unlikely, since the zinc-finger domain alone is unable to suppress transcription, although it binds to DNA. Rather, each protein interacts in a fundamentally different manner with the transcriptional machinery, involving hitherto unidentified co-factors.

Other genes involved in growth suppression have also been identified. For example, a gene called prohibitin has been isolated (BOYLAN and ZARBL 1991; NUELL et al. 1991). Prohibitin mRNA is expressed in the rat kidney and microinjection of synthetic prohibitin mRNA blocks entry into S-phase in fibroblasts, while antisense oligonucleotides stimulate entry into the S-phase (NUELL et al. 1991). Furthermore, the soluble lectin-like protein, murine β-galactoside-binding protein, has been shown to be a cell-growth-regulatory molecule exerting control during the G_0- and G_2-phases of the cell cycle (WELLS and MALLUCCI 1991). It is likely that many other genes with growth-suppressive abilities working together in an increasingly complex network of growth regulation will be identified in the 1990s.

9 Mechanisms of Apoptosis

Apoptosis is a distinct type of cell death, fundamentally different from necrosis, and is important in development and growth of adult tissue (ELLIS et al. 1991; FESUS et al. 1991). The term "programmed cell death" has also been applied to apoptosis. The apoptotic cell is, in contrast to necrosis, not characterized by marked inflammation and organelle swelling. Morphological changes of apoptosis are a reduction in nuclear size, condensation of chromatin at the nuclear periphery, and, finally, nucleolar disintegration with dissociation of the transcriptional complex from the fibrillar center (FESUS et al. 1991). Typical for apoptosis is an internucleosomal DNA fragmentation with double-strand cleavage of DNA, resulting in 180- to 200-bp fragments on agarose gels. This process requires energy, depends on protein synthesis, and involves the activation of one or more endonucleases, although the enzyme responsible for the fragmentation has not been identified. A 36-kD polypeptide with a single transmembrane region having homology to the tumor necrosis factor has been shown to mediate apoptosis (ITOH et al. 1991). This protein is encoded by the *Fas* gene, 1.9- and 2.7-kb RNAs of which are expressed in various cell lines (ITOH et al. 1991). Although the detailed functions of *Fas* are not known, it may act as a susceptibility gene for apoptosis. Interestingly, it has been demonstrated in immortalized fibroblasts that overexpression of the oncogene *c-myc* can induce apoptosis under special circumstances (EVAN et al. 1992). On the other hand, expression of the *bcl-2* gene, originally isolated from the breakpoint of the translation between chromosomes 14/18 found in lymphomas, suppresses apoptosis. Thus, cells may grow when normal apoptosis is suppressed by *bcl-2* expression (CLEARY et al. 1986; BISSONNETTE et al. 1992). Recent studies have identified apoptosis of tubular cells as a major contributor to cell death during the reperfusion phase of renal ischemia (GOBE et al. 1990; SCHUMER et al. 1992), as well as in experimental hydronephrosis (GOBE and AXELSEN 1987). Even more important, apoptosis seems to be a requirement for subsequent hyperplastic regeneration processes after tubular ischemia. Although data are still sparse, it is apparent that apoptosis is relevant to the fine tuning of growth regulation.

10 Mechanisms of Tubular Hypertrophy

In contrast to proliferation of tubular cells, cellular hypertrophy is a separate process with increases in cell size, RNA, and protein content without DNA replication (WOLF and NEILSON 1991; FINE 1986). In very particular situations, described mainly in liver tissue, cells may replicate their DNA during the S-phase but do not undergo mitosis, resulting in hypertrophy with polyploidy. Compared with hyperplasia, the mechanisms of which can be conveniently explained by the above-described gating of the cell cycle, much less is known about the regulatory elements controlling tubular hypertrophy. It is a matter of controversy whether cells undergoing hypertrophy remain arrested in the G_1-phase of the cell cycle or do not enter the cell cycle at all and stay in a special G_0-phase. Some authors have observed apparent differences in the expression of immediate early genes in proliferation and hypertrophy (KUJUBU et al. 1991; NORMAN et al. 1988), while others, including ourselves, have found similar expression patterns of those genes in the two growth responses, supporting the view that hypertrophic cells enter the G_1-phase and remain arrested there (NAKAMURA et al. 1992; OUELLETTE et al. 1990; WOLF and NEILSON 1990a). It is reasonable to assume that cellular hypertrophy may be caused by the parallel induction of stimulating and inhibiting growth factors. In such a scenario, a growth-stimulatory factor would push cells out of the quiescent state (G_0) into G. The progression toward mitosis would then be inhibited by a growth suppressor such as T6F-β_1 (MOSES et al. 1990; HOLLEY et al. 1980). Investigations into the hypertrophy of vascular smooth muscle cells indicate that a balance between growth stimulating and inhibiting factors indeed occurs (GIBBONS et al. 1992). We believe that a primary set of genes causally involved in the cell biology of hypertrophy exist. We have isolated several genes by differential hybridization from the ANG II-induced in vitro model of tubular hypertrophy (WOLF and NEILSON 1990b). Preliminary results indicate that one of these genes (called 22H) is expressed in the late G_1-phase of the cell cycle and is induced in the remnant kidney 6–24 h after uninephrectomy. In contrast, 22H transcripts were not increased in the proliferative model of folic acid-induced tubular necrosis in mice. These results suggest that a certain population of genes induces a genetic program leading to tubular enlargement. Further studies are necessary to identify the interface of these new genes with the above-described events controlling the cell cycle.

11 Summary

The study of tubular growth has certainly become more complex since Pierre-Rayers's time and is progressing toward a molecular dissection of regulatory events. Understanding the mechanisms of tubular growth is important, because these cells represent the bulk of the nephron, and there is convincing evidence of a link between tubular hypertrophy and the progression of renal disease with irreversible tubulointerstitial fibrosis as an end point. Two tubular growth responses can be distinguished: hypertrophy and hyperplasia. These fundamentally different patterns of growth indicate that diverse molecular mechanisms may be involved in inducing distinct growth responses. It is likely that cytokines and polypeptide growth factors play a role in tubular hypertrophy and hyperplasia. Probably, a combination of growth factors including inhibitory polypeptides like TGFβ, rather than a single factor, is necessary for differentiated tubular growth responses. Such factors bind to their receptors, and signals are transduced to the nucleus by various second messengers involving protein kinases, cyclic nucleotides, Ca^{++}, and inositolphosphates. The phosphorylation of nuclear trans-acting factors resulting in an expression of immediate early genes may be the common pathway of many of these mediators. Finally, whether the cell is to proliferate or to remain in the G_1-phase of the cell cycle is determined by the very complex cascade phosphorylation of kinases and their associations with different cyclins. How the induction of immediate early genes is linked to events of the cell cycle is currently incompletely understood. Negative regulation of growth through protein growth suppressors like the retinoblastoma gene product or the expression of special genes only during cell rest may be mandatory for the fine tuning of tubular growth.

References

Adams PD, Parker PJ (1992) Activation of mitogen-activated protein (MAP) kinase by a MAP kinase–kinase. J Biol Chem 267: 13135–13137

Almendral JM, Sommer D, McDonald-Bravo H, Burckhardt J, Perera J, Bravo R (1988) Complexity of the early genetic response to growth factors in mouse fibroblasts. Mol Cell Biol 8: 2140–2148

Angel P, Hattori K, Smeal T, Karin M (1988) The jun proto-oncogene is positively autoregulated by its product, jun/AP-1. Cell 55: 875–885

Arion D, Meijer L, Brizuela L, Beach D (1988) Cdc2 is a component of the M-phase-specific histone H1 kinase: evidence for identity with MPF. Cell 55: 371–378

Asselin A, Nepveu A, Marcu KB (1989) Molecular requirements for transcriptional initiation of the murine c-myc gene. Oncogene 4: 549–558

Asselin C, Marcu KB (1989) Mode of c-myc gene regulation in folic acid-induced kidney regeneration. Oncogene Res 5: 67–72

Averbukh A, Berman S, Weissgarten J, Cohn M, Golik A, Cohen N, Modai D (1992) Postnephrectomy mesangial cells secrete a factor(s) that stimulate(s) tubular cell growth in vitro. Nephron 60: 216–219

Baichwald VR, Tjian R (1990) Control of c-jun activity by interaction of a cell-specific inhibitor with regulatory domain d: differences between v- and c-jun. Cell 63: 815–825

Baichwald VR, Park A, Tjian R (1991) V-src and EJ ras alleviate repression of c-jun by cell-specific inhibitor. Nature 352: 165–168

Bailey A, Sanchez JD, Rigsby D, Roesel J, Alvarez R, Rodu B, Miller DM (1990) Stimulation of renal and hepatic c-myc and c-Ha-ras expression by unilateral nephrectomy. Oncogene Res 5: 287–293

Bandara LR, Adamczewski JP, Hunt T, La Thangue NB (1991) Cyclin A and the retinoblastoma gene product complex with a common transcription factor. Nature 352: 249–251

Banfic H (1990) Inositol lipid signaling during initiation of compensatory renal growth. Nephron 55: 237–241

Banfic H, Kukolja S (1988) Plasma from uninephrectomized rats stimulates production of inositol triphosphates and inositol tetrakiphosphate in renal cortical slides. Biochem J 255: 671–676

Bickmore WA, Oghene K, Little MH, Seawright A, van Heyningen V, Hastie ND (1992) Modulation of DNA-binding specificity by alternative splicing of the Wilms tumor wt1 gene transcript. Science 257: 235–237

Bishop JM (1983) Cellular oncogenes and retroviruses. Annu Rev Biochem 52: 301–354

Bissonnette RP, Echeverri F, Mahboubi A, Green DR (1992) Apoptotic cell death induced by c-myc is inhibited by bcl-2. Nature 359: 552–556

Blackwood EM, Eisenman RN (1991) Max: a helix-loop-helix zipper protein that forms a sequence-specific DNA-binding complex with myc. Science 251: 1211–1217

Blazer-Yost B, Watanabe M, Haverty TP, Ziyadeh FN (1992) Role of insulin and IGF 1 receptors in proliferation of cultured renal proximal tubule cells. Biochim Biophys Acta 1133: 329–335

Boettinger D (1989) Interaction of oncogenes with differentiation programs. In: Vogt PK (ed) Oncogenes. Selected reviews. Springer, Berlin Heidelberg New York, pp 31–78 (Current topics in microbiology and immunology, vol 147)

Bonventre JV, Sukhatme VP, Bamberger M, Ouellette AJ, Brown D (1991) Localization of the protein product of the immediate early growth response gene, Egr-1, in the kidney after ischemia and reperfusion. Cell Reg 2: 251–260

Boylan MO, Zarbl H (1991) Transformation effector and suppressor genes. J Cell Biochem 46: 199–205

Brenner BM (1985) Nephron adaptation to renal injury or ablation. Am J Physiol 249: F324–F337

Breyer MD, Redha R, Breyer JA (1991) Segmental distribution of epidermal growth factor binding sites in rabbit nephron. Am J Physiol 259: F553–F558

Broek D, Bartlett R, Crawford K, Nurse P (1991) Involvement of p34^{cdc2} in establishing the dependency of S-phase on mitosis. Nature 349: 388–393

Buchkovich K, Duffy LA, Harlow E (1989) The retinoblastoma protein is phoyphorylated during specific phases of the cell cycle. Cell 58: 1097–1105

Cantley LC, Auger KR, Carpenter C, Duckworth B, Graziani A, Kapeller R, Soltoff S (1991) Oncogenes and signal transduction. Cell 64: 281–302

Celano P, Berchtold CM, Kizer DL, Weeraratna A, Nelkin BD, Baylin SB, Casero RA (1992) Characterization of an endogeneous RNA transcript with homology to the antisense strand of the human c-myc gene. J Biol Chem 267: 15092–15096

Cisek LJ, Corden JL (1989) Phosphorylation of RNA polymerase by the murine homologue of the cell-cycle control protein cdc2. Nature 339: 679–684

Chavrier P, Lemaire P, Revelant O, Bravo R, Charnay P (1988) Characterization of a mouse multigene family that encodes zinc-finger structures. Mol Cell Biol 8: 1319–1326

Chiu IM, Reddy EP, Givol D, Robbins KC, Tronick SR, Aaronson SA (1984) Nucleotide sequence analysis identifies the human c-sis proto-oncogene as a structural gene for platelet-derived growth factor. Cell 37: 123–129

Chiu R, Boyle WJ, Meek J, Smeal T, Hunter T, Karin M (1988) The c-fos protein interacts with c-jun/AP-1 to stimulate transcription of AP-1 responsive genes. Cell 54: 541–552

Chou YH, Bischoff JR, Beach D, Goldman RD (1990) Intermediate filament reorganization during mitosis is mediated by p34^{cdc2} phosphorylation of vimentin. Cell 62: 1063–1071

Clarke PR, Karsenti E (1991) Regulation of p34^{cdc2} protein kinase: new insights into protein phosphorylation and the cell cycle. J Cell Sci 100: 409–414

Clearly ML, Smith SD, Sklar J (1986) Cloning and structural analysis of cDNAs for bcl-2 and a hybrid bcl-2/immunoglobulin transcript resulting from the t(14; 18) translocation. Cell 47: 19–28

Coccia EM, Cicala C, Charlesworth A, Ciccarelli C, Ross GB, Philipson L, Sorrentino V (1992) Regulation and expression of a growth-arrest-specific gene (gas5) during growth, differentiation, and development. Mol Cell Biol 12: 3514–3521

Cole MD (1991) Myc meets its max. Cell 65: 715–716

Conover CA, Liu F, Powell D, Rosenfeld RG, Hintz RL (1989) Insulin-like growth factor binding proteins from cultured human fibroblasts. Characterization and hormonal regulation. J Clin Invest 83: 852–859

Cowley BD, Chadwick LJ, Grantham JJ, Calvet JP (1989) Sequential proto-oncogene expression in regenerating kidney following acute renal injury. J Biol Chem 264: 8389–8393

Cowley BD, Chadwick LJ, Grantham JJ, Calvet JP (1991) Elevated proto-oncogene expression in polycystic kidneys of the C57/6J (cpk) mouse. J Am Soc Nephrol 1: 1048–1053

Cross F, Roberts J, Weintraub H (1989) Simple and complex cell cycles. Annu Rev Cell Biol 5: 341–395

Culpepper RM, Schoolwerth AC (1992) Remnant kidney oxygen consumption: hypermetabolism or hyperbole. J Am Soc Nephrol 3: 151–156

Cyert MS, Thorner J (1989) Putting it on and taking it off: phosphoprotein phosphatase involvement in cell cycle regulation. Cell 57: 891–893

Daughaday WH, Rotwein P (1989) Insulin-like growth factors I and II. peptide, messenger ribonucleic acid and gene structures, serum, and tissue concentrations. Endocr Rev 10: 68–91

DeCaprio JA, Ludlow JW, Lynch D, Furukawa Y, Griffn J, Piwnica-Worms H, Huang CM, Livingstone DM (1989) The product of the retinoblastoma susceptibility gene has properties of a cell cycle regulatory element. Cell 58: 1085–1095

Del Sal G, Ruaro ME, Philipson L, Schneider C (1992) The growth-arrest-specific gene, gas1, is involved in growth suppression. Cell 70: 595–607

Devoto SH, Mudryj M, Pines J, Hunter T, Nevins JR (1992) A cyclin a-protein kinase complex possesses sequence-specific DNA binding activity: $p33^{cdk2}$ is a component of the E2F-cyclin A complex. Cell 68: 167–176

Domin J, Rozengurt E (1992) Heterologous densensitization of platelet-derived growth factor-mediated arachidonic release and prostaglandin synthesis. J Biol Chem 267: 15217–15223

Dou QP, Markell PJ, Pardee AB (1992) Thymidine kinase transcription is regulated at G_1/S phase by a complex that contains retinoblastoma-like protein and a cdc2 kinase. Proc Natl Acad Sci USA 89: 3256–3260

Draetta G, Luca F, Westendorf J, Brizuele L, Ruderman J, Beach D (1989) Cdc2 protein kinase is complexed with both cyclin A and B: evidence for proteolytic inactivation of MPF. Cell 56: 829–838

Ellis RE, Yuan J, Horvitz HR (1991) Mechanisms and functions of cell death. Annu Rev Cell Biol 7: 663–698

El Nahas AM, Le Carpentier JE, Bassett AH (1990) Compensatory renal growth: role of growth hormone and insulin-like growth factor-I. Neprol Dial Transplant 5: 123–129

Evan GL, Wyllie AH, Gilbert CS, Littlewood TD, Land H, Brooks M, Waters CM, Penn LZ, Hancock DC (1992) Induction of apoptosis in fibroblasts by c-myc protein. Cell 69: 119–128

Fagin JA, Melmed S (1987) Relative increase in insulin-like growth factor I messenger ribonucleic acid levels in compensatory renal hypertrophy. Endocrinology 120: 718–724

Fesus L, Davies PJA, Piacentini M (1991) Apoptosis: molecular mechanisms in programmed cell death. Eur J Cell Biol 56: 170–177

Fine L, Holley RW, Nasri H, Badie-Dezfooly (1985) BSC-1 growth inhibitor transforms a mitogenic stimulus into a hypertrophic stimulus for renal proximal tubular cells: relationship to Na^+/H^+ antiport activity. Proc Natl Acad Sci USA 82: 6163–6166

Fine L (1986) The biology of renal hypertrophy. Kidney Int 29: 619–634

Flyvberg A, Frystyk J, Marshall SM (1990) Additive increase in kidney insulin-like growth factor I and initial renal enlargement in uninephrectomized diabetic rats. Horm Metab Res 22: 516–520

Flyvberg A, Marshall SM, Frystyk J, Rasch R, Bornfeldt KE, Arnquist H, Jensen PK, Pallesen PK, Pallesen G, Orskov H (1992) Insulin-like growth factor I in initial renal hypertrophy in potassium-depleted rats. Am J Physiol 262: F1032–F1031

Franza BR, Rauscher III FJ, Josephs SF, Curran T (1988) The fos complex and fos-related antigens recognize sequence elements that contain AP-1 binding sites. Science 238: 1150–1153

Freeman RS, Donoghue DJ (1991) Protein kinases and proto-oncogenes: biochemical regulators of the eukaryotic cell cycle. Biochemistry 30: 2293–2302

Galaktionov K, Beach D (1991) Specific activation of cdc25 tyrosine phosphatases by B-type cyclins: evidence for multiple roles of mitotic cyclins. Cell 67: 1181–1194

Gautier J, Norbury C, Lohka M, Nurse P, Maller J (1988) Purified maturation-promoting factor contains the product of a Xenopus homolog of the fission yeast cell cycle control gene $cdc2^+$. Cell 54: 433–439

Gautier J, Matsukawa T, Nurse P, Maller J (1989) Dephosphorylation and activation of *Xenopus* p34^{cdc2} protein kinase during the cell cycle. Nature 339: 626–629

Gentz R, Rauscher III FJ, Abate C, Curran T (1989) Parallel association of fos and jun leucine zippers juxtaposes DNA binding domains. Science 243: 1695–1699

Gibbons GH, Pratt RE, Dzau VJ (1992) Vascular smooth muscle cell hypertrophy vs. hyperplasia. Autocrine transforming growth factor-β expresssion determines growth response to angiotensin II. J Clin Invest 90; 456–461

Gilman MZ, Wilson RN, Weinberg RA (1986) Multiple protein-binding sites in the 5'-flanking region regulate *c-fos* expression. Mol Cell Biol 6: 4305–4316

Gille H, Sharrocks AD, Shaw PE (1992) Phosphorylation of transcription factor p62TCF by MAP kinase stimulates ternary complex formation at *c-fos* promoter. Nature 358: 414–417

Girard F, Strausfeld U, Fernandez A, Lamb NJC (1991) Cyclin A is required for the onset of DNA replication in mammalian fibroblasts. Cell 67: 1169–1179

Glotzer M, Murray AW, Kirschner MW (1991) Cyclin is degraded by the ubiquitin pathway. nature 349: 132–139

Gobe GC, Axelsen RA (1987) Genesis of renal tubular atrophy in experimental hydronephrosis in the rat. Role of apoptosis. Lab Invest 56: 273–281

Gobe GC, Axelsen RA, Searle JW (1990) Cellular events in experimental unilateral ischemic renal atrophy and in regeneration after contralateral nephrectomy. Lab Invest 63: 770–779

Goodyer PR, Kachera Z, Bell C, Rozen R (1988) Renal tubular cells are potential targets of epidermal growth factor. Am J Physiol 255: F1191–F1196

Golchini K, Norman J, Bohman R, Kurtz I (1989) Induction of hypertrophy in cultured proximal tubule cells by extracellular NH$_4$Cl. J Clin invest 84: 1767–1779

Gould KL, Nurse P (1989) Tyrosine phosphorylation of the fission yeast cdc2+ protein kinase regulates entry into mitosis. Nature 342: 39–44

Graziani A, Gramaglia D, Cantley LC, Comoglio (1991) The tyrosine-phosphorylated hepatocyte growth factors/scatter factor receptor associates with phosphatidylinositol 3-kinase. J Biol Chem 266: 22087–22090

Haber DA, Sohn RL, Buckler AJ, Pelletier J, Call Km, Housman DE (1991) Alternative splicing and genomic structure of the Wilms tumor gene WT1. Proc Natl Acad Sci USA 88: 9618–9622

Hammerman MR, Rogers S (1987) Distribution of IGF receptors in the plasma membrane of proximal tubular cells. Am J Physiol 253: F841–F847

Harding MA, Gattone II VH, Grantham JJ, Calvet JP (1992) Localization of overexpressed *c-myc* mRNA in polycystic kidneys of the *cpk* mouse. Kidney Int 41: 317–325

Harris H, Miller OJ, Klein G, Worst P, Tacibana T (1969) Suppression of malignancy by cell fusion. Nature 223: 363–368

Harris RH, Hise MK, Best CF (1983) Renotropic factors in urine. Kidney Int 23: 616–623

Haverty TP, Kelly CJ, Hines WH, Amenta PS, Watanabe M, Harper RA, Kefalides NA, Neilson EG (1988) Characterization of a renal tubular epithelial cell line which secretes the autologous target antigen of autoimmune experimental interstitial nephritis. J Cell Biol 107: 1359–1368

Herschman HR (1991) Primary response genes induced by growth factors and tumor promoters. Annu Rev Biochem 60: 281–319

Hipskind RA, Nordheim A (1991) In vitro transcriptional analysis of the human *c-fos* proto-oncogene. J Biol Chem 266: 19572–19582

Hofbauer R, Denhardt DT (1991) Cell cycle-regulated and proliferation stimulus-responsive genes. Crit Rev Eukaryotic Gene Exp 1: 247–300

Holley RW, Böhlen P, Fava R, Baldwin JH, Kleeman G, Armour R (1980) Purification of kidney epithelial cell growth inhibitors. Proc Natl Acad Sci USA 77: 5989–5992

Humes HD, Cieslinski DA, Coimbra TM, Messana JM, Galvao C (1989) Epidermal growth factor enhances tubule cell regeneration and repair and accelerates the recovery of renal function in postischemic acute renal failure. J Clin Invest 84: 1757–1761

Humes HD, Beals TF, Cieslinski DA, Sanchez IO, Page TP (1991) Effects of transforming growth factor-b, transforming growth factor-a, and other growth factors on renal proximal tubule cells. Lab Invest 64: 538–545

Igawa T, Kanda S, Kanetake H, Saitoh Y, Ichihara A, Tomita Y, Nakamura T (1991) Hepatocyte growth factor is a potent mitogen for cultured rabbit renal tubular epithelial cells. Biochem Biophys Res Commun 174: 831–838

Iguchi-Ariga SM, Okazaki T, Itani T, Ogata M, Sato Y, Ariga H (1988) An initiation site of DNA replication with transcriptional enhancer activity present upstream of the *c-myc* gene. EMBO J 7: 3135–3142

Irvine RF (1991) Inositol tetrakisphosphate as a second messenger: confusions, contradictions, and a potential resolution. Bioessays 13: 419–428

Irvine RF (1992) Inositol phosphates and Ca^{2+} entry: toward a proliferation or simplification. FASEB J 6: 3085–3091

Ishibashi K, Sasaki S, Sakamoto H, Nakamura Y, Hata T, Nakamura T, Marumo F (1992) Hepatocyte growth factor is a paracrine factor for renal epithelial cells: stimulation of DNA synthesis and Na, K-ATPase activity. Biochem Biophys Res Commun 182: 960–965

Itoh N, Yonehara S, Ishii A, Yonehara M, Mizushima SI, Sameshima, Hase A, Seto Y, Nagata S (1991) The polypeptide encoded by the cDNA for human cell surface antigen *fas* can mediate apoptosis. Cell 66: 233–243

Kakkis E, Riggs KJ, Gillespie W, Calame K (1989) A transcriptional repressor of *c-myc*. Nature 339: 718–721

Kanetake H, Yamamoto N (1981) Studies on the mechanisms of compensatory renal hypertrophy and hyperplasia in a nephrectomized animal model. I. Evidence for a renotropic growth-stimulating factor in uninephrectomized rabbit sera using tissue culture. J Urol 18: 326–330

Karin M (1992) Signal transduction from cell surface to nucleus in development and disease. FASEB J 6: 2581–2590

Kartha S, Sukhatme VS, Toback FG (1987) ADP activates proto-oncogene expression in renal epithelial cells. Am J Physiol 252: F1175–F1179

Kato GJ, Dang CV (1992) Function of the *c-myc* oncoprotein. FASEB J 6: 3065–3072

Kim SJ, Wagner S, Liu F, O'Reilly MA, Robbins PD, Green MR (1992) Retinoblastoma gene product activates expression of the human TGF-β_2 gene through transcription factor ATF-2. Nature 358: 331–333

Koff A, Giordano A, Desai D, Yamashita K, Harper JW, Elledge S, Nishimoto T, Morgan DO, Franza BR, Roberts JM (1992) Formation and activation of a cylin E-cdk2 complex during the G_1 phase of the human cell cycle. Science 247: 1689–1694

Kujubu DA, Fine LG (1989) Physiology and cell biology update: polypeptide growth factors and their relation to renal disease. Am J Kidney Dis 14: 61–73

Kujubu DA; Norman JT, Herschman HR, Fine LG (1991) Primary response gene expression in renal hypertrophy and hyperplasia: evidence for different growth initiation processes. Am J Physiol 260: F823–F827

Kuncio GS, Neilson EG, Haverty T (1991) Mechanisms of tubulointerstitial fibrosis. Kidney Int 39: 550–556

Laiho M, DeCapiro JA, Ludlow JW, Livingston DM, Massague J (1990) Growth inhibition by TGF-β linked to suppression of retinoblastoma protein phosphorylation. Cell 62: 175–182

Lajara R, Rotwein P, Bortz JD, Hansen VA, Sadow JL, Betts CR, Rogers SA, Hammerman MR (1989) Dual regulation of insulin-like growth factor I expression during renal hypertrophy. Am J Physiol 257: F252–F261

Lakshmanarao SS, Toole-Smith WE, Fattaey HK, Leach RJ, Johnson TC (1991) Identification of a cell surface component of Swiss 3T3 cells associated with an inhibition of cell division. Exp Cell Res 195: 412–415

Lee WH, Bookstein R, Hong F, Young LJ, Shew JY, Lee EYH (1987a) Human retinoblastoma susceptibility gene: cloning, identification, and sequence. Science 235: 1394–1399

Lee WH, Shew JY, Hong FD, Sery TW, Donoso LA, Young LJ, Bookstein R, Lee EYH (1987b) The retinoblastoma susceptibility gene encodes a nuclear phosphoprotein associated with DNA binding activity. Nature 329: 642–645

Lemley KV, Kriz W (1991) Anatomy of the renal interstitium. Kidney Int 39: 370–381

Levine AJ, Momand J, Finlay CA (1991) The p53 tumor suppressor gene. Nature 351: 453–455

Lewin B (1990) Driving the cell cycle: M-phase kinase, its partners, and substrates. Cell 61: 743–752

Lieske JC, Walsh-Reitz MW, Toback FG (1992) Calcium oxalate monohydrate crystals are endocytosed by renal epithelial cells and induce proliferation. Am J Physiol 262: F622–F630

Lin BTY, Gruenwald S, Morla AO, Lee WH, Wang JYJ (1991) Retinoblastoma cancer-suppressor gene product is a substrate of the cell cycle regulator cdc2 kinase. EMBO J 10: 857–864

Logan JL, Benson B (1990) Serum renotropic factor stimulates prostaglandin synthesis in primary cultures of rabbit kidney cells. Prostaglandins Leukot Essent Fatty Acids 41: 183–186

Logan JL, Benson B (1992) Studies on serum renotropic activity after uninephrectomy in rabbits. Nephron 60: 466–470

Lowndes NF, McInerny CJ, Johnson AL, Fantes PA, Johnston LH (1992) Control of DNA synthesis genes in fission yeast by the cell-cycle gene cdc10$^+$. Nature 355: 449–453

Lüscher B, Eisenman RN (1990) New light on *myc* and *myb*. Part I. *Myc*. Genes Dev 4: 2025–2035

Macara IG (1989) Oncogenes and cellular signal transduction. Physiol Rev 69: 797–820

Madden SL, Cook DM, Morris JF, Gashler A, Sukhatme VP, Rauscher FJ III (1991) Transcriptional repression mediated by the WT1 Wilms tumor gene product. Science 253: 1550–1553

Malt R (1983) Humoral factors in regulation of compensatory renal hypertrophy. Kidney Int 23: 611–615

Maller JL (1990) Xenopus oocytes and the biochemistry of cell division. Biochemistry 29: 3157–3166

Manfioletti G, Ruaro ME, Del Sal G, Philipson L, Schneider C (1990) A growth-arrest-specific (*gas*) gene codes for a membrane protein. Mol Cell Biol 10: 2924–2930

Manzano F, Esbrit P, Garcia-Ocana A, Garcia-Canero R, Jimenez-Clavero MA (1989) Partial purification and characterisation of a renal growth factor from plasma of uninephrectomized rats. Nephrol Dial Transplant 4: 334–338

Margolis B (1992) Proteins with SH2 domains: transducers in the tyrosine kinase signaling pathway. Cell Growth Differ 3: 73–80

Marshall CJ (1991) Tumor-suppressor genes. Cell 64: 313–326

Marshall SM, Flyvbjerg A, Frkiaer J, Orskov H (1991) Insulin-like growth factor I and renal growth following ureteral obstruction in the rat. Nephron 58: 219–224

McIntosh JR, Koonce MP (1989) Mitosis. Science 246: 622–628

Mercer WE, Shields MT, Lin D, Appella E, Ullrich SJ (1991) Growth suppression induced by wild-type p53 protein is accompanied by selective down-regulation of proliferating-cell nuclear antigen expression. Proc Natl Acad Sci USA 88: 1958–1962

Milanes Cl, Pernalete N, Starosta R, Perez-Gonzalez M, Paz-Martinez V, Bellorin-Font E (1989) Altered response of adenylate cyclase to parathyroid hormone during compensatory renal growth. Kidney Int 26: 802–809

Milburn MV, Tong L, DeVos A, Brünger A, Yamaizumi Z, Nishimura S, Kim SH (1990) Molecular switch for signal transduction: structural differences between active and inactive forms of proto-oncogenic *ras* proteins. Science 247: 939–945

Miller RT (1991) Transmembrane signalling through G proteins. Kidneys Int 39: 421–429

Miller SB, Rogers SA, Estes CE, Hammerman MR (1992) Increased distal nephron EGF content and altered distribution of peptide in compensatory renal hypertrophy. Am J Physiol 262: F1032–F1038

Mittnacht S, Weinberg RA (1991) G$_1$/S phosphorylation of the retinoblastoma protein is associated with an altered affinity for the nuclear compartment. Cell 65: 381–393

Momand J, Zambetti GP, Olson DC, George D, Levine AJ (1992) The *mdm-2* oncogene product forms a complex with the p53 protein and inhibits p53-mediated transactivation. Cell 69: 1237–1245

Moria AO, Draetta G, Beach D, Wang JYJ (1989) Reversible tyrosine phosphorylation of cdc2: dephosphorylation accompanies activation during entry into mitosis. Cell 58: 193–203

Moses HL, Yang EY, Pletenpol JA (1990) TGF-β stimulation and inhibition of cell proliferation: new mechanistic insights. Cell 63: 245–247

Muller WJ, Lee FS, Dickson C, Peters G, Pattengale P, Leder P (1990) The *int*-2 gene product acts as an epithelial growth factor in transgenic mice. EMBO J 9: 907–913

Mulroney SE, Haramati A, Roberts CT, LeRoith D (1991) Renal IGF-I mRNA levels are enhanced following unilateral nephrecomy in immature but not adult rats. Endocrinology 128: 2660–2662

Mulroney SE, Haramati A, Werner H, Bondy C, Roberts CT, LeRoith D (1992a) Altered expression of insulin-like growth factor-I (IGF-I) and IGF receptor genes after unilateral nephrectomy in immature rats. Endocrinology 130: 249–256

Mulroney SE, Lumpkin MD, Roberts CT, LeRoith D, Haramati A (1992b) Effect of a growth hormone-releasing factor antagonist on compensatory renal growth, insulin-like growth factor-I (IGF-I), and IGF-I receptor gene expression after unilateral nephrectomy in immature rats. Endocrinology 130: 2697–2702

Murray AW (1989) The cell cycle as a cdc2 cycle. Nature 342: 14–15

Nagaike M, Hirao S, Tajima H, Noji S, Taniguchi S, Matsumoto K, Nakamura T (1991) Renotropic functions of hepatocyte growth factor in renal regeneration after unilateral nephrectomy. J Biol Chem 266: 22781–22784

Nakabeppu Y, Nathans D (1989) The basic region of *fos* mediates specific DNA binding. EMBO J 8: 3833–3841

Nakamura H, Nemenoff RA, Gronich JH, Bonventre JV (1991) Subcellular characteristics of phospholipase A2 activity in the rat kidney. Enhanced cytosolic, mitochondrial, and microsomal phospholipase A2 enzymatic activity after renal ischemia and reperfusion. J Clin Invest 87: 1810–1818

Nakamura T, Ebihara I, Tomino Y, Koide H, Kikuchi K, Koiso K (1992) Gene expression of growth-related proteins and ECM constituents in response to unilateral nephrectomy. Am J Physiol 262: F389–F396

Nath KA, Hostetter MK, Hostetter TH (1985) Pathophysiology of chronic tubulo-interstitial disease in rats. Interactions of dietary acid load, ammonia and complement C3. J Clin Invest 76: 667–675

Nath KA (1992) Tubulointerstitial changes as a major determinant in the progression of renal damage. Am J Kidney Dis 20: 1–17

Neilson EG (1989) Pathogenesis and therapy of interstitial nephritis. Kidney Int 35: 1257–1270

Nepveu A, Levine RA, Campisi J, Greenberg ME, Ziff EB, Marcu KB (1987) Alternative modes of *c-myc* regulation in growth factor-stimulated and differentiating cells. Oncogene 1: 243–250

Nomata K, Igarashi H, Kanetake H, Miyamoto T, Saito Y (1990) Expression of *ras* gene family result of compensatory renal growth in mice. Urol Res 18: 251–254

Norman JT, Bohman RE, Fischmann G, Bowen JW, McDonough A, Slamon D, Fine LG (1988) Patterns of mRNA expression during early cell growth differ in kidney epithelial cells destined to undergo compensatory hypertrophy versus regenerative hyperplasia. Proc Natl Acad Sci USA 85: 6768–6772

Norman J, Tasu YK, Bacay A, Fine LG (1990) Epidermal growth factor accelerates functional recovery from ischaemic acute tubular necrosis in the rat: role of epidermal growth factor receptor. Clin Sci 78: 445–450

Nuell MJ, Stewart DA, Walker L, Friedman V, Wood CM, Owens GA, Smith JR, Schneider EL, Dell' Orco R, Lumpkin CK, Danner DB, McClung JK (1991) Prohibitin, an evolutionarily conserved intracellular protein that blocks DNA synthesis in normal fibroblasts and HeLa cells. Mol Cell Biol 11: 1372–1381

Nurse P (1990) Universal control mechanism regulating onset of M-phase. Nature 344: 503–507

Ottaviano Y, Gerace L (1985) Phosphorylation of the nuclear lamins during interphase and mitosis. J Biol Chem 260: 624–632

Ouellette AJ, Malt RA, Sukhatme VP, Bonventre JV (1990) Expression of two "immediate early" genes, *Egr-1* and *c-fos*, in response to renal ischemia and during compensatory renal hypertrophy in mice. J Clin Invest 85: 766–771

Pardee AB (1989) G_1 events and regulation of cell proliferation. Science 246: 603–608

Parker LL, Atherton-Fessler S, Piwnica-Worms H (1992) p107[wee1] is a dual-specificity kinase that phosphorylates p34[cdc2] on tyrosine 15. Proc Natl Acad Sci USA 89: 2917–2921

Pelech SL, Sanghera JS (1992) MAP kinases: charting the regulatory pathways. Science 257: 1355–1356

Pfeilschifter J (1989a) Cross-talk between transmembrane signalling systems: a prerequisite for the delicate regulation of glomerular haemodynamics by mesangial cells. Eur J Clin Invest 19: 347–361

Pfeilschifter J (1989b) Cellular signalling in the kidney: the role of inositol lipids. Renal Physiol Biochem 12: 1–31

Phillipson L, Sorrentino V (1991) From growth arrest to growth suppression. J Cell Biochem 46: 95–101

Pines J, Hunter T (1989) Isolation of a human cyclin cDNA: evidence for cyclin mRNA and protein regulation in the cell cycle and for interaction with p34[cdc2]. Cell 58: 833–836

Pulverer BJ, Kyriakis JM, Avruch J, Nikolakaki E, Woodgett JR (1991) Phosphorylation of *c-jun* mediated by MAP kinases. Nature 353: 671–674

Rankin CA, Grantham JJ, Calvet JP (1992) *c-fos* expression is hypersensitive to serum stimulation in cultured cystic kidney cells from the C57BL/6j-*cpk* mouse. J Cell Physiol 152: 578–586

Ransone LJ, Verma IM (1989) Association of nuclear oncoproteins *fos* and *jun*. Curr Opin Cell Biol 1: 536–540

Rauscher FJ III, Morris JF, Tournay OE, Cook DM, Curran T (1990) Binding of the Wilms' tumor locus zinc-finger protein to the *EGR-1* consensus sequence. Science 250: 1259–1262

Rayer PFO (1837–1841) Traite des maladies des reins et des alterations secretion urinaire. 3 volumes and atlas. Balliere, Paris

Reed SI (1991) G_1-specific cyclins: in search of an S-phase-promoting factor. TIG 7: 95–99

Ritz E, Zeier M, Lundin P (1989) French and German nephrologists in the mid-19th century. Am J Physiol 9: 167–172

Rocco MV, Chen Y, Goldfarb S, Ziyadeh FN (1992) Elevated glucose levels stimulate transforming growth factor-beta gene expression and bioactivity in murine proximal tubule cell culture. Kidney Int 41: 107–114

Rogers SA, Miller SB, Hammerman MR (1991) Insulin-like growth factor I gene expression in isolated rat renal collecting duct is stimulated by epidermal growth factor. J Clin Invest 87: 347–351

Rosenberg ME, Hostetter TH (1990) Effect of angiotensin II (A II) on early growth genes in the kidney. J Am Soc Nephrol 1: 426 (abstract)

Rosenberg ME, Paller MS (1991) Differential gene expression in the recovery from ischemic renal injury. Kidney Int 39: 1156–1161

Rozengurt E, Murray M, Zachary I, Collins M (1987) Protein kinase C activation enhances cAMP accumulation in Swiss 3T3 cells: inhibition by pertussis toxin. Proc Natl Acad Sci USA 84: 2282–2286

Russell P, Nurse P (1986) Cdc25$^+$ functions as an inducer in the mitotic control of fission yeast. Cell 45: 145–153

Russell P, Nurse P (1987) Negative regulation of mitosis by wee1$^+$, a gene encoding a protein kinase homolog. Cell 49: 559–567

Rysek RP, Hirai SI, Bravo R (1988) Transcriptional activation of c-jun during the G_0/G_1 transition in mouse fibroblasts. Nature 334: 535–537

Safirstein R, Price PM, Saggi SJ, Harris RC (1990) Changes in gene expression after temporary renal ischemia. Kidney Int 37: 1515–1521

Salido EC, Yen PH, Shapiro LJ, Fisher DA, Barajas L (1989) In situ hybridization of pre-pro-epidermal growth factor mRNA in the mouse kidney. Am J Physiol 256: F632–F638

Salihagic A, Mackovic H, Banfic H, Sabolic I (1988) Short-term and long-term stimulation of Na^+-H^+ exchange in cortical brush-border membranes during compensatory growth of the kidney. Eur J Physiol 413: 190–196

Sassone-Corsi P, Verma IM (1987) Modulation of c-fos gene transcription by negative and positive cellular factors. Nature 326: 507–510

Sassone-Corsi P, Sisson JC, Verma IM (1988) Transcriptional autoregulation of the proto-oncogene fos. Nature 334: 314–319

Sassone-Corsi P, Visvader J, Ferland L, Mellon PL, Verma IM (1988b) Induction of proto-oncogene fos transcription through the adenylate cyclase pathway: characterization of a cAMP-responsive element. Genes Dev 2: 1529–1538

Sawczuk IS, Olsson CA, Buttyan R, Nguyen-Huu MC, Zimmerman KA, Alt FW, Zakeri Z, Wolgemuth D, Reitelman C (1988) Gene expression in renal growth and regrowth. J Urol 140: 1145–1148

Sawczuk IS, Hoke G, Olsson CA, Connor J, Buttyan R (1989) Gene expression in response to acute unilateral ureteral obstruction. Kidney Int 35: 1315–1319

Sawczuk IS, Olsson CA, Hoke G, Buttyan R (1990) Immediate induction of c-fos and c-myc transcripts following unilateral nephrectomy. Nephron 55: 193–195

Schlondorff D, Weber H (1978) Evidence for altered cyclic nucleotide metabolism during compensatory renal hypertrophy and neonatal kidney growth. Yale J Biol Med 51: 387–392

Schneider C, King RM, Philipson L (1988) Genes specifically expressed at growth arrest of mammalian cells. Cell 54: 787–793

Schrier RW, Harris DCH, Chan L, Shapiro JI, Caramelo C (1988) Tubular hypermetabolism as a factor in the progression of chronic renal failure. Am J Kidney Dis 12: 242–249

Schumer M, Colombel MC, Sawczuk IS, Gobe G, Connor J, O'Toole KM, Olsson CA, Wise GJ, Buttyan R (1992) Morphologic, biochemical, and molecular evidence of apoptosis during the reperfusion phase after brief periods of renal ischemia. Am J Pathol 140: 831–838

Shirodkar S, Ewen M, DeCaprio JA, Morgan J, Livingston DM, Chittenden T (1992) The transcription factor E2F interacts with the retinoblastoma product and a p107-cyclin A complex in a cell cycle-regulated manner. Cell 68: 157–166

Smith R, Peters G, Dickson C (1988) Multiple RNAs expressed from the int-2 gene in mouse embryonal carcinoma cell lines encode a protein with homology to fibroblast growth factors. EMBO J 7: 1013–1022

Sporn MB, Roberts AB, Wakefield LM, Assoian RK (1986) Transforming growth factor-β: biological function and chemical structure. Science 233: 532–534

Stiles AD, Sosenko IR, D'ercole AJ, Smith BT (1985) Relation of kidney tissue somatomedin-C/insulin-like growth factor I to postnephrectomy renal growth in the rat. Endocrinology 117: 2397–2401

Stryer L, Bourne HR (1986) G proteins: a family of signal transducers. Annu Rev Cell Biol 2: 391–419

Studzinski GP, Brelvi ZS, Feldman SC, Watt RA (1986) Participation of *c-myc* protein in DNA synthesis of human cells. Science 234: 467–470

Stürzbecher HW, Maimets T, Chumakov P, Brain R, Addison C, Simanis V, Rudge K, Philp R, Grimaldi M, Court W, Jenkins JR (1990) p53 interacts with p34^{cdc2} in mammalian cells: implications for cell cycle control and oncogenesis. Oncogene 5: 795–801

Sukhatme VP, Kartha S, Toback GF, Taub R, Hoover RG, Tsai-Morris CH (1987) A novel early growth response gene rapidly induced by fibroblast, epithelial cell and lymphocyte mitogens. Oncogene Res 1: 343–355

Sukhatme VP, Cao X, Chang LC, Tsai-Morris CH, Stamenkovich D, Ferreira PCP, Cohen DR, Edwards SA, Shows TB, Curran T, Le Beau MM, Adamson ED (1988) A zinc-finger-encoding gene co-regulated with *c-fos* during growth and differentiation, and after cellular depolarization. Cell 53: 37–43

Sukhatme VP (1990) Early transcriptional events in cell growth: the *egr* family. J Am Soc Nephrol 1: 859–866

Taylor SS (1989) cAMP-dependent protein kinase. J Biol Chem 262: 8443–8446

Tisher CC, Madsen KM (1988) Anatomy of the renal interstitium. In: Nephrology, vol 1. Proceedings of the 10th international congress on nephrology. Bailliere Tindall, London, pp 587–598

Toback FG, Walsh-Reitz MM; Mendley SR, Kartha S (1990) Kidney epithelial cells release growth factors in response to extracellular signals. Pediatr Nephrol 4: 363–371

Toback FG (1992) Regeneration after acute tubular necrosis. Kidney Int 41: 226–246

Travali S, Koniecki J, petralia S, Baserga R (1990) Oncogenes in growth and development. FASEB J 4: 3209–3214

Tsai-Morris CH, Cao X, Sukhatme VP (1988) 5' Flanking sequence and genomic structure of *Egr-1*, a murine mitogen-inducible, zinc-finger-encoding gene. Nucleic Acid Res 16: 8835–8846

Trudel M, D'Agati V, Constantini F (1989) The *c-myc* oncogene induces kidney cysts in transgenic mice. Kidney Int 35: 364 (abstract)

Turner R, Tjian R (1989) Leucine repeats and an adjacent DNA-binding domain mediate the formation of functional *c-fos-c-jun* heterodimers. Science 243: 1689–1694

Uchida S, Tsutsumi O, Hise MK Oka T (1988) Role of epidermal growth factor in compensatory renal growth. Kidney Int 33: 387 (abstract)

Ullrich A, Schlesinger J (1990) Signal transduction by receptors with tyrosine kinase activity. Cell 61: 203–212

Ullrich SJ, Anderson CW, Mercer WE, Appella E (1992) The p53 tumor-suppressor protein, a modulator of cell proliferation. J Biol Chem 267: 15259–15262

Vogt PK, Tjian R (1988) *Jun*: a transcriptional regulator turned oncogenic. Oncogene 3: 3–7

Ward GE, Kirschner MW (1990) Identification of cell cycle-regulated phosphorylation sites on nuclear lamin C. Cell 61: 561–577

Weintraub SJ, Prater CA, Dean DC (1992) Retinoblastoma protein switches the E2F site from positive to negative element. Nature 358: 259–261

Wells A, Mallucci L (1991) Identification of an autocrine negative growth factor: mouse β-galactoside-binding protein is a cytostatic factor and cell growth regulator. Cell 64: 91–97

Wesson LG (1989) Compensatory growth and other growth responses of the kidney. Nephron 51: 149–184

Wolf G (1992) History of nephrology. Changing concepts of compensatory renal growth: from humoral pathology to molecular biology. Am J Nephrol 12: 369–373

Wolf G, Neilson EG (1990a) Angiotensin II induces cellular hypertrophy in cultured murine proximal tubular cells. Am J Physiol 259: F768–F777

Wolf G, Neilson EG (1990b) Angiotensin II (A II)-induced genes in murine proximal tubule cells: isolation and preliminary characterization. J Am Soc Nephrol 1: 429 (abstract)

Wolf G, Neilson EG (1991) Molecular mechanisms of tubulointerstitial hypertrophy and hyperplasia. Kidney Int 39: 401–420

Wolf G, Neilson EG (1993) Angiotensin II as a hypertrophogenic cytokine for proximal tubular cells. Kidney Int 43 [Suppl. 39]: S100–S107

Wolf G, Killen PD, Neilson EG (1991a) Intracellular signalling of transcription and secretion of type-IV collagen after angiotensin II-induced cellular hypertrophy in cultured proximal tubular cells. Cell Reg 2: 219–227

Wolf G, Heeger PS, Neilson EG (1991b) Proto-oncogenes as targets of hormone and growth-factor actions in the kidney. In: Goldfarb S, Ziyadeh FN (eds) Hormones, autacoids, and the kidney. Contemporary issues in nephrology. Churchill Livingstone, New York, pp 11–139

Wolg G, Neilson EG, Goldfarb S, Ziyadeh FN (1991c) The influence of glucose concentration on angiotensin II-induced hypertrophy of proximal tubular cells in culture. Biochem Biophys Res Commun 176: 902–909

Wolf G, Kuncio GS, Sun MJ, Neilson EG (1991d) Expression of homeobox genes in a proximal tubular cell line derived from adult mice. Kidney Int 39: 1027–1033

Yin Y, Tainsky MA, Bischoff FZ, Strong LC, Wahl GM (1992) Wild-type p53 restores cell cycle control and inhibits amplification in cells with mutant p53 alleles. Cell 70: 937–948

Ziegler A, Knesel J, Fabbro D, Nagamine Y (1991) Protein kinase C down-regulation enhances cAMP-mediated induction of urokinase-type plasminogen activator mRNA in LLC-PK$_1$ cells. J Biol Chem 266: 21067–21074

Morphometric Assessment
of Tubulointerstitial Damage in Renal Disease

R. Sinniah and T.N. Khan

1 General Introduction

In renal pathology glomerular changes have been studied in greater detail than the tubulointerstitium. Interest in the glomeruli was due to their function as the filtration barrier, and also they showed a variety of specific histological and immunohistochemical changes in various glomerulonephritides. In contrast, the tubulointerstitial changes in the majority of primary tubulointerstitial nephritides and secondary to glomerular diseases are strikingly similar. Therefore the tubulointerstitial component of the kidney in renal disease received little attention.

Damage to the tubulointerstitium in various glomerulonephritides became important when the glomerular filtration rate (GFR) was shown to be related to tubulointerstitial damage (TID). Early works on the correlation of tubulointerstitial structure to function highlighted the importance of TID in determining the GFR (Muehrcke et al. 1957; Rosenbaum et al. 1967; Risdon et al. 1968; Schainuck et al. 1970). These studies were based on quasi-quantitative analyses, and were either based on "persisting glomerulonephritides" (Rosenbaum et al. 1967) or unselective kidney tissue (Schainuck et al. 1970). However, convincing data on the significance of TID in renal function emerged only when morphometric methods were employed to quantitate renal injury.

A great variety of aetiological agents and several pathogenetic mechanisms lead to tubulointerstitial injury (CHURG et al. 1985). Tubulointerstitial nephritis can be primary damage or a component of various glomerulonephritides. This chapter reviews only the changes that occur in the tubulointerstitial component of the kidney, mainly in various primary and secondary glomerulonephritides. The relative contribution of glomerular structural changes in the impairment of renal functions is not discussed.

2 Morphometry in the Study of Renal Disease

The significance and correlation of structural changes to renal function is gaining importance. Renal pathologists can no longer just report the morphological changes, as structural damage leads to functional impairment which are facets of the same biological process. Morphological data has to be quantified to identify the functional correlates and to permit an understanding of its pathological significance. The obvious limitation in morphometry is that it cannot be used to study diseases which have unilateral or localised involvement of the kidney. Glomerular diseases and tubulointerstitial nephritides with bilateral involvement of kidneys lend themselves to morphometric analyses even if the involvement is focal.

2.1 Morphometric Methods Used in Renal Pathology

Several methods are available for estimating the relative volume of the various tissue components in renal tissue sections. These methods are based on the belief that the mean relative area of a component in a series of random sections through a tissue is a consistent estimate of its relative volume in the whole tissue. Keeping in view the complex biology of the disease process, this is often not true. The second problem is one of measuring area in a section, which can be done by the simple point-counting method (HALLY 1964). In morphometry it is desirable to know (a) how many points must be counted to achieve any given degree of accuracy; and (b) whether it is necessary to examine every slice of the organ tissues to obtain an accurate measurement of the quantity of damage in a disease condition. The larger the volume proportion to be estimated, the fewer is the number of points that need to be counted in order to obtain a given standard error of the estimate. Ideally, the whole organ should be sampled, by examining series of slices of equal thickness, in order to obtain reliable results (ANDERSON and DUNNIL 1965). Due to the limitations involved in the study of human renal tissues where only a small biopsy is available, various methods have been used to obtain the best possible estimates.

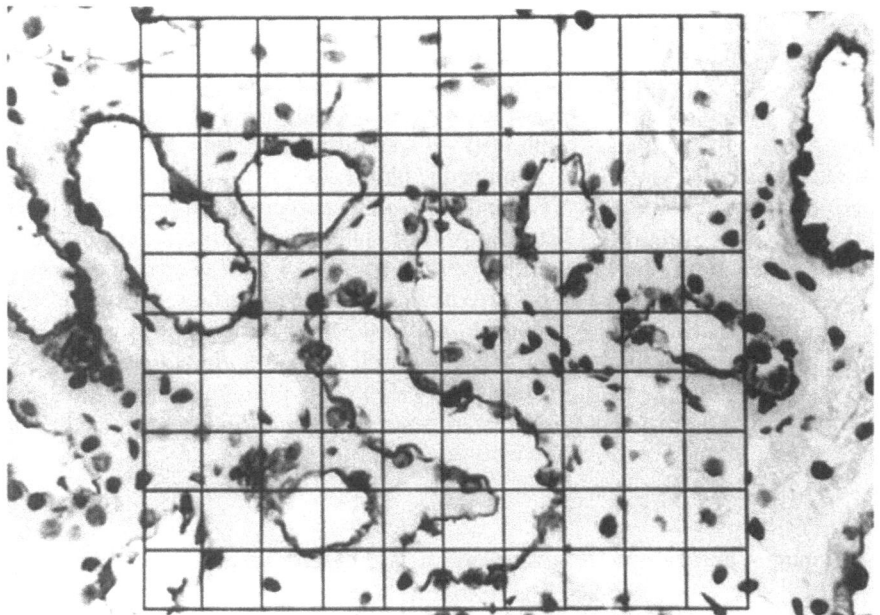

Fig. 1. Renal biopsy stained with Arachis hypogaea (PNA) lectin. The distal tubules are clearly outlined. This is overlaid by a square-lattice grid used in morphometric methods. Of the 77 points, 37 (48.05%) fall on distal tubules, 25 (32.47%) fall on the proximal tubules which are unstained, and 15 (19.48%) on the interstitium. × 345

2.1.1 Technique of Point Counting

Commonly an eyepiece graticule with a regular array of crosses or a square lattice is used (BENNETT et al. 1982; HOWIE et al. 1990; KHAN and SINNIAH 1993a). The centres of intersection of the lines or crosses are used as points for counting (Fig. 1). Alternatively, a projection microscope can be used with a point-lattice of 1 cm distance (MACKENSEN-HAEN et al. 1988). Five to nine visual fields per biopsy are counted to estimate the cortical interstitium (percentage interstitial volume). Glomeruli and large blood vessels are neglected (BENNETT et al. 1982; MACKENSEN-HAEN et al. 1988). The total surface area, epithelial surface area, and luminal surface area of 40 to 100 cross-sectioned tubules (BOHLE et al. 1987; MACKENSEN-HAEN et al. 1988) or percentage tubular volume per biopsy are calculated (KHAN and SINNIAH1993a).

2.1.2 Morphometric Method Based on Summation Average Graph

The number of fields to be counted is determined by a preliminary study of the cortex of normal kidneys with no evidence of renal damage or immune deposits on light and immunofluorescence microscopy. An eyepiece graticule is superimposed randomly and 30 fields are analyzed in each case, which yielded a count of 3630 points with a square lattice containing 121 points. For the study of TID the points are put into one of the following three categories: (1) those falling on proximal tubules; (2) those falling on distal tubules; (3) those falling on the interstitium. Points falling on glomeruli, blood vessels and cortical collecting ducts are recorded separately. From these counts, percentage of points falling on each of the above anatomical structures is calculated and referred to as *proximal tubular percentage, distal tubular percentage* and *interstitial percentage*. In each case, the cumulative means of proximal tubular percentage, distal tubular percentage and interstitial percentage are plotted after each field until the means remained steady on summation average graph (AHERNE and DUNNILL 1982a; HOWIE et al. 1990; KHAN and SINNIAH 1993a). The summation average graph method necessitates a large number of points to be counted and considerably lowers the standard error of the estimate.

2.2 Immuno- and Lectin-Histochemistry in Aid of Morphometry

In cases of TID it is not possible to clearly identify the anatomical segments of the tubules in the absence of a marker stain. Consecutive serial sections can be stained with peanutagglutin (PNA) and in phytohaemagglutinin-E (PHA-E) lectins using double labelling (Fig. 2). PNA lectin is used as a staining marker because of its usefulness in staining both the distal tubules and cortical collecting ducts (HOLTHOFER et al. 1981; KHAN and SINNIAH 1993a). It is also economical, less time consuming and stains even the severely atrophic tubules. The identification of the distal tubules can be confirmed by serial sections stained with Tamm-Horsfall glycoprotein. The proximal tubules are not stained by PNA lectin but by PHA-E lectin, which is specific for proximal tubules (TRUONG et al. 1988; KHAN and SINNIAH 1993b).

3 Regression and Correlation Analysis

Once the tubular damage has been quantified with morphometric techniques, it is important to assess this damage in terms of a functional parameter of renal function. The creatinine concentration (mg/100 ml) and clearances of creatinine, inulin and PAH (ml/min per $1.73\,m^2$), the most commonly used functional parameters, are recorded as near as possible to the day of obtaining the renal biopsies. Apart from the excretory function of the glomeruli, an important function of the kidney is its ability to concentrate urine, i.e. raise urine osmolality.

Relationships between morphometric findings are quantified by the product-moment correlation coefficients (ARMITAGE and BERRY 1987). Poly-

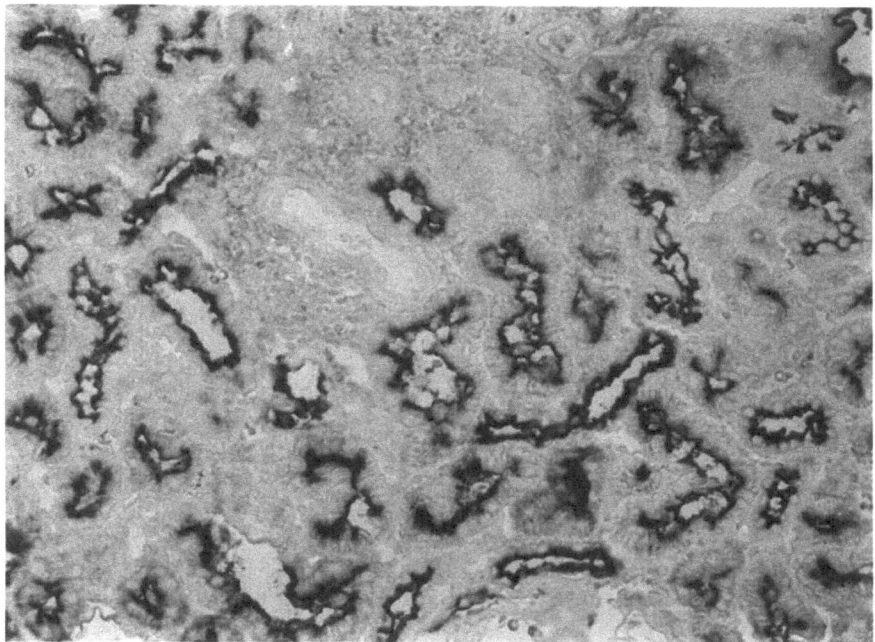

Fig. 2. Double labelling showing PHA-E lectin staining the brush border of the proximal tubules (blue) and PNA lectin staining the apical cell membrane of distal tubules (brown). × 200

nomial regression analysis is employed to obtain the best-fitting function between renal function (dependent variable) and independent (morphometric) variables (ARMITAGE and BERRY, 1987; FUNG and LEE 1991).

4 Morphometric Analysis in Glomerulonephritides

Bohle and colleagues (1987) performed a series of studies based on morphometric point counting in well-defined inflammatory and non- inflammatory glomerular diseases. They demonstrated that glomerular damage did not appreciably reduce GFR if the tubulointerstitium showed no pathological changes (Figs. 3a,b). However, the excretory functions of the glomeruli were detrimentally affected by interstitial fibrosis and tubular atrophy (BOHLE et al. 1987).

Table 1 summarises some of the important morphometric studies in various glomerular diseases. Convincing data emerged showing statistically significant correlations between TID and renal function, especially of interstitial widening with fibrosis, with serum creatinine. It was also shown that clearances of creatinine, inulin and PAH showed a significant correlation to the breadth of the renal cortical interstitium (BOHLE et al. 1987). It was further shown that as the

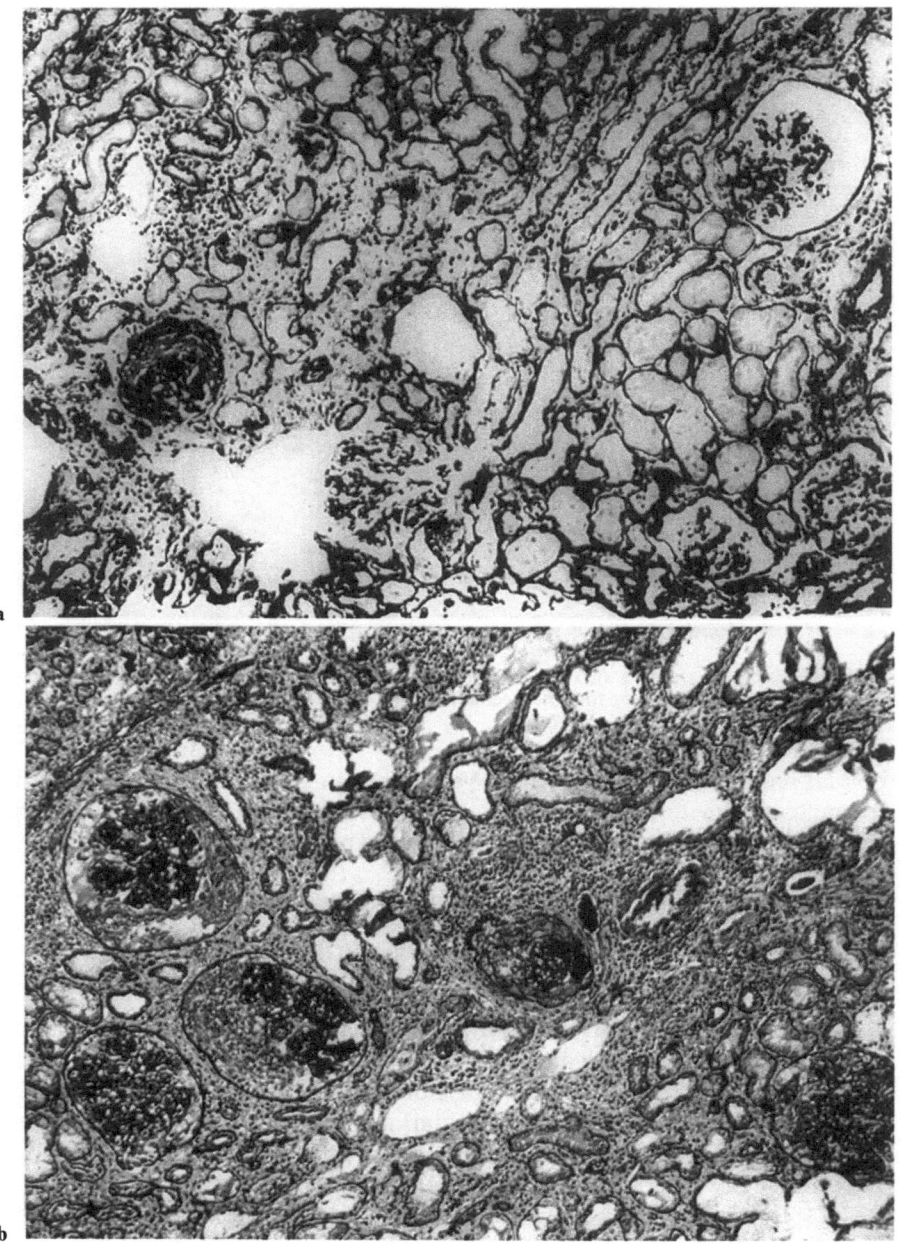

Fig. 3. a Renal biopsy from a patient with focal and segmental glomerulosclerosis and renal dysfunction. The section here shows minor changes in most glomeruli with one obsolescent glomerulus. There is patchy tubular atrophy and interstitial fibrosis. silver stain, X 100. **b** Renal biopsy from a patient with crescentic glomerulonephritis and renal dysfunction. The section shows extensive glomerular damage and tubular atrophy with interstitial fibrosis. silver stain, × 100

Table 1. Relation of tubulointerstitial structural changes to kidney functions in various glomerulonephritides

Type of glomerulonephritis	Tubulointerstitial structural changes	Relation to renal function	Reference
1. Primary glomerular diseases			
(a) Diffuse endocapillary glomerulonephritis	Tubular damage	Creatinine clearance	Lewy et al. 1971
	Interstitial widening/fibrosis	Serum creatinine	Bohle et al. 1977a
	Interstitial widening/fibrosis	Serum creatinine	Bohle et al. 1977b
(b) Diffuse mesangial proliferative glomerulonephritis			
(c) Focal and segmental glomerulosclerosis	Tubulointerstitial damage	Serum creatinine and poor prognosis	Wehrmann et al. 1990
(d) Diffuse membranous glomerulonephritis	Tubulointerstitial damage	Serum creatinine and poor prognosis	Wehrmann et al. 1989
(e) Diffuse membranoproliferative glomerulonephritis	Interstitial widening/fibrosis	Serum creatinine and poor prognosis[a]	Fishbach et al. 1977
	Interstitial widening/fibrosis	Serum creatinine and poor prognosis[a]	Mackensen-Haen et al. 1979
	Interstitial widening/fibrosis	Serum creatinine	Bohle et al. 1987
(f) Diffuse crescentic glomerulonephritis	Interstitial widening/fibrosis	Serum creatinine and poor prognosis[a]	Bohle et al. 1979
2. Glomerulonephritis of systemic disease			
(a) IgA Nephritis	Interstitial widening/fibrosis	Serum creatinine, Creatinine clearance and poor prognosis[a]	Bogenschütz et al. 1990
	Interstitial fibrosis	Independent prognostic indicator	D'Amico et al. 1986
	Percentage interstitial volume in serial biopsies	Dissociated with creatinine clearance	Bennett et al. 1982
	Interstitial widening/fibrosis (without acute renal failure)	Creatinine clearance and serum creatinine	Mackensen-Haen et al. 1988
(b) Nephritis of Henoch-Schönlein Purpura	Tubular atrophy and interstitial fibrosis	Serum creatinine	Bohle et al. 1989(a)
(c) Lupus Nephritis	Severe diffuse tubulointerstitial damage	Severe renal failure	Tron et al. 1979
	Interstitial widening/fibrosis	Serum creatinine	Bohle et al. 1989(b)
3. Glomerular lesions in metabolic diseases			
(a) Diabetic Nephropathy	Interstitial widening/fibrosis	Serum creatinine	Bader et al. 1980
(b) Amyloidosis of the kidney	Interstitial widening/fibrosis	Serum creatinine	Mackensen-Haen et al. 1977

[a]Poor prognosis indicates high percentage of renal death (patients who died as a result of their renal disease or those who developed end stage renal disease necessitating regular dialysis).

size of the renal cortical interstitium increases, the concentration ability of the kidney progressively decreases as manifested in the fall in urine osmolality.

Another interesting feature of these studies was the kidney survival rate as an indicator of prognosis, which was calculated in the form of survival curves in relation to various morphological and clinical parameters. Univariate and multivariate survivorship analyses showed that TID was an important morphological parameter associated with an increased risk of terminal renal failure or death due to renal causes in focal sclerosing glomerulonephritis (WEHRMANN et al. 1990), membranous glomerulonephritis (WEHRMANN et al. 1990) and IgA nephritis (BOGENSCHUTZ et al. 1990).

4.1 Relative Importance of Proximal and Distal Tubular Damage

Study of tubular injury showed that damage to the proximal tubules played a role in producing impaired GFR (Mackensen-Haen et al. 1992). Distal tubular damage is also potentially important because of its strategic location to the macula densa, and its important physiological role as the diluting segment of the tubules. The correlation of distal tubular damage to GFR is not clearly understood, and its importance as a morphometric parameter in determining GFR is beginning to be recognized (BOHLE et al. 1987; MACKENSEN-HAEN et al. 1992).

We observed that the distal tubules did not express antiproteinase response, and, hence, were vulnerable to proteolytic attack (KHAN and SINNIAH 1993c). In our recent study utilizing lectin histochemistry we observed that, in cases with TID, it was the distal tubules which showed damage more often than the adjoining proximal tubules (KHAN and SINNIAH 1993b). In the study of TID, the three important predictors of GFR are interstitial expansion, and proximal and distal tubular damage. It has not been clearly demonstrated which is the best predictor in determining the fall in GFR. It is important to analyze the degree of damage occurring in the two anatomical components of the tubules to establish the most extensively damaged segment. These aspects were analysed by us in a morphometric study (KHAN and SINNIAH 1993a).

We studied 45 renal biopsies from patients with various glomerulonephritides. The control group comprised ten normal renal tissues; five each were obtained from donor transplanted kidneys and nondiseased kidneys of road traffic accident victims. The disease group (45 cases) included biopsies from a variety of primary and secondary glomerulonephritides; five cases each with minimal change disease, focal and segmental sclerosing glomerulonephritis, diffuse mesangial proliferative glomerulonephritis, membranous glomerulonephritis, and diabetic nephropathy, 11 cases of IgA nephritis and nine cases of lupus nephritis. Based on the results of this morphometric study, a statistically significant correlation existed between the creatinine clearance and the percentage area occupied by the proximal (Fig. 4a) and distal tubules (Fig. 4b) and the cortical interstitium (Fig. 4c). Multiple regression analysis to determine the best

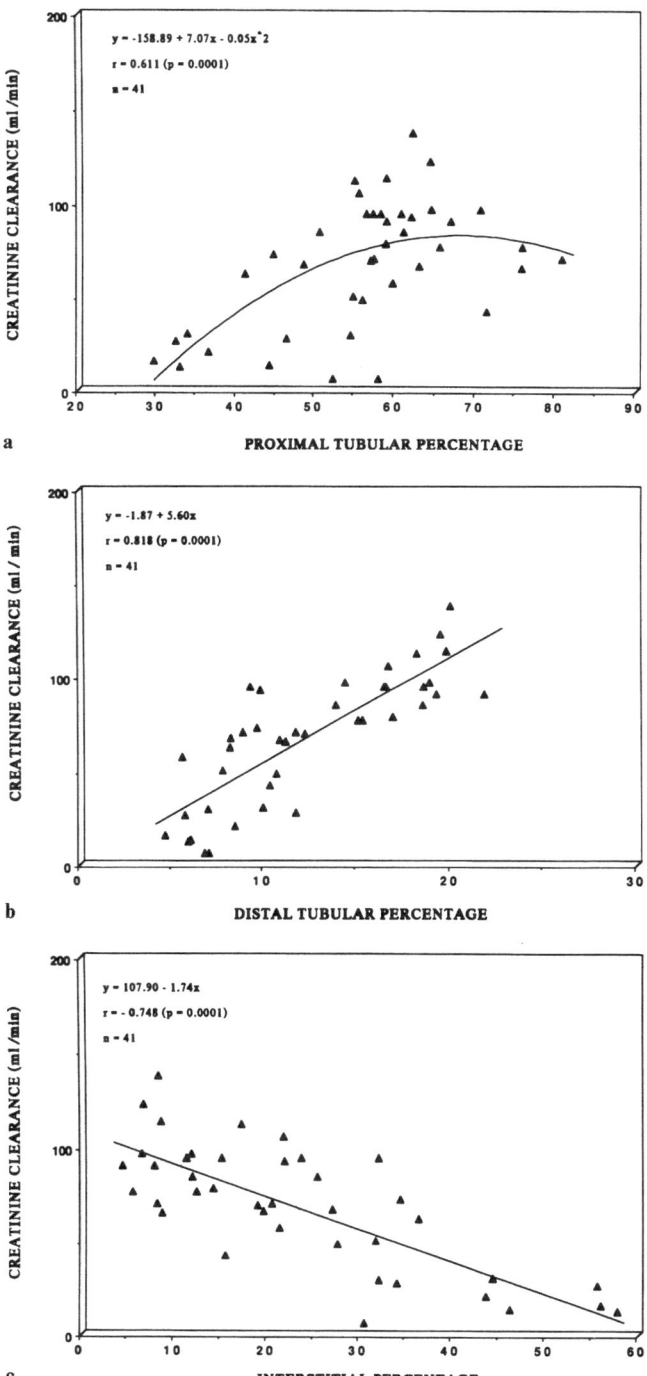

Fig. 4. a Regression of creatinine clearance on proximal tubular percentage in the disease group. **b** Regression of creatinine clearance on distal tubular percentage in the disease group. **c** Regression of creatinine clearance on interstitial percentage in the disease group. (From Khan and Sinniàh 1993a)

Table 2. Correlation matrix between creatinine clearance, proximal tubular percentage, distal tubular percentage and interstitial percentage

	Creatinine clearance (ml/min)	Proximal tubular percentage	Distal tubular percentage	Interstitial percentage
Creatinine clearance (ml/min)	—	r = 0.611[a] p = 0.0001	r = 0.818 p = 0.0001	r = −0.749 p = 0.0001
Proximal tubular percentage		—	r = 0.489 p = 0.0004	r = −0.901 p = 0.0001
Distal tubular percentage			—	r = −0.768 p < 0.0001

[a]The relation between proximal tubular percentage and creatinine clearance (ml/min) is significantly parabolic (from Khan and Sinniah 1993a)

Table 3. Relative mean difference in morphometric parameters of the disease group compared to the control group

Morphometric parameters	Control group		Disease group		Mean difference[b]	Relative mean difference[d]
	Mean	CV(%)[a]	Mean	CV(%)		
Proximal tubules	65.91	6.85	55.80	21.50	− 10.11 (0.0001)[c]	− 15.33
Distal tubules	15.54	18.28	12.31	40.45	− 3.83 (0.0492)[c]	− 21.29
Interstitium	10.51	20.83	23.46	62.53	12.95 (0.0001)[c]	123.21

[a]CV(%), computed by $(100 \times$ standard deviation)/mean, is the coefficient|of variation
[b]Mean difference is mean of disease group minus mean of control group
[c]p Values in brackets obtained from t test after performing arcsin transformation on the original data (Steel and Torrie 1980)
[d]Relative mean difference is the mean percentages of the parameters in the disease group expressed as a percent deviation from the mean percentages of these for the control group. For example, the relative mean difference for proximal tubules is $[(55.80–65.91)/65.91] \times 100 = - 15.33\%$ (Lee and Kolonel 1982). (From Khan and Sinniah 1993a)

predictor for creatinine clearance was not performed because a strong correlation also existed between the independent variables (Table 2), in which situation this statistical analysis is not recommended (Armitage and Berry 1987).

To compare the relative magnitude of the damage occurring in both types of tubules and interstitium in the disease group compared to controls, the "relative mean difference," in addition to "mean difference" for each variable under study was computed as shown in Table 3 (Lee and Kolonel 1982). The relative mean difference was the mean percentage of a parameter in the disease group expressed as a percent deviation from the mean percentage of the same parameter from the control group. On this basis, the disease-control group's difference was greater for the distal tubules than for the proximal tubules, though the mean difference of the proximal tubules was more than that of the distal tubules. This indicates a greater fall in the percentage area occupied by the distal tubules due to tubular damage compared to proximal tubules for which this value was the smallest. The difference was highest for the interstitium, as it represents an expansion relative to the extent of damage to both the proximal and distal tubules (Table 3).

5 Morphometry in Acute Renal Failure

The morphometric investigation of the proximal and distal tubules, the cortical interstitium, the intertubular capillaries, the renal corpuscles and juxtaglomerular apparatus (JGA) in oligoanuric, polyuric and normouric phases of human acute renal failure (ARF) revealed mainly swelling of the epithelial cells of the proximal and distal tubules. The interstitium of the cortex is significantly widened in most cases of ARF. Compared to controls the JGAs were significantly larger in the kidneys in the oligoanuric phase of ARF, while they were slightly smaller in the normouric and polyuric phases (Klingebiel et al. 1983; Bohle et al. 1990).

6 Morphometry in Chronic Sclerosing Interstitial Nephritides

It is known that long-term chronic diffuse interstitial nephritis leads to irreversible renal injury (ZOLLINGER 1966). This is seen in many cases of idiopathic sclerosing interstitial nephritides (MACKENSEN-HAEN et al. 1979), Balkan nephropathy (DAMMIN 1972) and drug-induced tubulointerstitial nephritis (MURRAY 1983). Morphometric study of different types of chronic sclerosing interstitial nephritis showed a statistically significant correlation between the breadth of the renal cortical interstitium and the level of serum creatinine concentration. With interstitial nephritis, it is evident that the serum creatinine concentration may be increased even when there is no glomerular pathology (MACKENSEN-HAEN et al. 1979).

7 Morphometric Studies Based on Electron Microscopy

Qualitative and quantitative structural changes of the tubules can also be analyzed by electron microscopy. Morphometric analysis can be carried out on montages of electron micrographs of randomly selected cortical areas and cross sections of individual proximal convoluted tubules (MOLLER et al. 1986). These experimental studies have shown that reduction in proximal tubular epithelial mitochondria and basolateral membrane changes precede the increase in cortical interstitium. The progression of tubular atrophy was concluded to follow impaired tubular function due to increased interstitial tissue and altered relationship between tubules and capillaries. The electron microscopy morphometry showed that even a slight increase in cortical interstitial volume by associated significant quantitative changes in tubular cell organelles leads to impaired tubular function (MOLLER and SKRIVER 1985). Electron microscopy morphometry has also been performed in spontaneously hypertensive rats. Measurements of the volume of mitochondria and other intracellular organelles suggest that reabsorption of substances at the beginning of the distal tubules is reduced but is intensified in the collecting ducts. The reabsorption of substances in the proximal tubules is essentially normal (Postnov and Perov 1977). These morphometric studies substantiate the importance of distal tubules which have been demonstrated in human patients (KHAN and SINNIAH 1993a).

In tubular damage another important morphometric correlate could be the TBM itself, as all the damaged tubules show thickening of the TBM. The relationship of TBM thickness to GFR has not been studied to date. This can be studied morphometrically from electron micrographs, as it is realized that in light microscopy it is difficult to separate the basal part of the tubular epithelium and adjoining interstitium from the TBM. Furthermore, the number of points falling on the TBM in a biopsy tissue on light microscopy will be very few and will yield a large standard error (SE) of the estimate (AHERNE and DUNNILL 1982b,c). The TBM is a metabolically active component of the renal tubules and shows significantly increased deposition of collagen type IV and laminin in TID (DOWNER et al. 1988). Morphological correlation with the GFR needs to be studied to explain the TBM thickening.

In most instances, tubular lesions coexist with interstitial lesions. The interstitium forms another important morphometric correlate of GFR as shown previously in several studies. Electron microscopy can be employed to study the interstitial banded collagen, and changes in cortical type I interstitial cells (ICs) in TID. It is believed that prostaglandins in lipid droplets of type I ICs exert an endocrine type antihypertensive action on the kidney (Muirhead 1980, 1988). The cortical type I ICs and the changes they undergo in TID have not been documented in human kidneys.

8 Video-Based System for Morphometry

There are a number of video-based systems used for quantitative histopathology which are commercially available. These systems comprise a microscope, a digitizer and a computer and are of varying degrees of sophistication. For computer-based morphometric analysis, there should be standardization of the histologic images for reproducibility. This would involve tissue processing, sectioning and staining, standardization and calibration of video camera and the sampling rate (pixels/micron rate). To minimize data-collection artifacts, parallel processing of control materials should be performed (JORDAN et al. 1988).

Specific algorithms have to be written to study the lesions in question. For the study of basement membrane structures in kidney electron micrographs, an adaptive window-based algorithm has been produced (ONG et al. 1993). This can measure the length and width of the glomerular basement membrane with minimal user interaction, and can easily be adapted to measure tubular basement membrane thickness.

9 Image Analysis and Cytochemical Stains in Renal Tissues

Cell organelles including lysosomes, renal brush border and mitochondria in human and rat kidney can be studied by specific cytochemical stains applied to light and electron microscopic materials. Densitometry and morphometry of subcellular structures in thin sections can be performed by automatic image analysis with software utilizing appropriate and specific algorithms (CORNELIS et al. 1985). These techniques are going to be utilized with greater frequency in the study of renal tubules and their functional relationship to other components of the kidney.

10 Relationship Between Tubulointerstitial Structures and Renal Function

It is established that the proximal and distal tubules maintain the electrolyte concentration and osmolality of urine. Their structural connection permit tubuloglomerular (TG) feedback control (SCHNERMANN and BRIGGS 1985), which is the major regulator of glomerular filtration (WRIGHT and OKUSA 1990). In TID, the mechanisms elicited by tubular damage and interstitial widening have been explained by Bohle and coworkers in several structure and function correlation studies (BOHLE et al. 1977a,b, 1979, 1981, 1987; MACKENSEN-HAEN et al. 1979, 1992; BOGENSCHÜTZ et al. 1990). They explained that the decrease in GFR in mild tubulointerstitial changes occurs via the renin-angiotensin axis. Deficient NaCl reabsorption occurs in the damaged renal tubules, leading to an increase in NaCl concentration at the macula densa, which then causes reduction in the activity of the renin-angiotensin axis, resulting in dilatation of the efferent arteriole (BAUMBACH and SKØTT 1986; LEYSSAC 1986). These events cause the fall in GFR, with resultant drop in creatinine clearance. This decline in GFR explains why excessive polyuria does not occur in spite of impaired concentrating ability (MACKENSEN-HAEN et al. 1992). In severe TID the fall in GFR is due to the reduction in the number and areas of postglomerular vessels (BOHLE et al. 1981, 1987).

In our recent study (KHAN and SINNIAH 1993a), both the distal and proximal tubular percentages correlated significantly with the fall in GFR. However, the

GFR correlated more strongly to the distal tubular damage than to proximal, raising the possibility that distal tubular damage may play a key role in the regulation of GFR. In another study in the same group of patients using lectin histochemistry (KHAN and SINNIAH 1993b), it was observed that the distal tubules, especially the thick ascending limb (TAL) rather than proximal tubules and cortical collecting ducts, were the initial sites of tubular damage and showed increased damage as TID progressed. The relative mean difference values computed from the morphometric results clearly support these observations (KHAN and SINNIAH 1993a). The relative mean difference for the distal tubules showed a higher value compared to the proximal tubules, indicating greater damage to them. The distal tubular system plays a key role in maintaining sodium homeostasis, and enables the kidney to concentrate and dilute urine. It also participates in the regulation of GFR and, most importantly, is the site where the final adjustment between sodium excretion and sodium intake is achieved (HIERHOLZER 1985).

In our opinion, damage to the proximal tubules, and consequent impaired reabsorption of NaCl in particular, can be compensated by the TAL of the distal tubules, which respond to increased delivery of sodium salt with a significant increase in its reabsorption, as observed in rats (MORGAN and BERLINER 1969; KHURI et al. 1975; HIERHOLZER 1985). Conceptually, this load-dependent reabsorption of sodium salt by the distal tubule, which functions normally as a diluting segment, can compensate for the decreased reabsorption by the proximal tubules. If the TAL of the distal tubules is damaged, then it may lead to an uncompensated increase in the NaCl concentration in the tubular fluid. The increase in the NaCl content of urine passing the macula densa becomes plasma-isotonic and leads to a fall in GFR due to TG feedback mechanisms (BOHLE et al. 1987; KHAN and SINNIAH 1993a).

The study of renal structure and function based on morphometric analyses have given us a better understanding of renal pathophysiology. These meticulous studies have shown that the tubules and the interstitium have an intimate and important relationship to renal function, both in primary tubulointerstitial diseases and secondary to various types of glomerular pathology. In many cases, tubulointerstitial involvement is a more important and sensitive index of renal dysfunction than glomerular damage. The introduction of image analysis systems and the creation of specific algorithms incorporated into software will produce both speedy and reproducible results in the study of the anatomy and function of different components of the kidney.

References

Aherne WA, Dunnill MS (1982a) Preparation of tissues. Sampling. In: Morphometry. Arnold, London, pp 27–28
Aherne WA, Dunnill MS (1982b) Statistical suggestions. In: Morphometry. Arnold, London, pp 181–186

Aherne WA, Dunnill MS (1982c) Point counting and the estimation of volume fraction. In: Morphometry. Arnold, London, pp 39–41

Anderson JA, Dunnill MS (1965) Observations on the estimation of the quantity of emphysema in the lung by the point-sampling method. Thorax 20: 462–466

Armitage P, Berry G (1987) Multiple measures. In: Statistical methods in medical research. Blackwell Scientific Publication, Oxford, pp 296–357

Bader R, Bader H, Grund KE, Mackensen-Haen S, Christ H, Bohle A (1980) Structure and function of the kidney in diabetic glomerulosclerosis. Correlations between morphological and functional parameters. Pathol Res Pract 167: 204–216

Baumbach L, Skott O (1986) Renin release from different parts of rat afferent arterioles in vitro. Am J Physiol 251: F12–F16

Bennett WM, Walker RG, Kincaid-Smith P (1982) Renal cortical interstitial volume in mesangial IgA nephropathy. Dissociation from creatinine clearance in serially biopsied patients. Lab Invest 4: 330–335

Bogenschütz O, Bohle A, Batz C, Wehrmann M, Pressler H, Kendziorra H, Gärtner HV (1990) IgA nephritis: On the importance of morphological and clinical parameters in the long-term prognosis of 239 patients. Am J Nephrol 10: 137–147

Bohle A, Bader R, Grund KE, Mackensen-Haen S, Neunhoeffer J (1977a) Serum creatinine concentration and renal interstitial volume. Analysis of correlations in endocapillary (acute) glomerulonephritis and in moderately severe mesangioproliferative glomerulonephritis. Virchows Arch [A] 375: 87–96

Bohle A, Grund KE, Mackensen-Haen S, Tolon M (1977b) Correlations between renal interstitium and level of serum creatinine. Virchows Arch [A] 373: 15–22

Bohle A, Christ H, Grund KE, Mackensen-Haen S (1979) The role of the interstitium of the renal cortex in renal disease. Contr Nephrol 16: 109–114

Bohle A, Von Gise H, Mackensen-Haen S, Stark-Jakob B (1981) The obliteration of the postglomerular capillaries and its influence upon the function of both glomeruli and tubuli. Functional interpretation of morphologic findings. Klin Wochenschr 59: 1043–1051

Bohle A, Mackensen-Haen S, Von Gise H (1987) Significance of tubulointerstitial changes in the renal cortex for the excretory function and concentration ability of the kidney. A morphometric contribution. Am J Nephrol 7: 421–433

Bohle A, Gärtner HV, Laberke HG, Krück F (1989a) The kidney. Structure and function, 1st edn. Schattauer, Stuttgart, pp 224–235

Bohle A, Gärtner HV, Laberke HG, Krück F (1989b) The kidney. Structure and function, 1st edn. Schattauer, Stuttgart, pp 236–260

Bohle A, Christensen J, Kokot F, Osswald H, Schubert B, Kendziorra H, Pressler H, Marcovic-Lipkovski J (1990) Acute renal failure in man: New aspects concerning pathogenesis. A morphometric study. Am J Nephrol 10: 374–388

Churg J, Cotran RS, Sinniah R, Sakaguchi H, Sobin LH and pathologists and nephrologists in 17 countries (1985) In: Renal disease. Classification and atlas of tubulo-interstitial diseases. Igaku-Shoin, Tokyo, pp 1–3

Cornelis A, Van Meerbeck D, Nyssen M, Roels F (1985) Specific cytochemical stains in the image analysis of subcellular organelles. Anal Quant Cytol Histol 7: 256–266

D'Amico G, Minetti L, Ponticelli C, Fellin G, Ferrario F, Barbiano di Belgioioso G, Imbasciati E, Ragni A, Bertoli S, Fogazzi G, Duca G (1986) Prognostic indicators in idiopathic IgA mesangial nephropathy. Q J Med 59: 363–378

Dammin GJ (1972) Endemic nephropathy in Yugoslavia. Arch Pathol 93: 372–374

Downer G, Phan SH, Wiggins RC (1988) Analysis of renal fibrosis in a rabbit model of crescentic nephritis. J Clin Invest 82: 998–1006

Fishbach HS, Mackensen-Haen S, Grund KE, Kellner A, Bohle A (1977) Relationship between glomerular lesions, serum creatinine and interstitial volume in membranoproliferative glomerulonephritis. Klin Wochenschr 55: 603–608

Fung KP, Lee J (1991) Basic program for polynomial regression and smoothing. Comput Appl Biosci 7: 103–104

Hally AD (1964) A counting method for measuring the volumes of tissue components in microscopical sections. Q J Microsc Sci 105: 503–517

Hierholzer K (1985) Sodium reabsorption in the distal tubular systems. In: Seldin DW, Giebisch G (eds) The kidney, vol II. Physiology and pathophysiology. Raven, New York, pp 1063–1096

Holthofer H, Virtanen I, Pettersson E, Tornroth T, Alfthan O, Linder E, Miettinen A (1981) Lectins as fluorescence microscopic markers for saccharides in the human kidney. Lab Invest 45: 391–399

Howie AJ, Gunson BK, Sparke J (1990) Morphometric correlates of renal excretory function. J Pathol 160: 245–253

Jordan SW, Brayer JM, Bartels PH, Anderson RE (1988) Video-based image collection for quantitative histopathology. Anal Quant Cytol Histol 10: 37–46

Khan TN, Sinniah R (1993a) Morphometric study showing the importance of distal tubular damage in impaired creatinine clearance. Am J Nephrol 13: 178–183

Khan TN, Sinniah R (1993b) Study of renal tubular glycoconjugates in tubulointerstitial damage using conjugated lectins. J Pathol 170: 187–196

Khan TN, Sinniah R (1993c) Renal tubular antiproteinase (α-1-antitrypsin and α-1-antichymotrypsin) response in tubulointerstitial damage. Nephron 65: 232–239

Khuri RN, Strieder N, Widerholt M, Giebisch G (1975) The effect of graded solute diuresis on renal tubular sodium transport in the rat. Am J Physiol 228: 1262–1268

Klingebiel TH, Gise HV, Bohle A (1983) Morphometric studies on acute renal failure in humans during the oligoanuric and polyuric phases. Clin Nephrol 20: 1–10

Laberke HG, Bohle A (1980) Acute interstitial nephritis: Correlations between clinical and morphological findings. Clin Nephrol 14: 263–273

Lee J, Kolonel LN (1982) Nutrient intakes of husbands and wives: implications for epidemiological research. Am J Epidemiol 115: 515–525

Lewy JF, Salinas-Madrigal L, Herdson PB, Pirani CL, Metoff J (1971) Clinico pathologic correlations in acute poststreptococcal glomerulonephritis. Medicine (Baltimore) 50: 453–501

Leyssac PP (1986) Changes in single nephron renin release are mediated by tubular fluid flow rate. Kidney Int 30: 332–339

Mackensen-Haen S, Grund KE, Bader R, Bohle A (1977) The influence of glomerular and interstitial factors on the serum creatinine concentration in renal amyloidosis. Virchows Arch [A] 375: 159–168

Mackensen-Haen S, Grund KE, Sindjic M, Bohle A (1979) Influence of renal cortical interstitium on the serum creatinine concentration in different chronic sclerosing interstitial nephritides. Nephron 24: 30–34

Mackensen-Haen S, Grund KE, Wschirmeister J, Bohle A (1979) Impairment of the glomerular filtration rate by glomerular and interstitial factors in membranoproliferative glomerulonephritis with normal serum creatinine concentration. Virchows Arch [A] 382: 11–19

Mackensen-Haen S, Eissele R, Bohle A (1988) Contribution on the correlation between morphometric parameters gained from the renal cortex and renal function in IgA nephritis. Lab Invest 59: 239–244

Mackensen-Haen S, Bohle A, Christensen J, Wehrmann M, Kendziorra H, Kokot F (1992) The consequences for renal function of widening of the interstitium and changes in the tubular epithelium of the renal cortex and outer medulla in various renal diseases. Clin Nephrol 37: 70–77

Moller JC, Skriver E (1985) Quantitative ultrastructure of human proximal tubules and cortical interstitium in chronic renal disease (hydronephrosis). Virchows Arch [A] 406: 389–406

Moller JC, Jorgensen TM, Mortensen J (1986) Proximal tubular atrophy: qualitative and quantitative structural changes in chronic obstructive nephropathy in the pig. Cell Tissue Res 244: 479–491

Morgan T, Berlinger RW (1969) A study by continuous microperfusion of water and electrolyte movements in the loop of Henle and distal tubule of the rat. Nephron 6: 388–405

Muehrcke RC, Kark RM, Pirani CL, Pollak VE (1957) Lupus nephritis: a clinical and pathologic study based on renal biopsies. Medicine (Baltimore) 36: 1–145

Muirhead EE (1980) Antihypertensive functions of the kidney: Arthur C. Corcoran memorial lecture. Hypertension 2: 444–464

Muirhead EE (1988) The renomedullary system of blood pressure control. Am J Med Sci 295: 231–233

Murray TG (1983) Drug-induced chronic tubulo-interstitial renal disease. In: Cotran RS, Brenner BM, Stein JH (eds) Contemporary issues in nephrology, vol 10. Tubulointerstitial nephropathies. Churchill Livingstone, New York, pp 188–209

Ong SH, Giam ST, Jayasooriah, Sinniah R (1993) Adaptive window-based tracking for the detection of membrane structures in kidney electron micrographs. Machine Vision Application 6: 215–223

Postnov YV, Perov YL (1977) Morphometric study of the ultrastructure of nephrons and collecting tubules in the kidney of rats with renal and spontaneous hypertension. Virchows Arch [B] 26: 175–185

Risdon RA, Sloper JAC, De Wardener HE (1968) Relationship between renal function and histological changes found in renal biopsy specimens from patients with persistent glomerulonephritis. Lancet ii: 363–366

Rosenbaum JL, Mikail M, Wiedmann F (1967) Further correlations of renal function with kidney biopsy in chronic renal disease. Am J Med Sci 254: 156–160

Schainuck LI, Striker GE, Luther RE, Benditt EP (1970) Structural-functional correlations in renal disease. II. The correlations. Hum Pathol 1: 631–641

Schnermann J, Briggs J (1985) Function of juxtaglomerular apparatus. Local control of glomerular haemodynamics. In: Seldin DW, Giebisch G (eds) The kidney, vol II. Physiology and pathophysiology. Raven, New York, pp 669–697

Steel RGD, Torrie JH (1980) Analysis of variance II. Multiway classification. In: Steel RDG, Torrie JH (eds) Principles and procedures of statistics. A biometric approach. McGraw-Hill, New York, pp 195–238

Tron F, Ganerval D, Droz D (1979) Immunologically mediated acute renal failure of non glomerular origin in the course of systemic lupus erythematosus (SLE). Am J Med 67: 529–532

Truong LD, Phung VT, Yoshikawa Y, Mattioli CA (1988) Glycoconjugates in normal human kidney. A histochemical study using 13 biotinylated lectins. Histochemistry 90: 51–60

Wehrmann M, Bohle A, Bogenschütz O, Eissele R, Freislederer A, Öhlschlegel C, Schumm G, Batz C, Gärtner HV (1989) Long-term prognosis of chronic idiopathic membranous glomerulonephritis. An analysis of 334 cases with particular regard to tubulo-interstitial changes. Clin Nephrol 31: 67–76

Wehrmann M, Bohle A, Held H, Schumm G, Kendziorra H, Pressler H (1990) Long-term prognosis of focal sclerosing glomerulonephritis. An analysis of 250 cases with particular regard to tubulointerstitial changes. Clin Nephrol 33: 115–122

Wright FS, Okusa MD (1990) Functional role of tubulo-glomerular feedback control of glomerular filtration. Adv. Nephrol 19: 119–133

Zollinger HU (1966) Chronic abuse of phenacetin and kidney lesions. In: Mostofi, Smith (eds) The kidney. International academy of pathology monograph. Williams and Wilkins, Baltimore, pp 523–528

Tubulitis in Renal Disease

B. IVÁNYI and S. OLSEN

1 Introduction

Tubulitis in the kidney is defined as the presence of inflammatory cells in the tubular wall (OOI et al. 1975). It is the hallmark of tubulointerstitial nephritis (OLSEN et al. 1986) and one of the important lesions in acute renal allograft rejection (SOLEZ et al. 1993). However, it may occur in other renal diseases as well, e.g., glomerulonephritis and acute tubular necrosis (OLSEN et al. 1981), systemic vasculitis affecting the kidney (AKISUSA et al. 1990), chronic renal ischemia (TRUONG et al. 1992). Knowledge of the clinical implications, pathogenesis, and consequences of tubulitis is limited due to the complex structural-functional relationships between the tubular epithelium, the peritubular interstitium, and the capillaries and the complicated segmental structure of the tubules. It seems likely that tubulitis is in most cases a result of a T-cell-mediated reaction. Studies of human renal allograft rejection (Sect. 7.1)

Current Topics in Pathology
Volume 88, S.M. Dodd (Ed.)
© Springer-Verlag Berlin Heidelberg 1995

and autoimmune nephritis in mice (KELLEY et al. 1993) led to the hypothesis that renal tubular epithelial cells may participate in the development of tubulitis, since they can be induced to express major histocompatibility complex (MHC) molecules and cell adhesion molecules, and present antigen to T cells (HAGERTY and ALLEN 1992).

This chapter will focus on the morphological features of tubulitis in the human kidney. Immunological and other aspects of tubulointerstitial disease which may be of importance for an understanding of tubulitis have been dealt with by CAMERON (1989, 1992), JONES and EDDY (1992), KELLY et al. (1991), McCLUSKEY (1992), NATH (1992), YEE et al. (1991), and WILSON (1991, 1992).

2 Definition of Tubulitis

The term tubulitis was used first by OOI et al. (1975) in a clinicopathological study of acute interstitial nephritis "to describe the infiltration of acute and/or chronic inflammatory cells in the peritubular regions or between the lining epithelial cells, with or without disruption of the tubular basement membrane." Their definition should be modified on the basis of subsequent observations. Peritubular accumulation of leukocytes does not eventually lead to the infiltration of these into the tubules. Rupture of the tubular wall, accumulation of leukocytes in the tubular lumen, and an increased rate of apoptosis in tubular epithelial cells may be present, but not always. Since the only constant feature of tubulitis in various renal disorders is the presence of leukocytes in the tubular walls, we and others (SOLEZ et al. 1993; TRUONG et al. 1991) define tubulitis simply as *a situation in which inflammatory cells are localized between tubular epithelial cells, and/or between these and the tubular basement membrane (TBM).*

3 Ultrastructure of Tubulitis

The electron-microscopic appearance of tubules infiltrated with inflammatory cells was studied in acute pyelonephritis and renal allograft rejection by IVÁNYI et al. (1983, 1988) and NÁDASDY et al. (1988). It was found that neutrophilic granulocytes, macrophages, and lymphocytes invaded the tubules in the same way. On the basis of a great number of electron micrographs, the following time sequence was presumed. Initially, the leukocytes are situated close to the outer side of the TBM. Eventually they open the TBM with a pseudopod and move first with their cytoplasm (Fig. 1) and then with their nuclei into the lateral space between two epithelial cells. After the passage, the TBM becomes a continuous layer again. The migration of leukocytes through the TBM must be fast because the study of a considerable number of thin sections and micrographs was necessary to find examples of passage through the TBM. Following invasion, the leukocyte is usually situated in the basal region of the tubular wall; it exhibits close cell-to-cell contacts with adjacent tubular epithelial cells and other emigrated leukocytes, and it is separated from the underlying TBM by a narrow layer of epithelial cytoplasm (Fig. 2). This appearance was common to acute pyelonephritis (IVÁNYI et al. 1983, 1988), allergic acute interstitial nephritis (IVÁNYI et al. 1992b), glomerulonephritis-associated tubulitis (unpublished observation, Fig. 3), and renal allograft rejection (NÁDASDY et al. 1988). The epithelial cytoplasm "protecting" the TBM and the close cell-to-cell contacts therefore seem to be important for maintainance of the integrity of the tubular wall infiltrated by inflammatory cells. In vitro, the close contacts have been shown to prevent leakage of tracers across penetration sites into the tubular wall (MILKS et al. 1983).

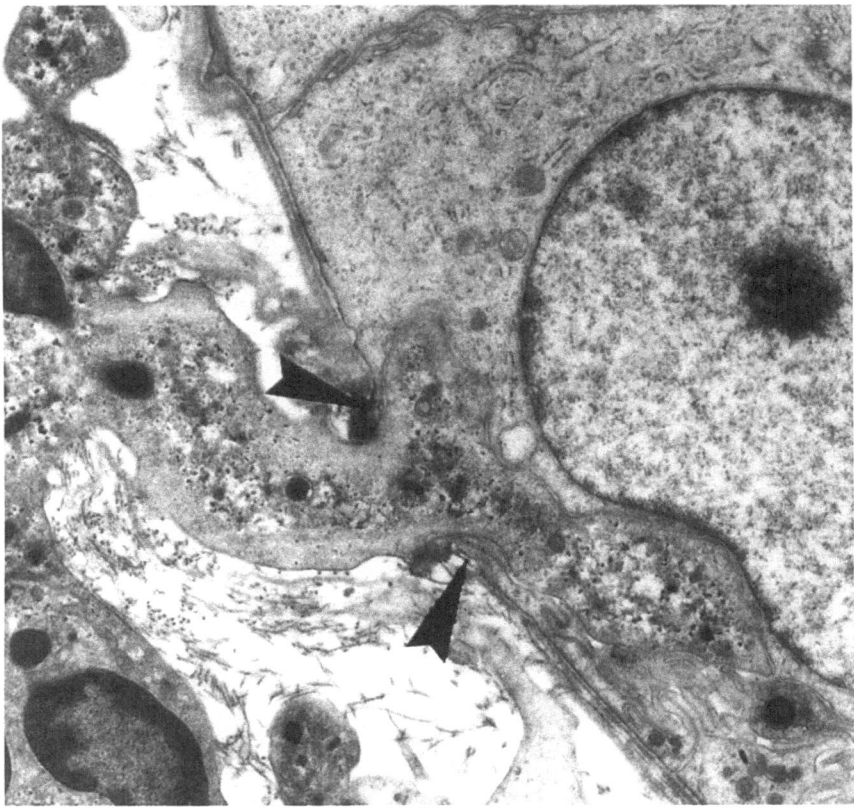

Fig. 1. Experimental acute pyelonephritis. The tubular basement membrane is opened (*arrowheads*), and the infiltrating pseudopod of a granulocyte is localized in the lateral intercellular space of two epithelial cells. × 11 500 (Reprinted from IVÁNYI et al. 1983, with permission)

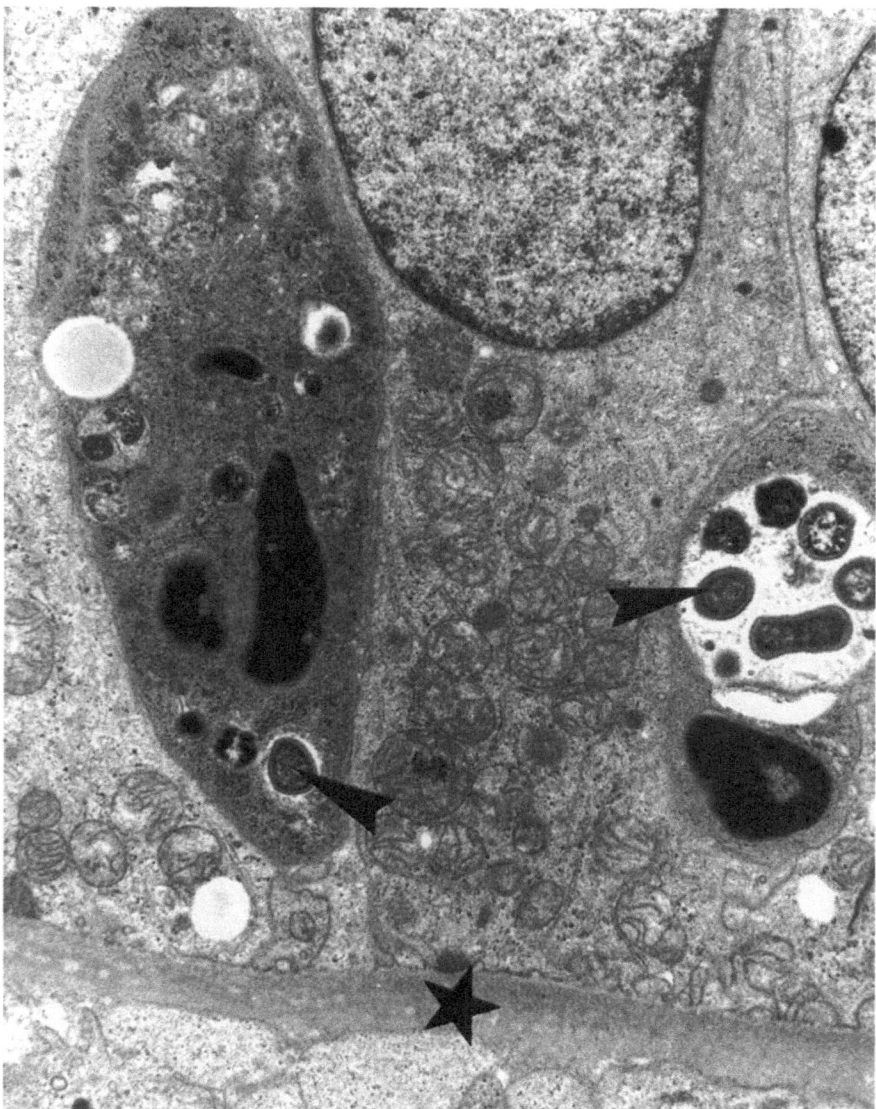

Fig. 2. Acute human pyelonephritis. Two neutrophilic granulocytes with phagocytosed bacteria (*arrowheads*) at the basal region of the lateral intercellular spaces between epithelial cells. The granulocytes are separated from the tubular basement membrane (TBM) by a narrow layer of epithelial cytoplasm. The TBM (*star*) is continuous. × 9000 (Reprinted from IVÁNYI et al. 1988, with permission)

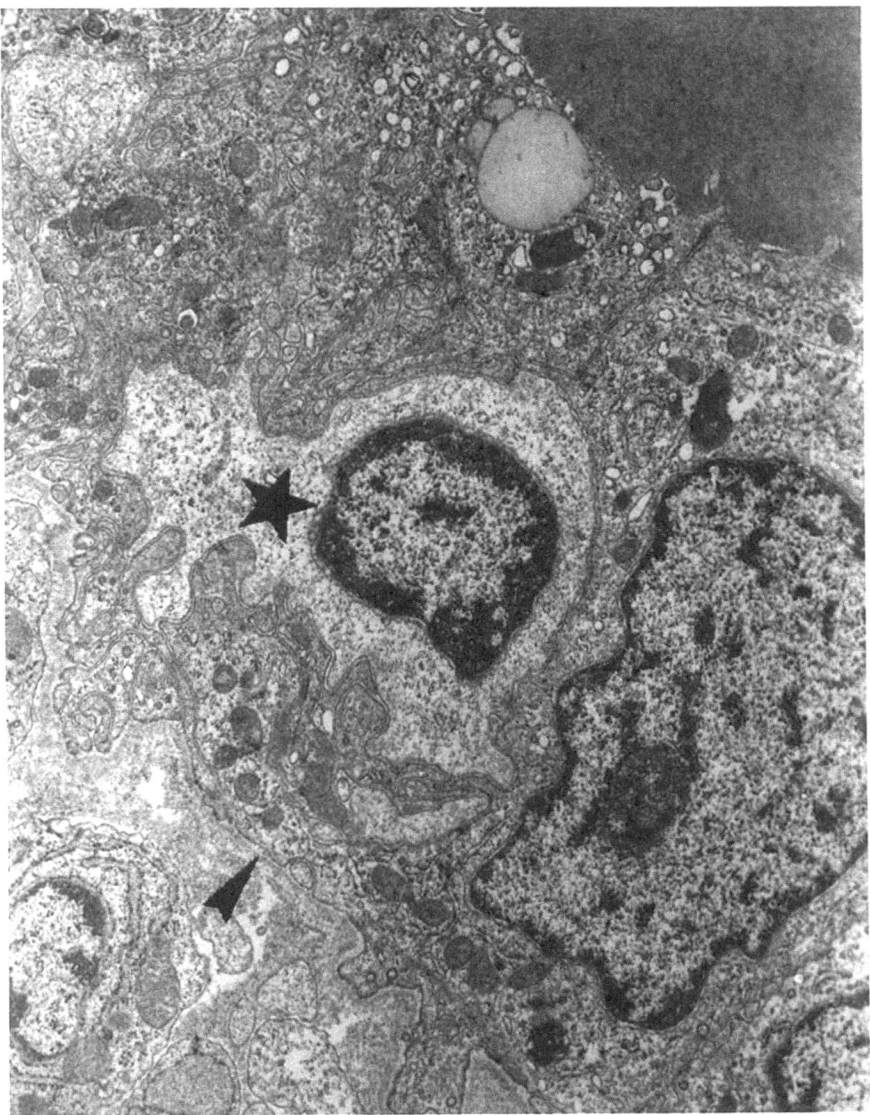

Fig. 3. Pauci-immune crescentic glomerulonephritis. The tubular wall-localized lymphocyte (*star*) is situated in the lateral intercellular space between adjacent epithelial cells and is separated from the tubular basement membrane (TBM) by a narrow layer of epithelial cytoplasm. The TBM (*arrowhead*) is continuous. × 4600

The adhesion of tubular epithelial cells to the TBM via integrin receptors (GOLIGORSKY et al. 1993; GOLIGORSKY and DIBONA 1993) appears to be so tight that the penetrating pseudopod is usually not able to separate the epithelial cell from the TBM. In some cases, however, the infiltrating cell may be located beneath the epithelium. We have seen this occasionally in acute allograft rejection. The loss of the basolateral expression of integrin receptors leading to the loosening of the contact between epithelium and TBM may conceivably be due to ischemia or cell-mediated cytotoxicity, or both.

The adhesion of tubular epithelial cells to their BM is obviously tighter than that between the peritubular capillary endothelial cells and their BM. In acute pyelonephritis and acute allograft rejection, we found that during the emigration of leukocytes from peritubular capillaries to the interstitium, the leukocytes often became localized in the capillary wall by lifting the endothelial cell body from the BM (OLSEN and BOHMAN 1979; IVÁNYI and THOENES 1987; IVÁNYI et al. 1992a).

4 Semiquantitative Estimation of Tubulitis

Tubulitis is a focal process. Its severity and extent differ from site to site, and from kidney to kidney. The semiquantitative estimation of tubulitis is therefore not easy. During work on the problem of the histological standardization of acute renal allograft rejection, a scheme was developed to score the severity of tubulitis (SOLEZ et al. 1993). The presence of tubular profiles with 1–4 leukocytes, 5–10 leukocytes, and more than 10 leukocytes in the most affected tubular profile was scored as T_1, T_2, and T_3, respectively. The minimum sampling standard was the presence of seven glomeruli in the biopsy. It is important that periodic acid-Schiff (PAS)-stained slides are used for scoring, since a clear definition of the TBM is required.

To describe tubulitis in glomerular disorders, diabetic nephropathy, renal amyloidosis and renal artery stenosis, we developed a grading system which combines the severity and extent of tubulitis. At a magnification of 40 x, tubular profiles were investigated for tubulitis. The severity (S) was scored according to SOLEZ et al. (1993). The extent (E) of tubulitis was assessed in a 3-mm^2 area of the biopsy specimen including the most severe focus of tubular inflammation. Four categories were distinguished: E_1: 1–10, E_2: 11–20, E_3: 21–30, and E_4: more than 30 tubular profiles with tubulitis. In nephrectomy specimens, a 9-mm^2 area was studied and the values were divided by three. E_1S_{2-3} and E_2S_1 cases were regarded as mild, E_2S_{2-3} and $E_{3-4}S_1$ as moderate, and $E_{3-4}S_2$ and E_3S_{3-4} as severe tubulitis "No" tubulitis included cases with E_1S_1 (IVÁNYI et al. 1995). AKISUSA et al. (1992) used the percentage of tubules with inflammatory cells in 20 high-power fields as a measure of the degree of tubulitis in renal biopsies with systemic vasculitis.

5 Methods for Studying the Segmental Localization of Tubulitis

Differences may exist in the distribution of tubulitis along the nephron. The electron microscope is not an ideal tool for studying this, because the epon-embedded material is too small, the number of blocks is limited, and it can be difficult to identify the segments, especially of the distal nephron. To solve the problem, we introduced a multiple immunolabeling method which allows the identification of renal cortical tubular segments in formalin-fixed, paraffin-embedded biopsy material. In this protocol, the PAS reaction stains the brush border of proximal tubules, and the anti-Tamm-Horsfall protein antibody the cytoplasm of distal straight tubules. The cytokeratin antibodies (clones AE1/AE3) stain the cytoplasm of the cells of the cortical collecting system (cortical collecting ducts and connecting tubules) in a mosaic staining pattern. The luminal binding pattern of peanut agglutinin (*Arachis hypogaea*) verifies the distal convoluted tubules (for color documentation see IVÁNYI and OLSEN 1991, IVÁNYI et al. 1992b, 1993). Using such multiply immunolabeled sections, we carried out stereological studies to describe tubulitis quantitatively. In allergic acute interstitial nephritis, the point-count method served to estimate the relative volume fraction of the inflammatory cell infiltrates within each category of tubular segments (IVÁNYI et al. 1992b). In acute renal allograft rejection (IVÁNYI et al. 1993) and anti-glomerular basement membrane (anti-GBM) nephritis (see Sect. 7.5.4), the relative intrasegmental length and the average intensity of tubulitis were determined using the stereological relationship between the number of isolated profiles and the length of the structure. The relative length of a tubular segment was estimated by dividing the number of profiles in the given tubular segment by the total number of tubular profiles. The *relative intraseg-mental length of tubulitis* was calculated by dividing the number of tubular profiles infiltrated by inflammatory cells in a given tubular segment by the total number of tubular profiles. The *average intensity of tubulitis* was calculated by dividing the total number of intraepithelial mononuclear cells in a given tubular segment by the total number of tubular profiles. The latter method disregards possible variations in absolute profile area.

Immunolabeled sections and the point-count method recently were used by MARCUSSEN et al. (1991), who analyzed tubulitis in renal biopsies from patients with transplant acute tubular necrosis, native acute tubular necrosis, and acute graft rejection.

6 Phenotypic Analysis of Tubulitis in the Native Kidney: Missing Data

A great number of publications have dealt with the phenotypic analysis of *interstitial* cell infiltrates in various renal disorders (ALEXOPOULOS et al. 1989a, 1989b, 1990; BENDER et al. 1984; BOLTON et al. 1987; BOUCHER et al. 1986;

Brunati et al. 1986; Caligaris-Cappio et al. 1985; Cheng et al. 1989; D'Agati et al. 1986; Gimenez and Mampaso 1986; Hooke et al. 1987; Husby et al. 1981; Li et al. 1990; Markovic-Lipkovski et al. 1990, 1991; Matsamura et al. 1988; Müller et al. 1988; Rosenberg et al. 1988; Sabadini et al. 1988; Stachura et al. 1984a,b; Takaya et al. 1985). These studies revealed that CD4$^+$ and CD8$^+$ T cells and macrophages are the major subgroups of inflammatory cells in the interstitium. The ratio of the CD4$^+$ and CD8$^+$ subsets varied in these studies. In general, T-helper/inducer cells predominated over T-cytotoxic/suppressor cells in chronic and idiopathic cases with tubulointerstitial nephritis and primary glomerulonephritides, whereas in drug-induced tubulointerstitial nephritis and lupus nephritis T-cytotoxic/suppressor cells were sometimes in the majority (Alexopoulos et al. 1989a, 1989b, 1990; Bender et al. 1984; Boucher et al. 1986; Cheng et al. 1989; D'Agati et al. 1986).

In all papers except one (Matsumura et al. 1988), the phenotypic analysis of tubular wall-localized inflammatory cells was not documented. Accordingly, we can only speculate about the immunological basis of tubulitis. The light- and electron-microscopic appearance of tubular wall-localized leukocytes and the cellular composition of *interstitial* infiltrates in the above-mentioned papers make it possible that, with the exception of acute pyelonephritis, T-cell mechanisms play a role in the development of tubulitis. It is uncertain whether delayed hypersensitivity (release of lymphokines from a few specifically sensitized T cells with a subsequent influx of leukocytes) or T-cell-mediated cytotoxicity is the basis of tubulitis. In the study of tubulointerstitial nephritis associated with Sjögren's syndrome by Matsumura et al. (1988), the lymphocytes invading the tubules were exclusively of the CD8$^+$ type.

The systematic determination of T-cell subsets in the tubular wall in various renal disorders, e.g., acute allergic interstitial nephritis, chronic pyelonephritis, Bence Jones cast nephropathy, crescentic glomerulonephritis, is an essential task for the future. It would also be important to study the activated state of the tubular wall-localized lymphocytes, as well as interactions between lymphocytes and tubular epithelial cells in culture. The expression of activation markers, i.e., granzyme B, perforin, interleukin-1 (IL-1)-beta, tumor necrosis factor (TNF)-alfa, may clarify whether tubulitis is a response of delayed hypersensitivity or T-cell-mediated cytotoxicity in these disorders. Granzyme B and perforin are markers for cytotoxic T cells (Hameed et al. 1991, 1992), and IL-1-beta and TNF-alfa positivity indicate delayed hypersensitivity (Lipman et al. 1992; Noronha et al. 1992). In culture conditions, the tubular epithelial cells and infiltrating T cells from the same biopsy specimen can be propagated. If cytotoxic T cells directed against renal tubular epithelium are present in the renal biopsy specimen, the culture T cells will lyse the epithelial cell line (Miltenburg et al. 1989).

7 Tubulitis in Renal Disorders

7.1 Tubulitis in Acute Renal Allograft Rejection

7.1.1 Inflammatory Cells in the Tubular Wall

The histopathology of acute renal allograft rejection includes interstitial mononuclear infiltrates, tubulitis (Fig. 4) and intimal arteritis (SOLEZ et al. 1993). An
electron-microscopic study of tubular changes revealed that the most frequent
inflammatory cell in the tubular wall was the lymphocyte, followed by the
macrophage and finally the granulocyte (NÁDASDY et al. 1988). Phenotypically,
the intratubular lymphocytes were predominantly T cells, mostly CD8[+] and
Leu-7[+] (CD57[+]) lymphocytes (BESCHORNER et al. 1985; SOLEZ et al. 1992).
Analysis of the in vitro outgrowth of T lymphocytes from needle biopsies
showed that the T cells were cytotoxic and donor specific, since they caused the
lysis of proximal tubular cell lines of donor origin (MILTENBURG et al. 1989; VAN
DER WOUDE et al. 1990). The cytotoxic cells were CD4[+] and CD8[+] (YARD et al.
1993).

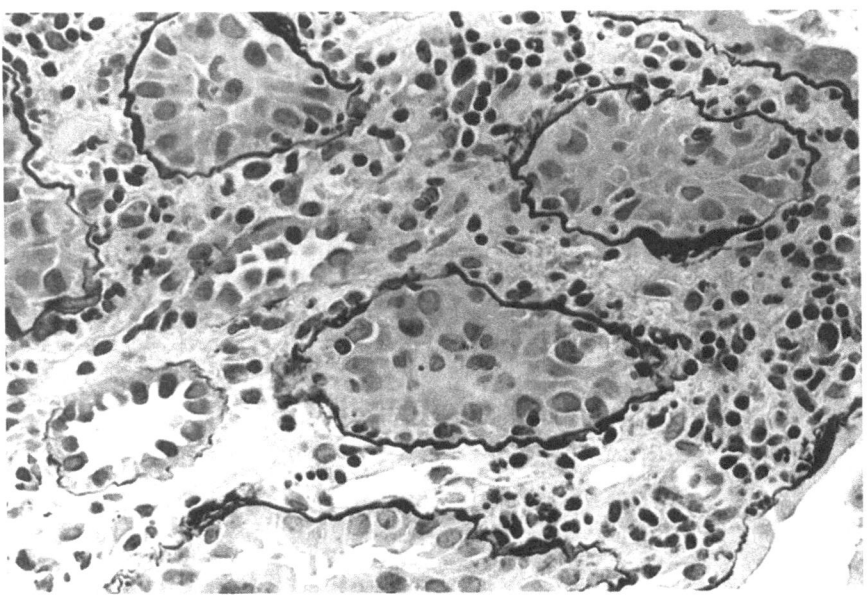

Fig. 4. Tubulitis in acute renal allograft reaction. Lymphocytes are present between the tubular
epithelial cells. PAS, × 340

7.1.2 Tubular Expression of MHC and Cell Adhesion Molecules

In the normal human kidney, tubular epithelial cells constitutively express HLA-ABC (class-I) antigens. The immunohistochemical reaction is confined to the cytoplasm of tubular cells. The proximal tubular cells express little if any HLA-DR (class-II) antigen. The weak immunohistochemical reaction (if present) is localized at the base of the cells (FUGGLE et al. 1983; HALL et al. 1984; RAFTERY et al. 1989). The distal tubules, collecting ducts, and loop of Henle do not express HLA-DR antigen. In acute rejection, the tubular expression of MHC class-I and -II molecules is markedly increased (MARKOVIC-LIPKOVSKI et al. 1992; FUGGLE et al. 1993). The increased expression of the HLA-DR molecule involved all tubules in the majority of cases (HALL et al. 1984; RAFTERY et al. 1989). The most intense reaction was seen in the proximal tubules (RAFTERY et al. 1989; MARKOVIC-LIPKOVSKI et al. 1992). Variable numbers of nonrejecting allografts also exhibited DR expression. In culture, renal tubular cells expressed HLA-ABC antigens, but not HLA-DR. Mixed lymphocyte supernatants and interferon-gamma (INF-gamma) increased the expression of both classes (BISHOP et al. 1986, 1988).

Intercellular adhesion molecule-1 (ICAM-1) is a ligand for all leukocytes via interaction with the lymphocyte function-related antigen-1 (LFA-1) (SPRINGER 1990). Normally, tubular epithelial cells express ICAM-1 not at all or only weakly (BISHOP and HALL 1989; FUGGLE et al. 1993). During acute rejection, there is a marked increase of ICAM-1 on tubular epithelial cells, which involves predominantly the proximal tubules and is very intense at the brush border (ANDERSEN et al. 1992; BISHOP and HALL 1989; BROCKMEYER et al. 1993; FAULL and RUSS 1989; FUGGLE et al. 1993; MARKOVIC-LIPKOVSKI et al. 1992; VON WILLEBRAND et al. 1993). In tissue culture, IFN-gamma and TNF-alfa induced tubular epithelial cells to express ICAM-1 (JEVNIKAR et al. 1990; KIRBY et al. 1993; NORONHA et al. 1992; SURANYI et al. 1991; WUTHRICH et al. 1990). In tissue sections, FUGGLE et al. (1993) and VON WILLEBRAND et al. (1993) found a correlation between the tubular expression of ICAM-1 and the presence of monocytoid and lymphoid cells in the interstitium. In contrast, there was no clear-cut association of cellular infiltrates with the tubular expression of ICAM-1 in another study (BROCKMEYER et al. 1993).

LFA-2 or CD2 is expressed on the T lymphocyte; its counter-receptor on the target cell is LFA-3. LFA-2 and -3 are members of the immunoglobulin family (SPRINGER 1990). Tubular cells in the normal kidney constitutively express LFA-3. The rate of expression was not found to be changed during rejection (BISHOP and HALL 1989).

Vascular cell adhesion molecule-1 (VCAM-1) is a ligand for lymphocytes, monocytes, and eosinophils via interactions with the VLA-4 (very late activation molecule-4, CD49d/CD29) receptor molecule (SPRINGER 1990). In normal kidneys, immunoreaction against VCAM-1 is localized on a few cells of the proximal tubules (BROCKMEYER et al. 1993). In other studies, VCAM-1 expression was variably seen on tubular profiles (BRISCOE et al. 1992; FUGGLE et al.

1993). The stain was patchy and concentrated towards the basolateral surface of the cells (BRISCOE et al. 1992). During rejection, increased tubular staining was observed by all groups. The increase involved both the number of tubules and the intensity of staining. The staining was focally distributed and included distal tubular segments. The tubular display of VCAM-1 did not reveal a strict correlation with infiltrating cells in the interstitium according to the report of BROCKMEYER et al. (1993), whereas FUGGLE et al. (1993) and BRISCOE et al. (1992) found an increased VCAM-1 expression in association with interstitial infiltrates.

The vascular endothelium and tubular epithelial cells of renal allografts are the targets of the rejection response (BISHOP et al. 1989; IVÁNYI et al. 1992a; RENKONEN et al. 1990). When responding to foreign antigen, the individual T cells simultaneously recognize an epitope of the foreign antigen and a determinant of the self-MHC complex expressed on the surface of the antigen-presenting cell. CD8$^+$ cytotoxic T cells recognize antigen in association with MHC class-I products, and CD4$^+$ helper/inducer or cytotoxic T cells recognize antigen in association with MHC class-II products. Antigen-independent interactions, such as LFA-1 and LFA-2, expressed by T lymphocytes, with LFA-3 and ICAM-1, expressed on antigen-presenting cells, lead to the transcription of T-cell-activation genes, the production of IL-2 and other cytokines, the formation of IL-2 receptors, and T-cell proliferation (KRENSKY et al. 1990; SPRINGER 1990; STROM 1992; SHERMAN and CHATTOPADHYAY 1993). It is conceivable that an increased expression of class-I antigen by tubular epithelial cells would render these cells more susceptible to cytotoxic injury by CD8$^+$ cytotoxic cells. Furthermore, cytokine-stimulated tubular epithelial cells, by expressing allo-class-II antigens and ICAM-1, may present antigen to T lymphocytes and directly activate resting allospecific lymphocytes which have infiltrated the graft tissue. Testing the latter theory in culture, KIRBY et al. (1993) found that cytokine-stimulated renal epithelial cells bound, but failed to initiate proliferation of resting allogenic lymphocytes. Their data indicate that the tubular expression of MHC and cell adhesion molecules seems to facilitate the interstitial accumulation of lymphocytes and monocytes in rejecting allografts. VCAM-1, expressed basolaterally, might play a role in the mediation of tubulitis, since the basolateral intercellular spaces are the sites of tubulitis. The role of ICAM-1 expression (which is localized immunohistochemically at the apical part of tubular epithelial cells) for the evolution of tubulitis is unclear at present.

7.1.3 Localization and Quantitative Characteristics of Tubulitis

In formalin-fixed kidney biopsy specimens from 15 patients with transplanted allografts undergoing acute rejection we investigated two parameters of tubulitis: the relative intrasegmental length and the average intensity of tubular inflammation (IVÁNYI et al. 1993). Tubulitis was most prominent in the distal convoluted tubules, followed by the cortical collecting system. The relative intrasegmental length of tubulitis was lowest in the proximal and distal straight tubules. The average intensity of tubulitis was lowest in the distal straight tubules, and this was statistically different from that found in the cortical collecting system and distal convoluted tubules. The average intensity of tubulitis was similar in the cortical collecting system and distal convoluted and proximal tubules. Using a point-count technique, MARCUSSEN et al. (1991) found a significant difference between the marked tubulitis in epithelial membrane antigen(EMA)-positive and the less affected EMA-negative (proximal) tubules. Tamm-Horsfall-positive (distal straight) tubules had the lowest values. These data indicate that the aberrant co-expression of MHC class-II antigens and cell adhesion molecules mainly by proximal tubular epithelial cells (Sect. 7.1.2) does *not* influence the distribution of tubulitis between cortical tubular segments in favor of proximal tubules.

7.2 Tubulitis Associated with Acute Tubular Necrosis in the Native and Grafted Kidney

In an early study of tubulitis in which different renal diseases were compared, OLSEN et al. (1981) described the presence of this lesion in ischemic acute renal failure (acute tubular necrosis) of the native kidney. MARCUSSEN et al. (1991) compared native and graft acute tubular necrosis and in both situations found a moderate but statistically significant increased number of LCA (leukocyte common antigen)-positive tubular wall-localized cells compared with control biopsies (baseline biopsies 1 h after revascularization of renal allotransplants). The degree of tubulitis was not as high as in acute graft rejection. In all groups, the tubulitis was more severe in distal than in proximal tubules.

7.3 Tubulitis in Allergic Acute Interstitial Nephritis

Allergic acute interstitial nephritis (acute tubulointerstitial nephritis) is usually caused by drugs or infections (HEPTINSTALL 1992; SOLEZ 1992). A hypersensitivity reaction may play a role in the pathogenesis, but direct evidence is lacking. In a minority of cases, TBM-drug conjugates may act as antigens, inducing anti-TBM antibodies (WILSON 1991). Morphologically, there is interstitial edema and a mononuclear cell infiltrate composed mainly of T lymphocytes. The lymphocytes invade the tubules, particularly in areas with marked interstitial inflammation. A recent study showed that tubulitis was mostly confined to the distal nephron segments and tended to spare the proximal convoluted tubules (IVÁNYI et al. 1992b). Silver staining of the TBM revealed its focal thinning or absence, which appeared not to be associated with the occurrence of tubulitis. Electron microscopically seen small and large lymphocytes invaded the tubules. Cytolytic injury was not seen in the epithelial cells adjacent to lymphocytes in the tubular wall. However, severe focal tubular damage was present in regions with interstitial infiltrates. The TBM became thin and eventually disappeared. The final stage was complete distintegration of the tubular wall with necrosis of tubular epithelial cells (OLSEN et al. 1986). The pathogenesis of tubular wall injury is still not clear, and the role of tubulitis in the process is not known.

SERON et al. (1991) investigated VCAM-1 and HLA-DR expression by tubular cells in five cases of nonsteroidal anti-inflammatory drug-induced acute interstitial nephritis. The number of proximal tubular profiles stained with anti-VCAM-1 antibody was very low in the normal kidney and markedly increased in interstitial nephritis. The number of VCAM-1-positive tubular cross-sections was higher in areas of activated leukocytes in the interstitium, indicating a relationship between the tubular display of VCAM-1 and the presence of interstitial infiltrates. There was no correlation between the number of tubular cross-sections expressing HLA-DR and the number of those expressing VCAM-1.

7.4 Tubulitis in Acute Pyelonephritis

Patchy suppurative interstitial inflammation, tubulitis with a neutrophilic granulocyte predominance, casts composed of neutrophils and a smaller number of macrophages, and tubular destruction are the histological hallmarks of acute pyelonephritis. It is likely that the transtubular passage of neutrophils and macrophages is a favorable route in the drainage of the interstitial suppurative inflammation, because the inflammatory cells containing bacteria leave the kidney with the urine. In vitro, neutrophils and monocytes are capable of traversing the renal tubular epithelial monolayer (CRAMER et al. 1980, 1986; MIGLIORISI et al. 1988; MILKS et al. 1983). The neutrophils migrate much faster than the monocytes (MIGLIORISI et al. 1988). The molecular pathology of the transtubular passage of leukocytes is not clear. The passage may be enhanced by the release of TNF-alfa from the migrating neutrophils (LLOYD and OPPENHEIM 1992) and monocytes, since TNF-alfa increases the permeability of tight junctions (MULLIN et al. 1992). In experimental pyelonephritis, microvascular perfusion defects were demonstrated in the renal parenchyma which led to severe tissue hypoxia (HILL and CLARK 1972; IVANYI 1991). Hypoxia may contribute to the opening of the tight junctions (MOLITORIS et al. 1989; MOLITORIS 1992).

We have had the opportunity to study five biopsy cases of acute pyelonephritis occurring in the native kidney. The indication for biopsy was acute uremia of unexplained origin. A unique feature of the tubulitis in these cases was that the proximal tubules around the glomeruli seemed to be relatively resistant to the inflammatory cell infiltration (Fig. 5). The granulocytes tended to infiltrate tubular segments without PAS-positive brush border. Three of these cases were examined electron microscopically; it was found that especially the collecting

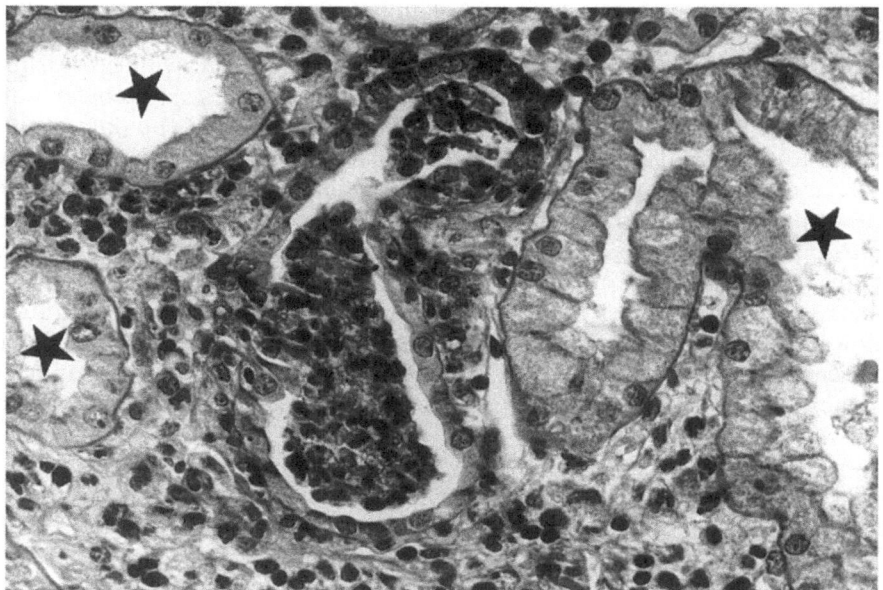

Fig. 5. Acute human pyelonephritis. The proximal tubules (*stars*) are resistant to the inflammatory cell infiltration. The collecting duct (*center*) exhibits tubular wall rupture and contains a pus cast. Pearse trichrome, × 360

ducts were affected by tubulitis, often associated with rupture of the tubular wall (Iványi et al. 1988). At present, no explanation is available for the preferential distal nephron involvement.

It is not established whether the attachment of bacteria to the luminal surface membrane of tubular epithelial cells, or even their incorporation into the lysosomes (Iványi et al. 1985, 1988), may evoke a transtubular migratory stimulus for granulocytes or not. Electron microscopy has demonstrated tubular profiles with intraluminal bacteria but not tubulitis.

7.5 Tubulitis in Nontubulointerstitial Renal Disease

7.5.1 Frequency, Grade, and Site of Tubulitis

We recently performed a semiquantitative light-microscopic pilot study of 274 renal biopsy and 12 nephrectomy specimens in order to assess the frequency, grade, and site of tubulitis in glomerular diseases, diabetic nephropathy, renal amyloidosis, and renal artery stenosis (Table 1). Tubulitis, mostly severe, was present in crescentic glomerulonephritis (linear, pauci-immune and granular) and renal artery stenosis (Fig. 6). The light-microscopic variant of dense deposit

Table 1. Frequency, grade, and site of tubulitis in nontubulointerstitial renal disease

	n	Grade[a] of tubulitis				Mostly in atrophic tubules
		none	mild	moderate	severe	
Crescentic GN, linear	15	0	0	0	15	2
Crescentic GN, pauci-immune	18	1	2	5	10	9
Crescentic GN, granular	5	0	0	0	5	1
Renal artery stenosis	11	0	2	0	9	11
Diabetic NP	30	11	8	7	4	16
IgA GN	50	32	11	4	3	15
Lupus nephritis, WHO IV	28	12	7	7	2	1
Henoch-Schönlein	12	10	1	0	1	0
MPGN, type I	16	10	2	1	3	1
Dense deposit disease	6	3	2	0	1[b]	1
Endocapillary GN	15	10	4	1	0	1
Focal segmental GS	15	12	1	0	2	2
Minimal change NP	21	20	0	1	0	0
Idiopathic membranous NP	27	25	0	1	1	1
Renal amyloidosis	17	11	4	2	0	4

[a]Tubulitis was graded according to severity and extent (see Sect. 4).
[b]Light microscopy: focal segmental necrotizing GN with crescents.
GN, Glomerulonephritis; *MP*, membranoproliferative; *GS*, glomerulosclerosis; *NP*, nephropathy

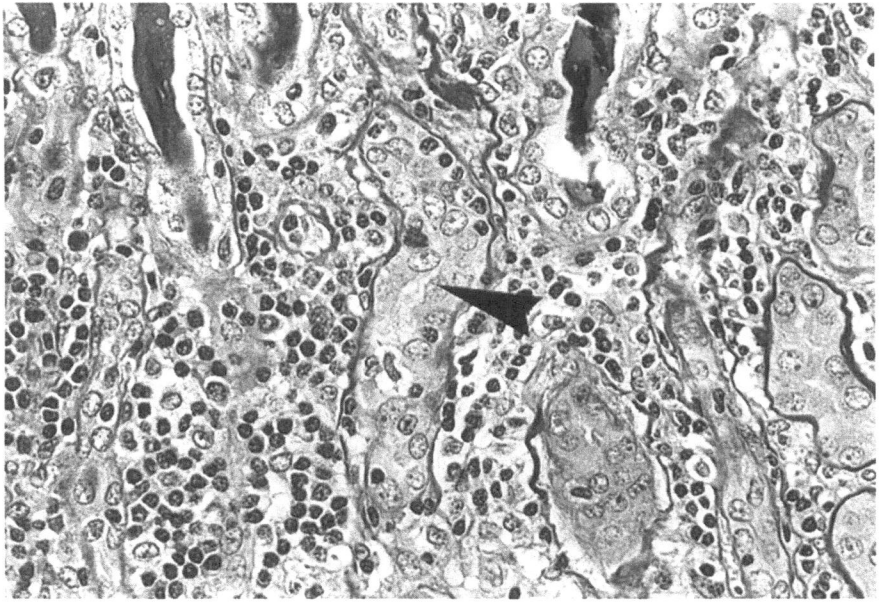

Fig. 6. Severe tubulitis in renal artery stenosis: more than ten lymphocytes within an atrophic tubule (*arrowhead*). The peritubular interstitium contains dense inflammatory cell infiltrate. PAS, × 700

disease, i.e., focal segmental necrotizing glomerulonephritis with crescents, was also associated with severe tubulitis, as described by SIBLEY and KIM (1984). Moderate or severe tubulitis was found in two fifths of the cases of diabetic nephropathy and in one quarter of the cases of membranoproliferative glomerulonephritis. Mild or moderate tubulitis occurred in half of the lupus nephritis cases. Tubulitis, mostly mild, was present in one third of the cases of IgA glomerulonephritis, and it was rare but moderate or severe in minimal change nephropathy and membranous nephropathy.

In most cases, small lymphocytes and larger mononuclear cells (probably also lymphocytes) were localized within the tubular walls. In crescentic and endocapillary glomerulonephritis, neutrophilic granulocytes occasionally also invaded the tubular wall. Tubulitis was found in both atrophic and nonatrophic tubules. In renal artery stenosis, diabetic nephropathy, and IgA glomerulonephritis, the tubulitis was localized predominantly to atrophic tubules (IVÁNYI et al. 1985).

AKISUSA et al. (1992) studied tubulointerstitial alterations in 18 renal biopsy cases of systemic vasculitis. Two indices, the number of interstitial inflammatory cells and the tubulitis percentage, were used to evaluate the changes quantitatively. Tubulointerstitial changes in systemic vasculitis seemed to be less prominent than those in drug-induced tubulointerstitial nephritis. However, six cases (33%) of systemic vasculitis were regarded as having developed pathological changes similar to drug-induced tubulointerstitial nephritis.

7.5.2 Tubular Target Antigens in Nontubulointerstitial Renal Disease

Little is known about tubular target antigens which may initiate an inflammatory reaction against the tubular wall. Immune complexes in the TBM usually do not give rise to tubulitis in lupus nephritis (SCHWARTZ et al. 1982; PARK et al. 1986). Tubulitis in anti-GBM nephritis may be attributed to the deposition of anti-TBM antibodies (ANDRES et al. 1978). The target antigen is localized in the TBM (BUTKOWSKI et al. 1989; YOSHIOKA et al. 1986; Sect. 7.5.5). It is possible that neo-antigens induced by renal ischemia play a role in the development of tubulitis in nontubulointerstitial renal disease. TRUONG et al. (1992) produced chronic renal ischemia in rats by clamping the renal artery and in this way was able to induce chronic tubulointerstitial nephritis. The atrophic tubular epithelium displayed the neo-expression of vimentin and keratin, indicating change in the antigenic profile. The authors concluded that ischemia-induced neo-antigens may initiate a cell-mediated immune response, leading to interstitial inflammation and tubulitis. This may be the explanation of the tubulitis in renal artery stenosis, diabetic nephropathy, and IgA glomerulonephritis, in which diseases it was confined predominantly to atrophic tubules. In this respect, it may be significant that tubulitis was most severe in renal artery stenosis, the condition most similar to experimental clamping of the renal artery. As shown in Table 1, tubulitis was also a feature of crescentic glomerulonephritis. By compressing the glomerular capillaries, crescents can slow or even stop the circulation in the postglomerular capillaries, leading to local ischemia, and in turn to tubulitis.

7.5.3 MHC, Cell Adhesion Molecule and Interleukin-6 Expression by Tubular Epithelial Cells in Nontubulointerstitial Renal Disease

Aberrant HLA class-II antigen expression has been on proximal tubular epithelial cells in variable numbers of cases of crescentic glomerulonephritis (MÜLLER et al. 1988), membranoproliferative glomerulonephritis (MÜLLER et al. 1989), and focal segmental glomerulosclerosis (MARKOVIC-LIPKOVSKI et al. 1991). The expression of ICAM-1 was observed on undamaged and damaged tubules in various types of glomerulonephritis, particularly in cases with crescent formation (CHOW et al. 1992; LHOTTA et al. 1991). An upregulated VCAM-1 expression of variable degree has been reported on proximal tubular epithelial cells in systemic vasulitis with crescents, minimal change nephropathy, IgA nephropathy, lupus nephritis, diabetic nephropathy, amyloidosis, and gout. The proximal tubule VCAM-1 expression correlated with the number of activated leukocytes in the interstitium (SERON et al. 1991). The significance of the aberrant co-expression of VCAM-1, ICAM-1, and HLA class-II antigens on tubular epithelial cells is not known.

Interleukin-6 (IL-6), (which plays a role in the differentiation of cytotoxic T cells, activation of macrophages, etc.) is not demonstrable in tubular epithelial cells in the normal kidney (FUKATSU et al. 1991). In IgA nephropathy and diabetic nephropathy, the co-localization of IL-6 and MHC molecules was found in the damaged and atrophic tubules adjacent to interstitial T-cell infiltrates, suggesting that tubular IL-6 may be involved in the pathogenesis of tubular injury seen in nontubulointerstitial renal disease (FUKATSU et al. 1993).

7.5.4 Localization and Quantitative Features of Tubulitis in Anti-GBM Nephritis

To obtain data about the segmental distribution and quantitative features of tubulitis in anti-GBM nephritis, two stereological parameters (the relative intrasegmental length and the average intensity of tubular inflammation) were investigated in a pilot study (not published) of formalin-fixed, paraffin-embedded renal biopsy specimens from 11 patients with anti-GBM nephritis.

The cortical tubular segments were identified with lectin and immuno-histochemical markers, all applied to the same section (IVÁNYI and OLSEN 1991; IVÁNYI et al. 1992b, 1993). Profiles of proximal convoluted tubules, proximal straight tubules, distal straight tubules, distal convoluted tubules, and the cortical collecting system with and without inflammatory cells were studied. Distal nephron segments not otherwise specified and profiles of tubules without segmental marker expression were also distinguished and investigated. The proximal straight tubules were recognized by their location in the medullary ray. The tubular wall-localized leukocytes were identified on the basis of their morphological appearance. For calculation of the relative intrasegmental length and the average intensity of tubulitis (Iványi et al. 1993), proximal convoluted tubules and proximal straight tubules were combined as proximal tubules. Differences between the tubular segments were analyzed with the paired Student's t-test. Statistical significance was accepted at a level of 5%.

The quantitative data on tubulitis are given in Table 2. In three cases, only 106, 140, and 155 tubular profiles were sampled. The relative intrasegmental length of tubulitis and the average intensity of tubulitis are plotted in Figs. 7 and 8, respectively. No significant difference was found between proximal tubules, distal convoluted tubules, and the cortical collecting system as concerns the relative intrasegmental length and average intensity of tubulitis. These parameters were lowest in the distal straight tubules (where they differed significantly from those in the proximal tubules), the proximal tubules, and the cortical collecting system. *The data indicate that the proximal tubular segments are not the main site of tubulitis.* The accessory immune functions of proximal tubular

Table 2. Quantitative analysis of tubulitis in anti-GBM nephritis

	Mean	range	
Number of sampled tubular profiles	225	106–309	
Relative length of tubular segments	Mean	range	
Proximal convoluted tubule	0.56	0.36–0.70	
Proximal straight tubule	0.01	0.00–0.05	
Distal straight tubule	0.05	0.01–0.11	
Distal convoluted tubule	0.03	0.00–0.09	
Cortical collecting system	0.11	0.06–0.20	
Distal nephron, not otherwise specified	0.11	0.03–0.24	
Tubule without segmental features	0.09	0.00–0.27	
Relative intrasegmental length of tubulitis	Mean	$\pm$ SD	Statistics: significantly different from:
Proximal tubule (convoluted + straight)	0.38	$\pm$ 0.19	DST
Distal straight tubule	0.23	$\pm$ 0.22	PT
Distal convoluted tubule	0.30	$\pm$ 0.23	
Cortical collecting system	0.34	$\pm$ 0.21	
Distal nephron, not otherwise specified	0.27	$\pm$ 0.13	
Tubule without segmental features	0.51	$\pm$ 0.38	
Average intensity of tubulitis	Mean	$\pm$ SD	
Proximal tubule (convoluted + straight)	0.99	$\pm$ 0.80	DST
Distal straight tubule	0.34	$\pm$ 0.35	PT, CCS, TWSF
Distal convoluted tubule	0.55	$\pm$ 0.50	
Cortical collecting system	0.70	$\pm$ 0.54	DST
Distal nephron, not otherwise specified	0.55	$\pm$ 0.28	
Tubule without segmental features	1.02	$\pm$ 0.95	DST

SD, Standard deviation; at 5% level; *DST*, distal straight tubule; *PT*, proximal tubule; *CCS*, cortical collecting system; *TWSF*, tubule without segmental features.

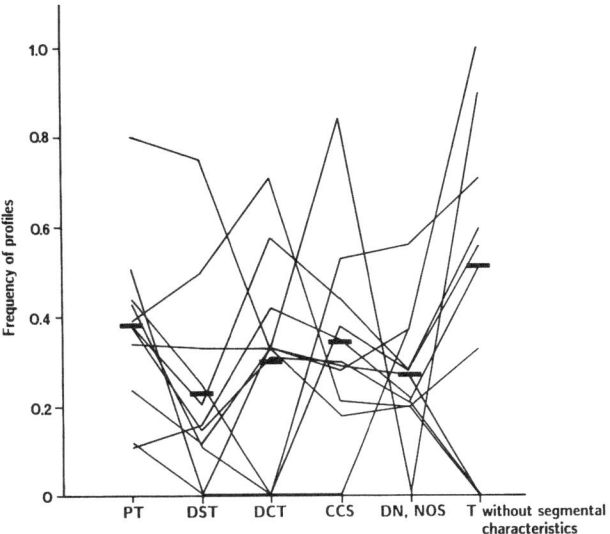

Fig. 7. Relative intrasegmental length of tubulitis in anti-GBM nephritis. Each *thin line* represents a single biopsy. No significant difference between values of proximal tubules (*PT*), distal convoluted (*DCT*), and cortical collecting system (*CCS*). Tubulitis was lowest in the distal straight tubules (*DST*). *DN*, *NOS*, distal nephron, not otherwise specified; *T*, tubule

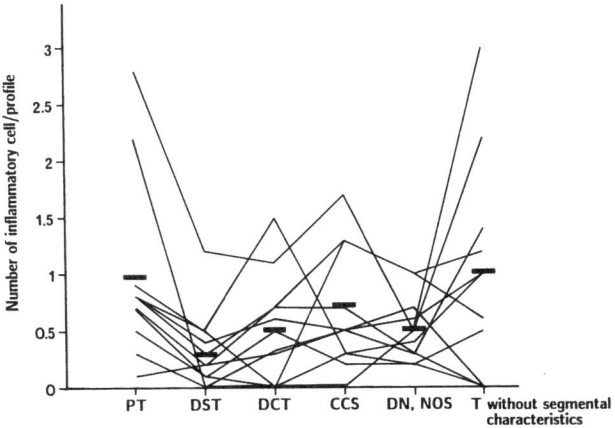

Fig. 8. Average intensity of tubulitis in anti-GBM nephritis: lowest in the distal straight tubules (*DST*). No significant difference between values of proximal tubules (*PT*), distal convoluted tubules (DCT), and cortical collecting system (*CCS*). *DN*, *NOS*, Distal nephron, not otherwise specified; *T*, tubule

epithelial cells (KELLEY et al. 1993; Sect. 7.1.2 and 7.5.3) would suggest that tubulitis in anti-GBM nephritis preferentially involves the proximal tubules and spares the segments of the distal nephron. Our results *do not* support this assumption.

7.5.5 Pathogenesis of Tubulitis and Tubular Damage in Anti-GBM Nephritis

The primary target of anti-GBM antibodies seems to be the 28-kD non-collagenous C-terminal domain of the alfa$_3$ chain of type-IV collagen (HUDSON et al. 1989; KLEPPEL et al. 1989; SAVIGE and GALLICCHIO 1991). The glomerular inflammation is accompanied by tubulointerstitial nephritis in 85% of cases (COHEN and GLASSOCK 1989). Tubulitis in anti-GBM nephritis may be related to the deposition of anti-TBM antibodies, which occur in 70% of patients with anti-GBM antibodies (WILSON 1992). The target antigen of anti-TBM antibodies is localized in type-IV collagen of the TBM. The TBM antigen was analyzed with antibodies to subunits of the globular domains of BM collagen by BUTKOWSKI et al. (1989). One staining pattern exhibited the staining of all renal basement membranes and the mesangial matrix. The other staining pattern was characterized by staining of the GBM as well as Bowman's capsule and distal tubule BM. In another study, eluted antibodies from the kidney of a patient with Goodpasture's syndrome bound strongly to the GBM of normal kidney, and also to Bowman's capsule and some distal TBM (SAVAGE et al. 1986; PUSEY et al. 1987). ANDRES et al. (1978) examined eight cases of anti-GBM nephritis with linear deposits of IgG in the GBM and TBM. The tubular deposits were localized mainly in the BM of the proximal convoluted tubules. Four kidneys were available for elution study. All four eluates contained antibodies reacting with the GBM, and only two eluates reacted with the TBM. These observations suggest that there is selectivity in the distribution and/or expression of TBM antigens in anti-GBM nephritis, and the localization of eluted antibodies may differ from that seen in the renal biopsy specimens. However, since tubulointerstitial nephritis can occur in anti-GBM nephritis without anti-TBM antibodies as well (ANDRES et al. 1978; COHEN and GLASSOCK 1989), other factors may also play a role as regards the mediation of tubulitis in anti-GBM nephritis. Renal ischemia induced by glomerular crescents (Sect. 7.5.2) may alter the antigenic profile of the tubular epithelium, and this change may be associated with the inflammatory infiltration of the tubules.

The tubular histopathology of tubulointerstitial nephritis in anti-GBM nephritis includes focal thickening, thinning, gaps, or complete disappearance of the TBM and tubulitis. Extensive tubular atrophy is frequent in patients with advanced disease (ANDRES et al. 1978). The mechanism by which tubular damage develops in anti-GBM nephritis and how tubulitis contributes to this damage is not known.

8 Significance and Possible Consequences of Tubulitis in Renal Disease

Definitive evidence for a specific injury to tubular cells by tubular wall-localized leukocytes is sparse. In Sjögren's syndrome, manifest tubular dysfunction (renal tubular acidosis, nephrogenic diabetes insipidus, etc.) is present in a small percentage of patients (POKORNY et al. 1989; VIERGEVER and SWAAK 1991), and chronic renal insufficiency seldom develops. CD8⁺ T cells within renal tubules (MATSUMURA et al. 1988, Sect. 6) may conceivably disturb the tubular function.

It is tempting to speculate that infiltration with inflammatory cells leads to persistent tubular damage, at least in some conditions. The high relative number of atubular glomeruli demonstrated in several types of chronic tubulointerstitial renal disease (MARCUSSEN 1992) could therefore be explained by tubular damage due to tubulitis. The aggressive tubulitis present in some types of glomerulonephritis, which usually takes a progressive course, might also be the cause of the marked tubular atrophy characteristic of the late stages of these diseases. Support for the hypothesis could be found in acute allergic interstitial nephritis, which is characterized by the severe destruction of tubular segments, as demonstrated by electron microscopy. In acute interstitial nephritis with acute renal failure, the renal function does not always normalize and the follow-up biopsies performed have shown some degree of interstitial fibrosis and tubular atrophy. In acute renal allograft rejection, infiltrating leukocytes seem to collect in the tubular walls due to immune reactions involving cytotoxic lymphocytes (Sect. 7.1.1). Chronic rejection is often a long-term result of one or more rejection episodes of severe grade. It is therefore conceivable that cytotoxic damage to the tubular epithelium is partly responsible for the tubular atrophy present in chronic rejection. In some cases of lupus nephritis and drug-induced acute tubulointerstitial nephritis, CD8⁺ T cells predominate in the *interstitial* T-cell population. In these cases, CD8⁺ T cells may also infiltrate the tubular walls, eventually leading to tubular damage.

It is clear, however, that these observations comprise at most circumstantial evidence. There are other data which speak directly against or are less consistent with this hypothesis.

The severe focal destruction of tubules in acute interstitial nephritis (OLSEN et al. 1986) may have other explanations than the direct cytotoxic action of lymphocytes. The destruction of tubular segments seems to be a late phenomenon in the sequence of events leading to this damage. The presence of lymphocytes in tubules is therefore compatible with the entirely normal ultrastructure of adjacent epithelial cells (IVÁNYI et al. 1992b). In previous studies on the segmental localization of tubulitis in allergic acute interstitial nephritis (IVÁNYI et al. 1992b), acute allograft rejection (IVÁNYI et al. 1993; MARCUSSEN et al. 1991), and in anti-GBM nephritis (Sect. 7.5.4), the proximal tubules were not found to be the main site of tubulitis. *These findings indicate that the capacity of proximal tubular epithelial cells to facilitate interactions with T cells does not appear to influence the location of tubulitis significantly.* Co-stimulatory immune functions have not been observed in the epithelial cells of the distal nephron. It should further be remembered that in most diseases with tubulitis it is not known whether the infiltrating cells are T-helper or T-cytotoxic lymphocytes. It may also be significant that tubulitis is often most pronounced in tubules which have already become atrophic (IVÁNYI et al. 1995; Sect. 7.5.1).

The molecular pathological basis of tubulitis remains an enigma, and current knowledge does not permit a clear-cut answer to the problem of the importance of tubulitis as concerns tubular atrophy in end-stage renal disease. Future investigations must decide whether tubulitis is a pathogenetically important lesion or an innocent epiphenomenon.

Acknowledgement. The studies of Dr. Iványi summarized in this chapter were supported in part by grants of OTKA 2736, ETT T-69/1990 and ETT T-06 585/1993, Budapest, Hungary.

References

Akisusa B, Irabu N, Matsumura R, Tsuchida H (1990) Tubulointerstitial changes in systemic vasculitic disorders: a quantitative study of 18 biopsy cases. Am J Kidney Dis 16: 481–486

Alexopoulos E, Seron D, Hartley RB, Nolasco F, Cameron JS (1989a) The role of interstitial infiltrates in IgA nephropathy: a study with monoclonal antibodies. Nephrol Dial Transplant 4: 187–195

Alexopoulos E, Seron D, Hartley RB, Nolasco F, Cameron JS (1989b) Immune mechanisms in idiopathic membranous nephropathy: the role of the interstitial infiltrates. Am J Kidney Dis 13: 404–412

Alexopoulos E, Seron D, Hartley RB, Cameron JS (1990) Lupus nephritis: correlation of interstitial cells with glomerular function. Kidney Int 37: 100–109

Andersen CB, Blaehr H, Ladefoged S, Larsen S (1992) Expression of the intercellular adhesion molecule-1 (ICAM-1) in human renal allografts and cultured human tubular cells. Nephrol Dial Transplant 7: 147–154

Andres G, Brentjens J, Kohli R, Anthone R, Anthone S, Baliah T, Montes M, Mookerjee BK, Prezyna A, Sepulveda M, Venuto R, Elwood C (1978) Histology of human tubulo-interstitial nephritis associated with antibodies to renal basement membranes. Kidney Int 13: 480–491

Bender WL, Whelton A, Beschorner WE, Darwish MO, Hall-Craggs M, Solez K (1984) Interstitial nephritis, proteinuria, and renal failure caused by nonsteroidal anti-inflammatory drugs. Am J Med 76: 1006–1011

Beschorner WE, Burdick JF, Williams GM, Solez K (1985) Phenotypic identification of in-traepithelial lymphocytes (IEL) in acute renal allograft rejection. Kidney Int 27: 204

Bishop GA, Hall BM, Suranyi MG, Tiller DJ, Horvath JS, Duggin GG (1986) Expression of HLA antigens on renal tubular cells in culture. I. Evidence that mixed lymphocyte culture supernatants and gamma interferon increase both class-I and class-II HLA antigens. Transplantation 42: 761–679

Bishop GA, Waugh JA, Hall BM (1988) Expression of HLA antigens on renal tubular cells in culture. II. Effect of increased HLA antigen expression on tubular cell stimulation of lymphocyte activation and on their vulnerability to cell-mediated lysis. Transplantation 46: 303–310

Bishop GA, Hall BM (1989) Expression of leucocyte and lymphocyte adhesion molecules in the human kidney. Kidney Int 36: 1078–1085

Bishop GA, Waugh JA, Landers DV, Krensky AM, Hall BM (1989) Microvascular destruction in renal transplant rejection. Transplantation 48: 408–414

Bolton WK, Innes DJ, Sturgill BC, Kaiser DL (1987) T-cells and macrophages in rapidly progressive glomerulonephritis: clinicopathologic correlations. Kidney Int 32: 869–876

Boucher A, Droz D, Adafer E, Noël LH (1986) Characterization of mononuclear cell subsets in renal cellular interstitial infiltrates. Kidney Int 29: 1043–1049

Briscoe DM, Pober JS, Harmon WE, Cotran RS (1992) Expression of vascular cell adhesion molecule-1 in human renal allografts. J Am Soc Nephrol 3: 1180–1185

Brockmeyer C, Ulbrecht M, Schendel DJ, Weiss EH, Hillebrand G, Burkhardt K, Land W, Gokel MJ, Riethmüller G, Feucht HE (1993) Distribution of cell adhesion molecules (ICAM-1, VCAM-1, ELAM-1) in renal tissue during allograft rejection. Transplantation 55: 610–615

Brunati C, Brando B, Confalonieri R, Belli LS, Lavagni MG, Minetti L (1986) Immunophenotyping of mononuclear cell infiltrates with renal disease. Clin Nephrol 26: 15–20

Butkowski RJ, Wieslander J, Kleppel M, Michael AF, Fish AJ (1989) Basement membrane collagen in the kidney: regional localization of novel chains related to collagen IV. Kidney Int 35: 1195–1202

Caligaris-Cappio F, Bergui L, Tesio L, Ziano R, Camussi G (1985) HLA-Dr + T cells of the Leu 3 (helper) type infiltrate the kidneys of patients with systemic lupus erythematosus. Clin Exp Immunol 59: 185–189

Cameron JS (1989) Immunologically mediated interstitial nephritis: primary and secondary. Adv Nephrol 18: 207–248

Cameron JS (1992) Tubular and interstitial factors in the progression of glomerulonephritis. Pediatr Nephrol 6: 292–303

Cheng HF, Nolasco F, Cameron JS, Hildreth G, Neild G, Hartley B (1989) HLA-DR display by renal tubular epithelium and phenotype of infiltrate in interstitial nephritis. Nephrol Dial Transplant 4: 205–215

Chow J, Hartley RB, Jagger C, Dilly SA (1992) ICAM-1 expression in renal disease. J Clin Pathol 45: 880–884

Cohen AH, Glassock RJ (1989) Anti-GBM glomerulonephritis including Goodpasture's syndrome. In: Tisher CC, Brenner BM (eds) Renal pathology with clinical and functional correlations. Lippincott, Philadelphia, pp 494–521

Cramer EB, Milks LC, Ojakian GK (1980) Transepithelial migration of human neutrophils: an in vitro model system. Proc Natl Acad Sci USA 77: 4069–4073

Cramer EB, Milks LC, Brontoli MJ, Ojakian GK, Wright SD, Showell HJ (1986) Effect of human serum and some of its components on neutrophil adherence and migration across an epithelium. J Cell Biol 102: 1868–1877

D'Agati V, Appel GB, Estes D, Knowles DM, Pirani CL (1986) Monoclonal antibody identification of infiltrating mononuclear leukocytes in lupus nephritis. Kidney Int 30: 573–581

Faull RJ, Russ GR (1989) Tubular expression of intercellular adhesion molecule-1 during renal allograft rejection. Transplantation 48: 226–230

Fuggle SV, Errasti P, Daar AS, Fabre JW, Ting A, Morris PJ (1983) Localization of major histocompatibility complex (HLA-ABC and DR) antigens in 46 kidneys. Transplantation 35: 385–390

Fuggle SV, Sanderson JB, Gray DWR, Richardson A, Morris PJ (1993) Variation in expression of endothelial adhesion molecules in pretransplant and transplanted kidneys—correlation with intragraft events. Transplantation 55: 117–123

Fukatsu A, Matsuo S, Tamai H, Sakamoto N, Matsuda T, Hirano T (1991) Distribution of interleukin-6 in normal and diseased human kidney. Lab Invest 65: 61–66

Fukatsu A, Matsuo S, Yuzawa Y, Miyai H, Futenma A, Kato K (1993) Expression of interleukin 6 and major histocompatibility complex molecules in tubular epithelial cells of diseased human kidneys. Lab Invest 69: 58–67

Giménez A, Mampaso F (1986) Characterization of inflammatory cells in drug-induced tubulointerstitial nephritis. Nephron 43: 239–240

Goligorsky MS, DiBona GF (1993) Pathogenetic role of Arg-Gly-Asp-recognizing integrins in acute renal failure. Proc Natl Acad Sci USA 90: 5700–5704

Goligorsky MS, Lieberthal W, Racusen L, Simon EE (1993) Integrin receptors in renal tubular epithelium: new insights into pathophysiology of acute renal failure. Am J Physiol 264 (Renal Fluid Electrolyte Physiol 33): F1–F8

Hagerty DT, Allen PM (1992) Processing and presentation of self- and foreign antigens by the renal proximal tubule. J Immunol 148: 2324–2330

Hall BM, Bishop GA, Duggin GG, Horvath JS, Philips J, Tiller DJ (1984) Increased expression of HLA-DR antigens on renal tubular cells in renal transplants: relevance to the rejection response. Lancet 2: 247–251

Hameed A, Truong LD, Price V, Kruhenbuhl O, Tschopp J (1991) Immunohistochemical localization of granzyme B antigen in cytotoxic cells in human tissues. Am J Pathol 138: 1069–1075

Hameed A, Olsen KJ, Cheng L, Fox WM, Hruban RH, Podack ER (1992) Immunohistochemical identification of cytotoxic lymphocytes using human perforin monoclonal antibody. Am J Pathol 140: 1025–1030

Heptinstall RH (1992) Interstitial nephritis. In: Heptinstall RH (ed) Pathology of the kidney, 4th edn. Little, Brown, Boston, pp 1315–1368

Hill GS, Clark RL (1972) A comparative angiographic, microangiographic, and histologic study of experimental pyelonephritis. Invest Radiol 7: 33–47

Hooke DH, Gee DC, Atkins RC (1987) Leukocyte analysis using monoclonal antibodies in human glomerulonephritis. Kidney Int 31: 964–972

Hudson BG, Wieslander, Wisdom BJ, Noelken ME (1989) Biology of disease. Goodpasture syndrome: molecular architecture and function of basement membrane antigen. Lab Invest 61: 256–269 (Erratum Lab Invest 61: 690)

Husby G, Tung KSK, Williams RC (1981) Characterization of renal tissue lymphocytes in patients with interstitial nephritis. Am J Med 70: 31–38

Iványi B (1991) Hypoxic damage to tubules due to blockage of perfusion in acute hematogenous E. coli pyelonephritis of rats. Acta Morphol Hung 39: 239–248

Iványi B, Olsen TS (1991) Immunohistochemical identification of tubular segments in percutaneous renal biopsies. Histochemistry 95: 351–356

Iványi B, Marcussen N, Olsen TS (1995) Tubulitis in primary vascular and glomerular renal disease. Path Res Pract (accepted)

Iványi B, Thoenes W (1987) Microvascular injury and repair in acute human bacterial pyelonephritis. Virchows Arch [A] 411: 257–265

Iványi B, Ormos J, Lantos J (1983) Tubulointerstitial inflammation, cast formation, and renal parenchymal damage in experimental pyelonephritis. Am J Pathol 113: 300–308

Iványi B, Krenács T, Petri S (1985) Phagocytosis of bacteria by proximal tubular epithelium in experimental pyelonephritis. Virchows Arch [B] 50: 59–70

Iványi B, Rumpelt HJ, Thoenes W (1988) Acute human pyelonephritis: leukocytic infiltration of tubules and localization of bacteria. Virchows Arch [A] 414: 29–37

Iványi B, Hansen HE, Olsen TS (1992a) Postcapillary venule-like transformation of peritubular capillaries in acute renal allograft rejection. Arch Pathol Lab Med 116: 1062–1067

Iványi B, Marcussen N, Kemp E, Olsen TS (1992b) The distal nephron is preferentially infiltrated by inflammatory cells in acute interstitial nephritis. Virchows Arch [A] 420: 37–42

Iványi B, Hansen HE, Olsen S (1993) Segmental localisation and quantitative characteristics of tubulitis in kidney biopsies from patients undergoing acute rejection. Transplantation 56: 581–585

Jevnikar AM, Wuthrich RP, Takei F, Xu HW, Brennan DC, Glimcher LH, Rubin-Kelley VE (1990) Differing regulation and function of ICAM-1 and class-II antigens on renal tubular epithelial cells. Kidney Int 38: 417–425

Jones CL, Eddy AA (1992) Tubulointerstitial nephritis. Pediatr Nephrol 6: 572–586

Kelly CJ, Roth DA, Meyers CM (1991) Immune recognition and response to the renal interstitium. Kidney Int 31: 518–530

Kelley VR, Diaz-Gallo C, Jevnikar AM, Singer GG (1993) Renal tubular epithelial and T-cell interactions in autoimmune renal disease. Kidney Int 43 [Suppl 39]: S-108–S-115

Kirby JA, Rajasekar MR, Lin Y, Proud G, Taylor RMR (1993) Interaction between T lymphocytes and kidney epithelial cells during renal allograft rejection. Kidney Int 43 [Suppl 39]: S-124–S-128

Kleppel MM, Kashtan C, Santi PA, Wieslander J, Michael AF (1989) Distribution of familial nephritis antigen in normal tissue and renal basement membranes of patients with homozygous and heterozygous Alport familial nephritis. Lab Invest 61: 278–289

Krensky AM, Weiss A, Crabtree G, Davis MM, Parham P (1990) T-lymphocyte-antigen interactions in transplant rejection. N Engl J Med 322: 510–517

Lhotta K, Neumayer HP, Joannidis M, Geissler D, König P (1991) Renal expression of intercellular adhesion molecule-1 in different forms of glomerulonephritis. Clin Sci 81: 477–481

Li H-L, Hancock WW, Hooke DH, Dowling JP, Atkins RC (1990) Mononuclear cell activation and decreased renal function in IgA nephropathy with crescents. Kidney Int 37: 1552–1556

Lipman ML, Stevens C, Bleackley C, Helderman JH, McCune TR, Harmon WE, Shapiro ME, Rosen S, Strom TB (1992) The strong correlation of cytotoxic T lymphocyte-specific serine protease gene transcripts with renal allograft rejection. Transplantation 53: 73–79

Lloyd AR, Oppenheim JJ (1992) Poly's lament: the neglected role of the polymorphonuclear neutrophil in the afferent limb of the immune response. Immunol Today 13: 169–172

Marcussen N (1992) Atubular glomeruli and the structural basis for chronic renal failure. Lab Invest 66: 265–284

Marcussen N, Lai R, Solez S, Solez K (1991) Morphometric and immunohistochemical investigation of renal biopsies from patients with transplant ATN, native ATN, or acute graft rejection. XVI World Congress of Anatomic and Clinical Pathology, 27 June, 1991. Vancouver, Abstracts, p 20

Markovic-Lipkovski J, Müller CA, Risler T, Bohle A, Müller GA (1990) Association of glomerular and interstitial mononuclear leukocytes with different forms of glomerulonephritis. Nephrol Dial Transplant 5: 10–17

Markovic-Lipkovski J, Müller CA, Risler T, Bohle A, Müller GA (1991) Mononuclear leukocytes, expression of HLA class-II antigens and intercellular adhesion molecule 1 in focal segmental glomerulosclerosis. Nephron 59: 286–293

Markovic-Lipkovski J, Müller CA, Engler-Blum G, Strutz F, Kühn W, Risler T, Lauchart W, Müller GA (1992) Human cytomegalovirus in rejected kidney grafts; detection by polymerase chain rejection. Nephrol Dial Transplant 7: 865–870

Matsumura R, Kondo Y, Sugiyama T, Sueishi M, Koike T, Takabayashi K, Tomioka H, Yoshida S, Tsuchida H (1988) Immunohistochemical identification of infiltrating mononuclear cells in tubulointerstitial nephritis associated with Sjögren's syndrome. Clin Nephrol 30: 335–340

McCluskey RT (1992) Immunologic aspects of renal disease. In: Heptinstall RH (ed) Pathology of the kidney, 4th edn. Little, Brown, Boston, pp 169–260

Migliorisi G, Folkes E, Cramer EB (1988) Differences in the ability of neutrophils and monocytes to traverse epithelial occluding junctions. J Leukoc Biol 44: 485–492

Milks LC, Brontoli MJ, Cramer EB (1983) Epithelial permeability and the transepithelial migration of human neutrophils. J Cell Biol 96: 1241–1247

Miltenburg AMM, Meijer-Paape ME, Daha MR, van Bockel JH, Weening JJ, van Es LA, van der Woude FJ (1989) Donor-specific lysis of human kidney proximal tubular epithelial cells by renal allograft-infiltrating lymphocytes. Transplantation 48: 296–302

Molitoris BA (1992) The potential role of ischemia in renal disease progression. Kidney Int 41 [Suppl 36]: S21–25

Molitoris BA, Dahl RH, Falk SA (1989) Ischemia-induced loss of epithelial polarity. Role of the tight junction. J Clin Invest 84: 1334–1339

Mullin JM, Laughlin KV, Marano CW, Russo LM, Soler AP (1992) Modulation of tumor necrosis factor-induced increase in renal (LLC-PK$_1$), transepithelial permeability. Am J Physiol 263 (Renal Fluid Electrolyte Physiol 32): F915–F924

Müller GA, Müller CA, Markovic-Lipkovski J, Kilper RB, Risler T (1988) Renal major histocompatibility complex antigens and cellular components in rapidly progressive glomerulonephritis identified by monoclonal antibodies. Nephron 49: 132–139

Müller CA, Markovic-Lipkovski J, Risler T, Bohle A, Müller GA (1989) Expression of HLA-DQ, -DR, and -DP antigens in normal kidney and glomerulonephritis. Kidney Int 35: 116–124

Nádasdy T, Ormos J, Stiller D, Csajbók E, Szenohradszky P (1988) Tubular ultrastructure in rejected human renal allografts. Ultrastruct Pathol 12: 195–207

Nath KA (1992) Tubulointerstitial changes as a major determinant in the progression of renal damage. Am & Kidney Dis 20: 1–17

Noronha IL, Eberlein-Gonska M, Hartley B, Stephens S, Cameron JS, Waldherr R (1992) In situ expression of tumor necrosis factor-alpha, interferon-gamma, and interleukin-2 receptors in renal allograft biopsies. Transplantation 54: 1017–1024

Olsen S, Bohman S-O (1979) Renal allograft rejection. In: Johannesen JV (ed) Urogenital system and breast, McGraw-Hill, New York, pp 128–142 (Electron microscopy in human medicine, vol 9)

Olsen S, Hansen ES, Jepsen FL (1981) The prevalence of focal tubulo-interstitial lesions in various renal diseases. Acta Pathol Microbiol Scand [A] 89: 137–145

Olsen TS, Wassef NF, Olsen HS, Hansen HE (1986) Ultrastructure of the kidney in acute interstitial nephritis. Ultrastruct Pathol 10: 1–16

Ooi BS, Jao W, First MR, Mancilla R, Pollak VE (1975) Acute interstitial nephritis. Am J Med 59: 614–629

Park MH, D'Agati V, Appel GB, Pirani CL (1986) Tubulointerstitial disease in lupus nephritis: relationship to immune deposits, interstitial inflammation, glomerular changes, renal function, and prognosis. Nephron 44: 309–319

Pokorny GY, Sonkodi S, Iványi B, Mohácsi G, Csáti S, Iványi T, Ormos J (1989) Renal involvement in patients with primary Sjögren's syndrome. Scand J Rheumatol 18: 231–234

Pusey CD, Dash A, Kershaw MJ, Morgan A, Reilly A, Rees AJ, Lockwood (1987) A single autoantigen in Goodpasture's syndrome identified by a monoclonal antibody to human glomerular basement membrane. Lab Invest 56: 23–31

Raftery MJ, Seron D, Koffman G, Hartley B, Janossy G, Cameron JS (1989) The relevance of induced class-II HLA antigens and macrophage infiltration in early renal allograft biopsies. Transplantation 48: 238–243

Renkonen R, Turunen JP, Rapola J, Häyry P (1990) Characterization of high-endothelial-like properties of peritubular capillary endothelium during acute renal allograft rejection. Am J Pathol 137: 643–651

Rosenberg ME, Schendel PB, McCurdy FA, Platt JL (1988) Characterization of immune cells in kidneys from patients with Sjögren's syndrome. Am J Kidney Dis 11: 20–22

Sabadini E, Castiglione A, Colasanti G, Ferrario F, Civardi R, Fellin G, D'Amico G (1988) Characterization of interstitial infiltrating cells in Berger's disease. Am J Kidney Dis 12: 307–315

Savage COS, Pusey CD, Kershaw MJ, Cashman SJ, Harrison P, Hartley B, Turner DR, Cameron JS, Evans DJ, Lockwood CM (1986) The Goodpasture antigen in Alport's syndrome: studies with a monoclonal antibody. Kidney Int 30: 107–112

Savige JA, Gallicchio M (1991) The non-collagenous domains of the alpha 3 and 4 chains of type IV collagen and their relationship to the Goodpasture antigen. Clin Exp Immunol 84: 454–458

Schwartz MM, Fennell JS, Lewis EJ (1982) Pathologic changes in the renal tubule in systemic lupus erythematosus. Hum Pathol 13: 534–547

Seron D, Cameron JS, Haskard DO (1991) Expression of VCAM-1 in the normal and diseased kidney. Nephrol Dial Transplant 6: 917–922

Sherman LA, Chattopadhyay S (1993) The molecular basis of allorecognition. Annu Rev Immunol 11: 385–402

Sibley RK, Kim Y (1984) Dense intramembranous disease: new pathologic features. Kidney Int 25: 660–670

Solez K (1992) Renal complications of therapeutic and diagnostic agents, analgesic abuse, and addiction to narcotics. In: Heptinstall RH (ed) Pathology of the kidney, 4th edn. Little, Brown, Boston, pp 1369–1431

Solez K, Marcussen N, Flynn GJ, Beschorner WE, Racusen LC, Burdick JF (1992) Pathology of acute tubular necrosis and acute rejection. In: Burdick JF, Racusen LC, Solez K, Williams GM (eds) Kidney transplant rejection, 2nd edn. Dekker, New York, pp 373–392

Solez K, Axelsen RA, Benediktsson H, Burdick JF, Cohen AH, Colvin RB, Croker BP, Droz D, Dunnill MS, Halloran PhF, Häyry P, Jenette JCh, Keown PA, Marcussen N, Mihatsch MJ, Morozumi K, Myers BD, Nast CC, Olsen S, Racusen LC, Ramos EL, Rosen S, Sachs DM, Salomon DR, Sanfilippo F, Verani R, von Willebrand E, Yamaguchi Y (1993) International standardization of criteria for the histologic diagnosis of renal allograft rejection: the Banff working classification of kidney transplant pathology. Kidney Int 44: 411–422

Springer TA (1990) Adhesion receptors of the immune system. Nature 346: 425–434

Stachura I, Si L, Madan E, Whiteside T (1984a) Mononuclear cell subsets in human renal disease. Enumeration in tissue sections with monoclonal antibodies. Clin Immunol Immunopathol 30: 362–373

Stachura I, Si L, Whiteside T (1984b) Mononuclear-cell subsets in human idiopathic crescentic glomerulonephritis (ICGN): analysis in tissue sections with monoclonal antibodies. J Clin Immunol 4: 202–208

Strom TB (1992) Molecular immunology and immunopharmacology of allograft rejection. Kidney Int 42 [Suppl 38]: S182–187

Suranyi MG, Bishop GA, Clayberger C, Krensky AM, Leenaerts P, Aversa G, Hall BM (1991) Lymphocyte adhesion molecules in T-cell-mediated lysis of human kidney cells. Kidney Int 39: 312–319

Takaya M, Ichikawa Y, Shimizu H, Uchiyama M, Taniguchi R, Tomino Y, Arimori S (1985) T-lymphocyte subsets of the infiltrating cells in the salivary gland and kidney of a patient with Sjögren's syndrome associated with interstitial nephritis. Clin Exp Rheumatol 3: 259–263

Truong L, Mawad A, Haineed A, Farhood A (1991) Tubulitis in renal disease. Lab Invest 64: 99a

Truong LD, Farhood A, Tasby J, Gillum D (1992) Experimental chronic renal ischemia: morphologic and immunologic studies. Kidney Int 41: 1676–1689

Viergever PP, Swaak TJG (1991) Renal tubular dysfunction in primary Sjögren's syndrome: clinical studies in 27 patients. Clin Rheumatol 10: 23–27

von Willebrand E, Loginov R, Salmela K, Isoniemi H, Häyry P (1993) Relationship between intercellular adhesion molecule-1 and HLA class-II expression in acute cellular rejection of human kidney allografts. Transplant Proc 25: 870–871

Wilson CB (1991) Nephritogenic tubulointerstitial antigens. Kidney Int 39: 501–517

Wilson CB (1992) Immunologic aspects of renal disease. JAMA 268: 2904–2909

van der Woude FJ, Daha MR, Miltenburg AMM, Meyer-Paape ME, Bruyn JA, van Bockel HJ, van Es LA (1990) Renal allograft-infiltrated lymphocytes and proximal tubular epithelial cells: further analysis of donor-specific lysis. Hum Immunol 28: 186–192

Wuthrich RP, Jevnikar AM, Takei F, Glimcher LH, Kelley VE (1990) Intercellular adhesion molecule-1 (ICAM-1) expression is upregulated in autoimmune murine lupus nephritis. Am J Pathol 136: 441–450

Yard BA, Daha MR, Kooymans-Couthino, Bruijn JA, Paape ME, Schrama E, van Es LA, van der Woude FJ (1992) IL-1-alfa stimulated TNF-alfa production by cultured human proximal tubular epithelial cells. Kidney Int 42: 383–389

Yard BA, Kooymans-Couthino M, Reterink T, van der Elsen P, Paape ME, Bruyn JA, van Es LA, Daha MR, van der Woude FJ (1993) Analysis of T-cell lines from rejecting renal allografts. Kidney Int 43 [Suppl 39]: S-133–S-138

Yee J, Kuncio GS, Neilson EG (1991) Tubulointerstitial injury following glomerulonephritis. Semin Nephrol 11: 361–366

Yoshioka K, Morimoto Y, Iseki T, Maki S (1986) Characterization of tubular basement membrane antigens in human kidney. J Immunol 136: 1654–1660

Note Added in Proof: These recent papers contain further data in connection with tubulointerstitial inflammation:

Alpers ChE, Hudkins KL, Davis CL, Marsh ChL, Riches W, McCarty JM, Benjamin ChD, Carlos TM, Harlan JM, Lobb R (1993) Expression of vascular cell adhesion molecule-1 in kidney allograft rejection. Kidney Int 44: 805–816

Brady HR (1994) Leukocyte adhesion molecules and kidney diseases. Kidney Int 45: 1285–1300

Bruijn JA, Dinklo NJCM (1993) Distinct patterns of expression of intercellular adhesion molecule-1, vascular cell adhesion molecule-1, and endothelial-leukocyte adhesion molecule-1 in renal disease. Lab Invest 69: 329–335

Buysen JGM, Houthoff HJ, Krediet RT, Arisz L (1990) Acute interstitial nephritis: a clinical and morphological study in 27 patients. Nephrol Dial Transplant 5: 94–99

Couser WG, Johnson RJ (1994) Mechanisms of progressive renal disease in glomerulonephritis. Am J Kidney Dis 23: 193–198

D'Agati VD, Theise ND, Pirani CL, Knowles DM, Appel GB (1989) Interstitial nephritis related to nonsteroidal anti-inflammatory agents and β-lactam antibiotics: a comparative study of the interstitial infiltrates using monoclonal antibodies. Modern Pathol 2: 390–396

Giachelli CM, Pichler R, Lombardi D, Denhardt DT, Alpers ChE, Schwartz SM, Johnson RJ (1994) Osteopontin expression in angiotensin II-induced tubulointerstitial nephritis. Kidney Int 45: 515–524

Mampaso F, Sanchez-Madrid F, Marcen R, Molina A, Pascual J, Bricio T, Martin A, Alvarez V (1993) Expression of adhesion molecules in allograft renal dysfunction. Transplantation 56: 687–691

Ong ACM, Fine LG (1994) Tubular-derived growth factors and cytokines in the pathogenesis of tubulointerstitial fibrosis: implications for human renal disease progression. Am J Kidney Dis 23: 205–209

Pichler R, Giachelli CM, Lombardi D, Pippin J, Gordon K, Alpers ChE, Schwartz SM, Johnson RJ (1994) Tubulointerstitial disease in glomerulonephritis. Potential role of osteopontin (uropontin). Am J Pathol 144: 915–926

Rahilly MA, Fleming S (1993) The specificity of integrin-ligand interactions in cultured human renal epithelium. J Pathol 170: 297–303

Strutz F, Neilson EG (1994) The role of lymphocytes in the progression of interstitial disease. Kidney Int 45 [Suppl 45]: S-106–S-110

Takemura T, Yoshioka K, Murakami K, Akano N, Okada M, Aya N, Maki S (1994) Cellular localization of inflammatory cytokines in human glomerulonephritis. Virchows Archiv 424: 459–464

Atubular Glomeruli in Chronic Renal Disease

N. Marcussen

1 Background

Quite different types of renal injury often lead to a common histopathological pattern. The histopathological changes that may be detected are interstitial fibrosis, glomerulosclerosis, and tubular atrophy. Even after the original etiological factor has ceased to act, the chronic renal disorders may continue to progress toward the end stage (KLAHR et al. 1988). Several possible mechanisms responsible for progression and pathogenesis of chronic renal failure have been

Current Topics in Pathology
Volume 88, S.M. Dodd (Ed.)
© Springer-Verlag Berlin Heidelberg 1995

proposed. Some of these hypotheses have been limited to specific diseases while others have tried to cover all conditions leading to end-stage renal failure.

Bright was one of the first physicians who described a relationship between pathological features of chronic renal disease and the clinical abnormalities of the uremic state (BRIGHT 1827–1831). Oliver, using microdissection, showed that the nephrons in chronic renal failure comprised a very heterogeneous population: some nephrons were hypertrophied, some consisted only of a tubule (aglomerular tubule), and in others only the glomerulus remained (atubular glomerulus) (OLIVER 1939). At the time of Oliver's work it was thought that the diseased kidney was transformed into a disorganized population of nephrons which varied from one disease to another and that the functional disturbances were due to this heterogeneity. This view made it difficult to establish any general principle that might apply to all patients. BRICKER and others in the late 1950s formalized "the intact nephron hypothesis", which proposed that the majority of damaged nephrons do not contribute to the formation of urine (BRICKER et al. 1960; BRICKER and FINE 1981; FRANKLIN and MERRILL 1960). This shifted the emphasis away from the diseased tubular sites. The remaining functioning nephrons were exposed to a greater solute load and had to respond with increased tubular reabsorption or excretion.

The partial nephrectomy model has often been used to investigate chronic renal disease. Rats deprived of more than five sixths of their kidney mass invariably develop glomerulosclerosis and progressive renal failure (SHIMAMURA and MORRISON 1975). Based on this crucial observation, HOSTETTER et al. (1981) proposed that glomerular hyperfiltration might be responsible for progressive renal disease. The concept was generalized to cover several types of renal disease and to explain the final common pathway for deterioration of renal function. However, in a large number of renal diseases, renal function, measured by parameters dependent on glomerular filtration, is not as closely related to structural glomerular changes as to lesions of the tubulointerstitial system (BOHLE et al. 1987; SCHAINUCK et al. 1970). These apparently divergent facts and the original ideas and findings of Oliver led us to perform studies on the occurrence of disconnection between structurally relatively intact renal corpuscles and the tubular system (atubular glomeruli). Authors other than Oliver have assumed the existence of such a disconnection in specific renal diseases, because they demonstrated either a lack of proximal tubules in traditional histological sections or their occasional presence by nephron dissection (HEPTINSTALL et al. 1963; SCHAINUCK et al. 1970).

The atubular glomerulus is deprived of its connection to a proximal tubule. Perhaps the most correct term would be "atubular corpuscle", because it is Bowman's capsule that is not connected to the proximal tubule. However, in this chapter, and in accordance with general consensus, the term glomerulus is here applied for the corpuscle. The atubular glomeruli are difficult to demonstrate and quantitate. As in other situations involving relationships between structure and function, quantitative data are of the utmost importance. Although it is possible in a single section to evaluate whether the interstitial fibrosis is slight, moderate,

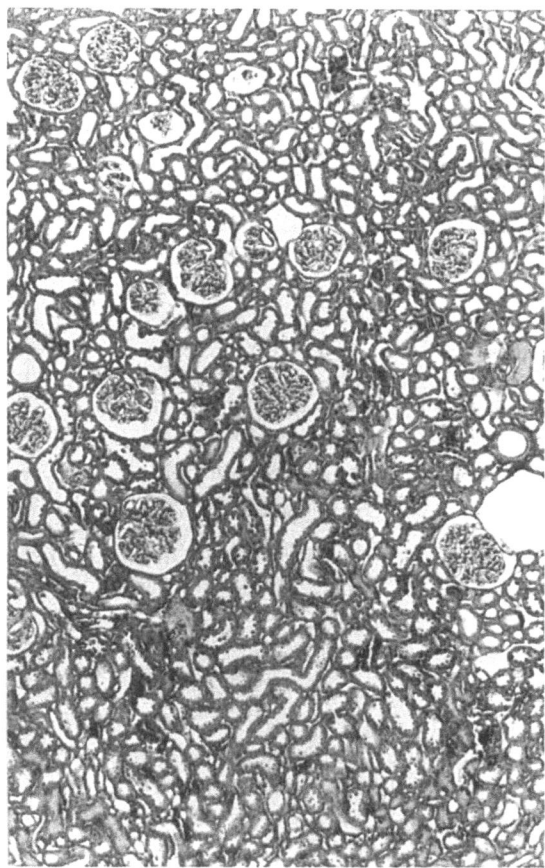

Fig. 1. Perfusion-fixed kidney from normal rat. Some events are detectable only in three dimensions; here no tubular pole is found in the glomeruli although the vast majority or all of the glomeruli have normal proximal tubules. PAS, × 80

or severe, these data do not correlate as well with renal function as absolute values for interstitial fibrosis. Furthermore, in a single section it is not possible to assess whether many atubular glomeruli are present or not (Fig. 1). Quantitative data are essential in the discussion of pathogenesis in chronic renal failure.

This chapter covers atubular glomeruli in chronic renal disease and emphasizes the importance of quantitative data obtained by stereological or morphometrical methods in the investigation of chronic nephropathy.

2 Methods for Direct Detection of Atubular Glomeruli

The detection of atubular glomeruli requires that the entire capsule of Bowman be investigated for the presence or absence of tubular connection. The three methods that have been used are: serial sections, microdissection, and scanning electron microscopy.

2.1 Serial Sections

Serial sections through a specimen containing cortical tissue enable the investigator to estimate by appropriate stereological methods the number or percentage of atubular glomeruli. It is necessary that the entire capsule of Bowman be included in the sections to determine whether a glomerulus is atubular or not. The number of sections required is high because the diameter of a human Bowman's capsule is on the order of 140 μm. The disector principle makes it possible to sample without bias and estimate the numer of glomeruli (STERIO 1984). The disector is a stereological sampling device with which randomly selected sections pairs are used to count and sample particles (glomeruli). In these correctly sampled glomeruli the connection between the glomerulus and the proximal tubule can be investigated, and in the same glomeruli the volume can be estimated using the Cavalieri principle. The Cavalieri method is based upon the estimation of the area of the glomerular profile in each section, summation of the areas, and multiplication of the sum with the mean section thickness, which is then equal to the volume of the glomerulus.

2.2 Microdissection

Microdissection has been widely used to study single nephrons under normal conditions and in various chronic and acute renal diseases (BAXTER 1965; BIBER et al. 1968; KRAMP et al. 1974; OLIVER 1953). With this technique, the part of the nephron that is damaged by the disease process can be identified, and it is possible to see whether a glomerulus is connected to a normal tubule or an atrophic tubule, or is atubular. With microdissection it is difficult to sample the nephrons without bias. If the tubules are atrophic, or if interstitial fibrosis is present microdissection may be complicated because there is considerable risk of artificial damage to the nephron due to mechanical manipulation and heavy maceration with strong acids or enzymes. The identification of glomeruli which have been disconnected from the tubules is difficult, because the attachment of the tubule to its corpuscle is weak and may fracture during dissection (OLIVER 1939).

2.3 Scanning Electron Microscopy

The technique of scanning electron microscopy may be used to investigate Bowman's capsule for the presence or absence of tubular connection. The major limitations of this method are the expensive equipment needed, the sampling of glomeruli, the difficulty in applying stereological methods, and the time required.

3 Evidence for the Presence of Atubular Glomeruli

3.1 Indirect Evidence

3.1.1 Light Microscopy

It is not possible in ordinary sections to see whether a glomerulus is atubular or not. However, some hints may be found. If the glomerulus is lying in a severely fibrotic area with no tubules present, or if the glomerulus is in a tumor-infiltrated area, the glomerulus may be atubular. In nonfunctioning renal allografts, glomeruli can be seen lying closely together surrounded by interstitial tissue where tubules are no longer detectable (BOHLE et al. 1989b). After single nephron obstruction, glomerular changes develop more slowly than the atrophy of the tubules; this shows that the glomerulus can exist despite severe atrophy of its connected tubule (TANNER et al. 1989). Also in renal cell carcinomas and other renal tumors, glomeruli are sometimes surrounded by tumor tissue where no tubules are seen, indicating that these glomeruli are atubular.

3.1.2 Enzyme- and Immunohistochemistry

Enzyme histochemistry is used to localize different tubular enzymes and to identify different tubular segments (BURSTONE 1962; JACOBSEN et al. 1967). These relatively simple stains have provided useful information regarding pathogenetic mechanisms, and the stains can be used to localize the target of injury (HOWIE et al. 1990; IVÁNYI and OLSEN 1991; MARCUSSEN 1991; SCHERBERICH et al. 1989). SCHERBERICH et al. (1989) have demonstrated by immunohistochemistry in end-stage chronic renal failure the existence of apparently enlarged glomeruli with increased enzyme activity surrounded by a completely destroyed tubular apparatus and fibrotic tissue. In cisplatin-induced nephropathy, after repeated staining of tubular enzymes only scattered clusters of intact staining tubules were found (MARCUSSEN and JACOBSEN 1992). Because no sclerotic glomeruli were found, these findings may indicate the presence of atubular glomeruli.

3.1.3 Functional Investigations

Raaschou noted that the inulin clearance fell in cases of chronic, nonobstructive pyelonephritis, although autopsy revealed completely intact glomeruli (RAASCHOU 1948). A poor correlation exists in various renal diseases between glomerular abnormalities and functional impairment, and SCHAINUCK et al. (1970) suggested, as one of several explanations, that atubular glomeruli might be present. In experimental chronic pyelonephritis in the rat the single nephron glomerular filtration rate has been found to be similar in diseased kidneys and in control kidneys, whereas the glomerular filtration rate was decreased in the pyelonephritic kidneys (LUBOWITZ et al. 1969). A selection bias for the sampling of nephrons may quite likely be present in such a study, but it does provide some evidence that the number of functioning nephrons is decreased. In rats with chemically induced chronic renal failure investigated by microdissection and micropuncture some nephrons had no filtration, and totally atrophic tubules were found attached to normal appearing glomeruli (KRAMP et al. 1974). At least functionally, this study also indicated the presence of atubular glomeruli.

DAMADIAN et al. (1965) investigated the presence of nonfunctioning, non-urine-forming nephrons in pyelonephritic kidneys in the dog. A double-marker technique was used for the simultaneous in vivo detection of glomerular perfusion and glomerular filtration. In the dogs 6–31% of the perfused glomeruli did not filter. In two of the dogs with pyelonephritis, microdissection of nephrons was performed and showed many glomeruli without tubular attachment. The authors concluded "that routine histologic examination of the diseased kidney cannot distinguish accurately between nephrons that contribute to urine formation and those that do not." In lithium-treated rats it was suggested that the decrease in the effective filtration fraction was caused by the presence of atubular glomeruli (CHRISTENSEN et al. 1992).

3.2 Direct Evidence

3.2.1 Stereological and Morphometrical Methods

Atubular glomeruli have been demonstrated in both man and animals with the use of serial sections (Table 1). Kidneys from 11 patients with chronic pyelonephritis were investigated by stereological methods (MARCUSSEN and OLSEN 1990).

Table 1. The percentages of atubular glomeruli and of glomeruli with normal proximal tubules in experimental and human chronic nephropathies

	Atubular glomeruli (%)	Glomeruli with normal proximal tubules (%)
Lithium nephropathy in rats (Marcussen et al. 1989)	36.1 ± 13.5[a]	48.1 ± 19.0
Cisplatin for 10 weeks (Marcussen and Jacobsen 1992)	35.3 ± 13.7	27.7 ± 15.7
Cisplatin for 10 weeks followed by 10 weeks without (Marcussen and Jacobsen 1992)	40.4 ± 18.2	28.7 ± 22.2
Human chronic pyelonephritis (Marcussen and Olsen 1990)	35.4 ± 19.6	49.9 ± 26.4
Human renal artery stenosis (Marcussen 1991)	52.0 ± 19.2	8.1 ± 13.1
Human long-term diabetes mellitus (Marcussen 1992)	8.8 ± 15.2	57.1 ± 31.0
Normal human kidneys (Marcussen 1991)	2.5 ± 4.8	95.9 ± 5.8

[a] Values and mean ± SD.

Glomeruli with little or no sclerosis were sampled without bias by the disector and followed in serial sections. Only 50% of the glomeruli were connected to normal proximal tubules, 35% were atubular, and the remaining 15% were connected to atrophic tubules. In the controls fewer than 3% of the glomeruli were not connected to normal proximal tubules. In areas of the kidneys with the most severe degree of fibrosis the number of atubular glomeruli was greatest. A negative correlation was found between the percentage of glomeruli without connection to normal proximal tubules and the volume fraction of proximal tubules.

In renal artery stenosis atrophy of the tubules takes place, whereby the glomeruli appear crowded in normal histological sections (HEPTINSTALL 1983). Using serial sections, the percentage of atubular glomeruli in 15 kidneys with stenosis of the renal artery was 52%, whereas only 8% were found to be connected to a normal proximal tubule; the remaining 40% were connected to an atrophic tubule (MARCUSSEN 1991).

Diabetic nephropathy has been investigated with regard to the presence of atubular glomeruli (MARCUSSEN 1992). Ten kidneys from patients with proteinuria and moderately elevated serum creatinine and seven kidneys from patients on dialysis were examined. Only glomeruli with no or slight glomerulosclerosis were sampled. In three of the kidneys from the dialysis group the glomerular sclerosis was so diffuse that these kidneys had to be excluded from further study. In the four kidneys from the group of patients on dialysis that were investigated, 14% of still-open glomeruli had not tubular connection. The ten kidneys from patients with comparatively well preserved function had 8–9% atubular glomeruli; a figure not significantly different from the 2–3% found in the controls. In the two groups, the volumes of glomeruli connected to atrophic tubules and of atubular glomeruli were lower than the volumes of the glomeruli with normal proximal tubules. The volume fractions of tubules were decreased and the relative interstitial volume increased, compared with the controls in both groups. The relative volumes were most increased, as expected, in the group on dialysis.

Atubular glomeruli have been demonstrated in different tubulointerstitial diseases in *experimental animals*. In rabbits with pyelonephritis, the proximal tubules had either disappeared or become atrophic and many tubules consisted only of a thickened basement membrane. Glomeruli had either a normal histological appearance or showed a dilated capsular space (HEPTINSTALL and GORRILL 1955). Bowman's membrane was frequently thickened. In some kidneys 6–7 months after initiation of pyelonephritis there were few glomerular changes, despite heavy loss of tubules (HEPTINSTALL et al. 1960). In another study, kidneys from rabbits were investigated by histology and microdissection 6 months after induction of pyelonephritis. Proximal tubules were not seen, and only a few collecting tubules were present. The glomerular changes varied from very small changes in the tuft to complete hyalinization (SHIMAMURA and HEPTINSTALL 1963). Nephron dissection revealed that the glomeruli had no attached proximal tubules, apart from short, thin strands seen on occasional glomeruli. Many

microdissected collecting ducts were also found to end blindly. By serial sectioning as well many glomeruli from rats who had had chronic pyelonephritis for
6 months were found to be without tubular connection (HEPTINSTALL et al.
1963).

In lithium-induced nephropathy in rats the atubular glomerulus was investigated by serial sectioning (MARCUSSEN et al. 1989, 1990, 1991). When lithium
was given to newborn rats for 8–16 weeks, about 35–40% of the glomeruli
became atubular and only one third were found to be connected to normal
proximal tubules (MARCUSSEN et al. 1989, 1991). The atubular glomeruli were
characterized by small volumes, amounting to only about one third of the
glomerular volume in control rats (Table 2). By contrast, the glomeruli connected to normal proximal tubules in lithium-treated animals were hypertrophic
(Fig. 2). A third of the glomeruli were seen to be connected to atrophic tubules.
The volumes of glomeruli connected to such atrophic tubules were in general
slightly larger than the atubular glomeruli (MARCUSSEN et al. 1991).

In cisplatin-induced nephropathy in adult rats the percentage of atubular
glomeruli correlated with the total dose of cisplatin when cisplatin was administered in repeated doses (MARCUSSEN and JACOBSEN 1992). After a total of
20 mg/kg body weight of cisplatin, administered over 10 weeks, 35% of the
glomeruli were found to be atubular. The percentage of atubular glomeruli
increased only slightly when the rats were followed up for a further 10 weeks
without administration of cisplatin (Table 1).

Table 2. The volumes of the different types of glomeruli in experimental lithium and cisplatin
nephropathy

	Volume of all glomeruli ($10^6\,\mu m^3$)	Volume of atubular glomeruli ($10^6\,\mu m^3$)	Volume of glomeruli with normal proximal tubules ($10^6\,\mu m^3$)
Lithium for 8 weeks followed by 8 weeks without (Marcussen et al. 1991)	0.64 ± 0.08	0.24 ± 0.08	1.04 ± 0.21
Lithium for 8 weeks followed by nephrectomy (total duration 16 weeks) (Marcussen et al. 1991)	0.62 ± 0.12	0.24 ± 0.07	1.78 ± 1.05
Cisplatin for 10 weeks (Marcussen and Jacobsen 1992)	0.89 ± 0.11	0.68 ± 0.11	1.27 ± 0.23
Cisplatin for 10 weeks followed by 10 weeks without (Marcussen and Jacobsen 1992)	0.85 ± 0.24	0.61 ± 0.14	1.33 ± 0.33

Values are means $\pm$ SD.

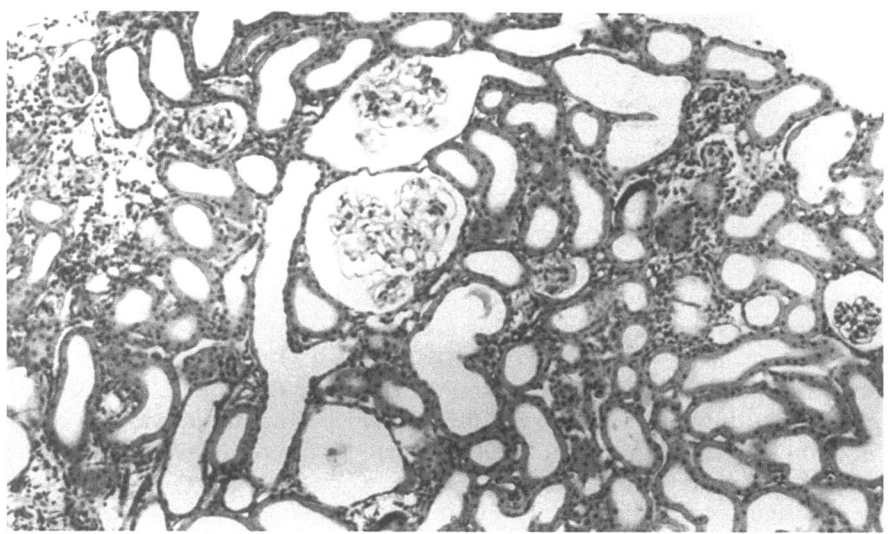

Fig. 2. Kidney from a rat treated with lithium from time of birth for 8 weeks, uninephrectomized and followed for 8 additional weeks. Two hypertrophic glomeruli are seen. Many small glomeruli (likely atubular) were present. PAS, × 250

3.2.2 Microdissection

The presence of the atubular glomerulus was demonstrated in 1939 by OLIVER, based on microdissection studies of human kidneys (OLIVER 1939). Some of the glomeruli described by Oliver had an avascular tuft, and some were described as small. Oliver also emphasized the heterogeneity of the nephrons and aglomerular tubules in chronic renal disease (OLIVER 1950; OLIVER et al. 1941). HEPTINSTALL and co-workers (1963) also demonstrated the presence of atubular glomeruli using microdissection, as described earlier. They also measured seven enzymes by histochemistry in microdissected control glomeruli and glomeruli from pyelonephritic scars; no difference in enzyme staining intensity was found. The atubular glomeruli from pyelonephritic scars, however, had higher DNA concentration, indicating cytoplasmic shrinkage rather than cellular loss.

3.2.3 Scanning Electron Microscopy

GIBSON et al. (1993) have used this technique to investigate the glomeruli and Bowman's capsule in glomerular cysts. He found that the atubular glomeruli consisted mainly of an atrophic tuft in a severely dilated Bowman's capsule. In Bowman's capsule, the authors often noted proteinaceous material and saw that parietal podocytes frequently lined the wall of the cysts; this is partly in contrast to the normal glomerulus, where the podocytes preferentially are found close to the vascular pole (GIBSON et al. 1992).

4 The Atubular Glomerulus

4.1 Light-Microscopic Features

The atubular glomerulus has open capillaries, but some atubular glomeruli may have narrow capillaries. The atubular glomeruli showed no alterations after hypertension in the rat (HEPTINSTALL et al. 1963). This is in contrast to the normal glomerulus, where nodular lesions have been described. No glomerular sclerosis was found in studies of atubular glomeruli in lithium-induced and in cisplatin-induced chronic nephropathy, where rats were treated with either of these drugs for up to 16 weeks.

No signs of damage were found in the juxtaglomerular apparatus in the atubular glomeruli in rat kidneys with experimental pyelonephritis or in glomeruli whose tubular continuity had been interrupted by localized traumatic lesions to the renal papilla (TRIBE and HEPTINSTALL 1964). Following adrenalectomy, the juxtaglomerular apparatus in the atubular glomeruli was capable of hyperplasia.

When lithium-treated rats received a high-protein diet, or when nephrectomy of the contralateral kidney was performed, atubular glomeruli were not able to respond to this extra load with an increase in glomerular volume (MARCUSSEN et al. 1991). Only glomeruli connected to normal proximal tubules were able to respond in this way.

4.2 Stereological Parameters Including Capillary Numbers

At the light-microscopic level the main stereological parameters that have been investigated in kidneys where atubular glomeruli are present include the glomerular volume and the number of capillaries. Investigations have also been performed in the interstitium and tubules. Changes in the tubules and interstitium are of course of the greatest importance in the investigation of atubular glomeruli, and some of these results will be dealt with later.

In lithium and cisplatin nephropathy the glomerular volumes have been estimated. The disector was used for the sampling of glomeruli and the Cavalieri principle for the estimation of individual glomerular volumes. With the same serial sections it was investigated whether Bowman's capsule was connected to a normal proximal tubule or not. From the volumes of individual glomeruli, the mean volume of normal glomeruli, atubular glomeruli, or hypertrophic glomeruli were calculated. In lithium nephropathy, the distribution of glomerular volumes revealed that all the small glomeruli were either atubular or connected to an atrophic tubule, and the large ones were all connected to a normal-appearing proximal tubule (Fig. 3). The atubular glomeruli had a volume about one third that of glomeruli in the controls. The hypertrophic glomeruli (connected to normal proximal tubules) had a volume up to five times normal values (Fig. 3). Nephrectomy and high-protein diet also increased the volume of glomeruli with normal tubular connections (Fig. 4). The volumes of atubular glomeruli in cisplatin nephropathy were about half those of control glomeruli. No hypertrophy of glomeruli with normal attachment to tubules was seen in the cisplatin-treated group. The number of glomeruli in cisplatin-induced nephropathy was not different from the number found in untreated rats. In cisplatin- and lithium-treated rats the decrease in proximal tubules and the increase in interstitial fibrosis paralleled the increase in the percentage of glomeruli with no or atrophic tubules (MARCUSSEN 1990; MARCUSSEN and JACOBSEN 1992).

The mean volume of glomeruli in a group of patients with pyelonephritis and in a control group was not significantly different. A much larger variation of the glomerular volumes was found in the pyelonephritic kidneys, and glomeruli without connections to normal proximal tubules had only half the volume of those connected to normal tubules (MARCUSSEN and OLSEN 1990). The mean volume of the atubular glomeruli in renal artery stenosis in man was only half of that of glomeruli with normal attachments to proximal tubules (MARCUSSEN 1991). The mean number of glomeruli was estimated in six kidneys with renal artery stenosis at $441\,000 \pm 194\,000$ and in eight controls at $564\,000 \pm 225\,000$; differences were not statistically significant.

An unbiased stereological method based on the topological definition of a capillary may be used to estimate the number of glomerular capillaries (NYENGAARD and MARCUSSEN 1993). In lithium nephropathy, the method was used to estimate the glomerular capillary number in glomeruli with no or atrophic tubules, in hypertrophic glomeruli connected to normal proximal tubules, and in control glomeruli. The estimation was done on 1-μm serial sections. On the same sections other stereological parameters were estimated as well. The mean number of capillaries in normal, hypertrophic, and atrophic glomeruli was $188 \pm 26 \ (\pm SD)$, 271 ± 32, and 65 ± 12, respectively (MARCUSSEN et al. 1994). The total length of the capillaries per glomerulus was increased in hypertrophic glomeruli and decreased in atrophic glomeruli compared with normal glomeruli. The **mean** capillary length of 48.3 ± 3.7 μm and 53.0 ± 11.3 μm in the hypertrophic and atrophic glomeruli, respectively, was significantly higher than the 41.0 ± 4.6 μm in the controls. This study demonstrates that hypertrophy of glomeruli takes place primarily by increase in the number of capillaries. The atubular glomeruli have a significantly lower capillary number, which could be due to atrophy or simply lack of development of these glomeruli. This last possibility exists, because the rats were treated with lithium from time of birth, and in the normal rat the capillary number per glomerulus is much lower at time of birth than later in its life (NYENGAARD 1993).

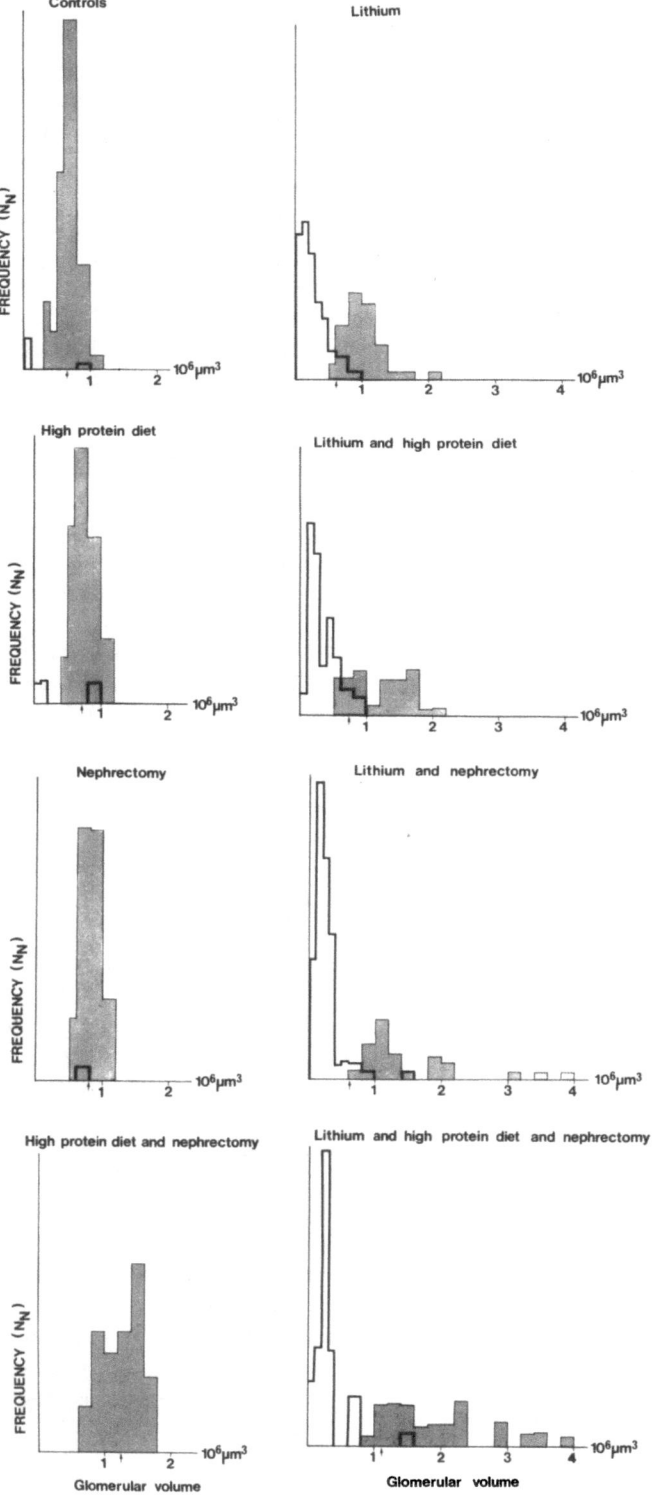

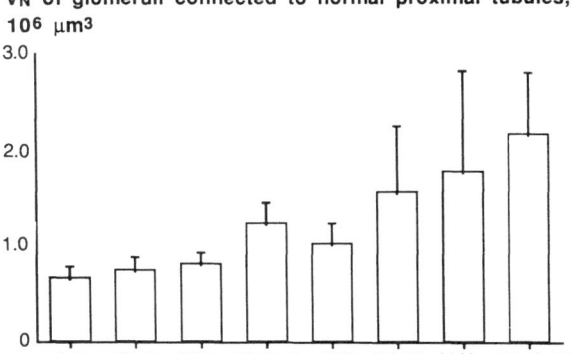

Fig. 4. Mean volume of glomeruli (*vN*) connected to normal proximal tubules in control rats (*C*) and in rats treated with lithium for 8 weeks from time of birth (*Li*). *HP*, rats received a high-protein diet from week 9 to 16; *Nx*, uninephrectomy at 8 weeks of age. The rats were followed up to 16 weeks of age. (Data from Marcussen et al. 1991)

4.3 Electron-Microscopic Features and Morphometry at the EM Level

Ultrastructurally, the atubular glomeruli in the lithium-treated rats seemed to have an increase in the mesangium and somewhat smaller capillary lumina, and the nuclei of the endothelial cells were in a more peripheral position than in the normal glomeruli, where the nuclei of the endothelial cells are positioned along the mesangial part of the capillary wall (Fig. 5). The urinary space was diminished. In some parts of the capillary loops the basement membrane seemed to be thickened and it appeared wrinkled in other parts. Ultrastructural morphometric investigation confirmed that the atubular glomeruli had increased volume fractions of mesangium, peripheral basement membrane, and epithelial cells. The absolute quantities were decreased, however, due to the decreased volume of these glomeruli (MARCUSSEN et al. 1990). The mean cross-sectional area of the capillaries was $40 \, \mu m^2$ in the controls and $24 \, \mu m^2$ in atubular glomeruli. The mean thickness of the peripheral basement membrane was increased by 31% in the atubular glomeruli. The foot processes had a normal mean width, but their distribution was abnormal with loss of the normal bimodality of the curve. In contrast, the relative volumes of mesangium and basement membrane were normal in the hypertrophic glomeruli. The relationships between changes in

◀───

Fig. 3. Distribution of glomerular volume in lithium nephropathy in rats. Newborn rats were treated with lithium for 8 weeks; thereafter they were nephrectomized or received a high-protein diet for an additional 8 weeks (*right column*). Non-lithium-treated rats represented in *left column*. *Open histograms*, show distributions of volumes of atubular glomeruli or glomeruli connected to atrophic proximal tubules; *hatched histograms*, show distributions of volumes of glomeruli connected to normal proximal tubules. *Arrows*, mean glomerular volume for all glomeruli. (Reproduced with permission from Marcussen et al. 1991)

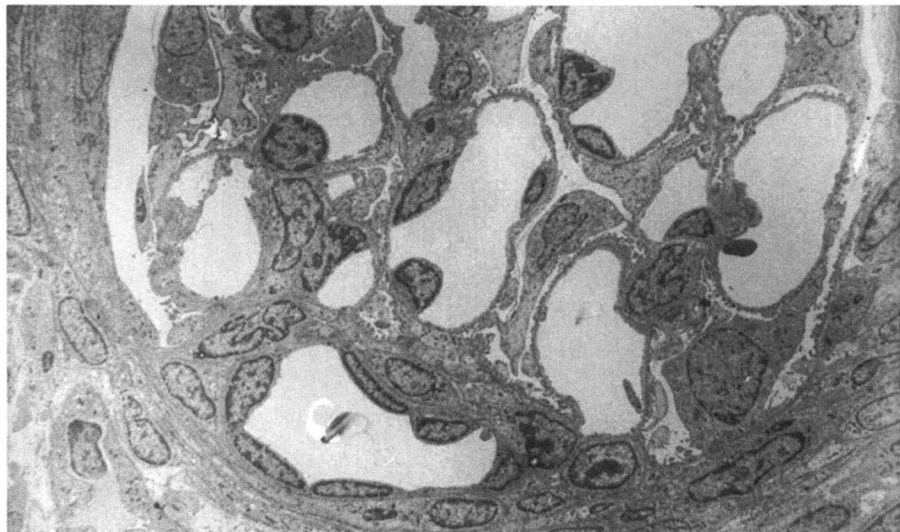

Fig. 5. Ultrastructural appearance of atubular glomerulus. × 3000

different structures was stereologically estimated as coefficients of isomorphic change (MARCUSSEN et al. 1990). The estimation of these coefficients revealed that in the hypertrophic glomeruli the peripheral filtration surface and capillary length were increased proportional to the increase in glomerular volume, whereas the atubular glomeruli showed a disproportionately large decrease in these structures. The disproportionate changes in the atubular glomeruli might be explained by the atubular glomeruli having no used for their filtration surface.

4.4 Pathogenesis of the Disconnection

The formation of atubular glomeruli must be due to tubular atrophy or destruction, although in lithium-induced nephropathy a developmental defect might be responsible, since in this model the toxic agent is administered in the immature, developing kidney. It is also likely that in kidneys of adult rats with toxic-induced injury the destruction of specific segments of the tubules is followed by retrograde tubular atrophy and breakdown, leading to the formation of atubular glomeruli. This was clearly illustrated by enzyme histochemical staining in the rats with cisplatin nephropathy, where the primary destruction of tubules after administration of two doses of cisplatin (4 mg/kg body weight) took place in the outer stripe of the outer medullary zone (MARCUSSEN and JACOBSEN 1992). After more doses of cisplatin the staining for tubular segmental markers (enzymes) became weak or absent in more proximal parts of the proximal tubules (Fig. 6), and after ten doses the tubules were severely decreased and only scattered clusters of tubular profiles showing enzyme staining were visible. These clusters of stained tubular profiles probably represented a few intact nephrons. The changes were accompanied by interstitial fibrosis. The changes involved the entire cortex, but the inner cortex was most severely affected; only 29% of the glomeruli were connected to normal proximal tubules in the inner one third of the cortex, compared with 48% in the outer one third of the cortex.

By light and electron microscopy and microdissection it was demonstrated that one day after blocking of the proximal tubule with wax all the proximal cells distal to the block were injured (EVAN et al. 1986). Atrophy of the tubules was seen 1 month after obstruction. The atrophy might be either due to a changed distribution of blood to the blocked tubule, causing local hypoxia, or disuse atrophy by interruption of normal activity. The proximal part of the blocked tubule also showed atrophic changes, but they developed more slowly than the distal changes (TANNER et al. 1989).

The mechanism by which glomerular cysts arise in kidneys in patients on chronic dialysis have been explained as tubular occlusion with fibrous thickening of Bowman's capsule (OGATA 1990). The tuft was described to disappear with increasing size of the cyst. However, it is important to realize that with increasing cyst size a small tuft will be seen in only a few sections, and in most sections through the cysts it will not be present. Serial sections are therefore required to prove the disappearance of the tuft.

Another possibility is that the primary injury is followed by interstitial changes, which could lead to focal ischemia and tubular atrophy. In human and experimental chronic pyelonephritis, Heptinstall suggested that the tubular destruction was the consequence of direct action of the causative micro-organism and associated inflammatory response (HEPTINSTALL et al. 1960; HEPTINSTALL 1983). Ischemia may also play a significant role, since renal artery stenosis is associated with severe tubular atrophy. In stenosis of the renal artery the tubular loss with "formation" of atubular glomeruli is due to ischemia affecting predominantly the proximal tubules (MARCUSSEN 1991). It is interesting, however, that in renal artery stenosis and in other diseases including primary glomerulonephritis a significant element of tubulitis is often found (IVÁNY et al. 1994). By tubulitis is understood the presence of inflammatory cells in the tubular wall. Tubulitis was originally described in acute pyelonephritis, acute interstitial nephritis, and acute renal allograft rejection. In renal artery stenosis, diabetic nephropathy, and IgA nephritis tubulitis is found predominantly in atrophic tubules (IVÁNYI et al. 1994). The tubular atrophy and interstitial inflammation is thought to be due to ischemia in nontubulointerstitial diseases (SILVA and HOGG 1989). Thus, tubulitis may, in renal artery stenosis, IgA nephritis, and diabetic nephropathy, be related to the ischemia, but it may also by itself lead to destruction of the tubules. It is more obvious that affected tubules may be destroyed by tubulitis in acute pyelonephritis and in acute allograft rejection. The importance of tubulitis for the glomerulo-tubular disconnection needs to be investigated further. Research into the relationship between the intertubular capillaries and the tubules may add

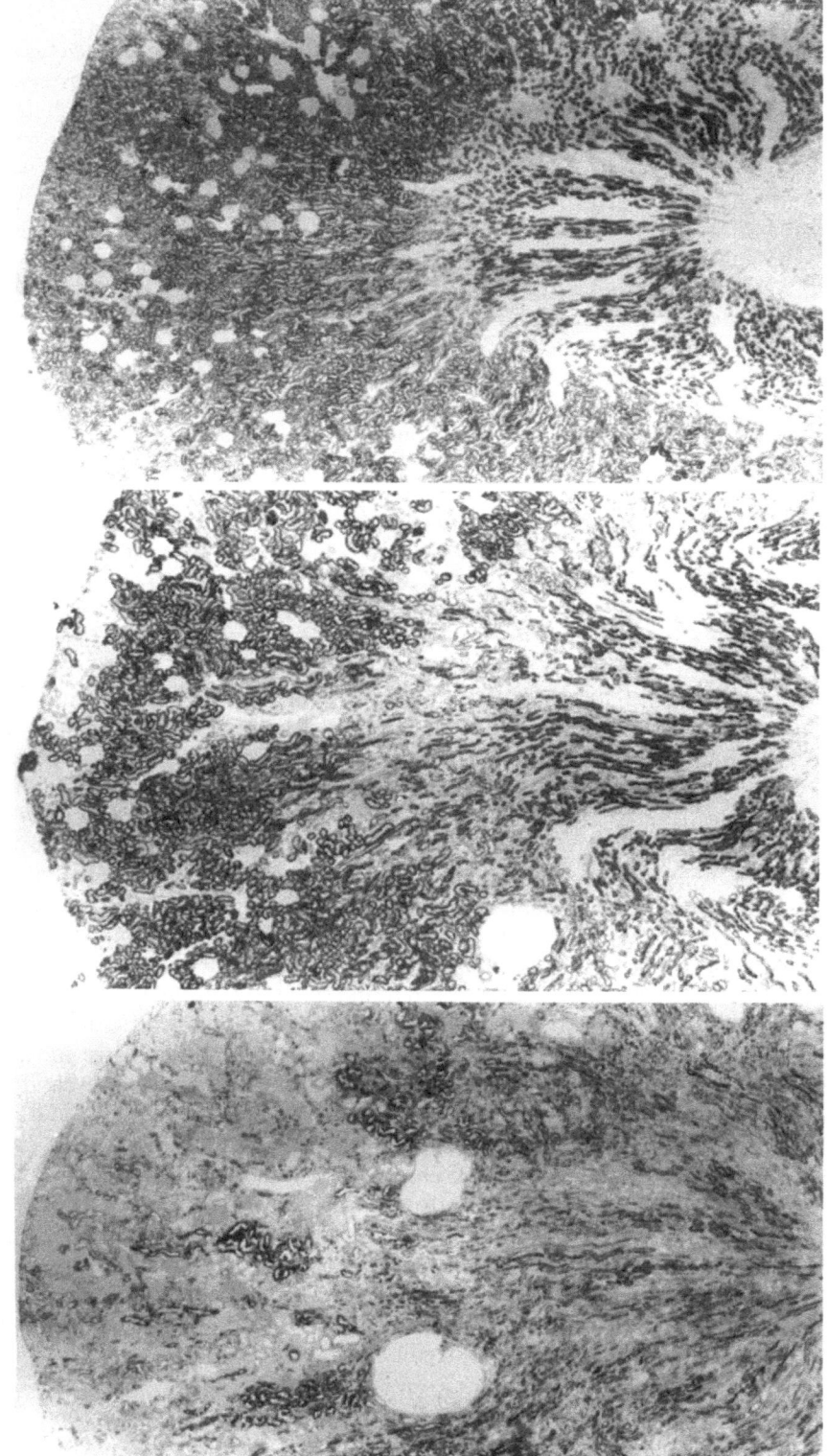

further to the knowledge of pathogenetic factors in the development of tubular atrophy (and the formation of atubular glomeruli).

5 Other Lesions in Chronic Nephropathy and Their Relation to Decreased Renal Function

5.1 Glomerular Lesions

Glomerulonephritis and diabetic nephropathy are common causes of glomerular injury. In several different types of glomerulonephritis no correlation has been described between the glomerular lesion and the glomerular filtration, and often renal failure is not present even in cases with quite marked changes in the glomeruli (BOHLE et al. 1977, 1989b; FISCHBACH et al. 1977; MUEHRKE et al. 1957; RISDON et al. 1968; ROSENBAUM et al. 1967; SCHAINUCK et al. 1970; WEHRMANN et al. 1990). Only in the final stage of glomerulonephritis with widespread glomerulosclerosis is the renal function decreased due to the lower number of functioning glomeruli.

Progressive glomerular injury has been studied in models of partial nephrectomy, in which one kidney and a part of the remaining kidney were removed. After 3/4 or 5/6 ablation in rats most of the animals developed hypertension, arteriolar lesions, and uremia accompanied by focal and later diffuse glomerular sclerosis (KOLETSKY and GOODSIT 1960; WOOD and ETHRIDGE 1933). Ultrastructurally, mesangial matrix increase was seen, eventually obliterating the capillary lumens (SHIMAMURA and MORRISON 1975). The extent of proteinuria and glomerulosclerosis was correlated with the amount of kidney mass removed (HOSTETTER et al. 1986). In a normotensive rat kidney model no glomerulosclerosis was present although significant proteinuria occurred, which is in accordance with the findings that proteinuria may take place from structurally intact glomeruli (BINDANI et al. 1990; YOSHIOKA et al. 1988). In studies on lithium-induced or cisplatin-induced chronic nephropathy, no glomerulosclerosis has been demonstrated up to 20 weeks after the beginning of treatment (MARCUSSEN 1990; MARCUSSEN et al. 1989, 1991; MARCUSSEN and JACOBSEN 1992). When one is evaluating glomerulosclerosis in experimental models, it should also be taken into consideration that most rat strains do develop glomerulosclerosis with ageing (COUSER and STILMANT 1975), and that the severity of glomerulosclerosis may be different in male and female rats and from one rat strain to another (GROND et al. 1986; HOEDEMAEKER and WEENING 1989). In human beings the

Fig. 6. Kidneys from normal rat (*right*), from rat treated with cisplatin for 6 weeks (*middle*), and from rat treated with cisplatin for 10 weeks (*left*). Sections are stained for succinate dehydrogenase (SDH), an enzyme that stains the entire nephron with some segmental differences in the normal kidney. In the 6-week group destruction of the S_3-segment of the proximal tubules is noted, whereas in the 10-week group only scattered clusters of tubules stain. SDH, $\times$ 15

percentage of sclerotic glomeruli is small up to the age of 50–60 years (Kaplan et al. 1975; Kappel and Olsen 1980; Smith et al. 1989). The glomerular volumes have a larger variation in many experimental and human tubulointerstitial diseases and in kidneys with adriamycin-induced glomerular changes than in the normal kidney (Marcussen et al. 1989, 1991; Marcussen 1990, 1991; Marcussen and Jacobsen 1992; Remuzzi et al. 1990).

Compensatory hypertrophy of the remaining renal tissue after renal ablation has been described, including overall hypertrophy of the glomeruli (Lombet et al. 1989; Marcussen et al. 1991; Olivetti et al. 1977; Seyer-Hansen et al. 1980, 1985). A circulating "renotropin" has been proposed to mediate the renal hypertrophy (Malt 1983; Yoshida et al. 1989). Factors other than the "renotropin" could be of importance in the chronically diseased kidney.

5.2 Tubular, Interstitial, and Vascular Lesions

Glomerular sclerosis has not often been considered an important component of the decreased renal function. Smith (1951) noted that in chronic pyelonephritis "the histological preservation of the glomeruli is not a reliable sign of function; patients may die in uraemia with completely normal-appearing glomeruli." Oliver used microdissection and showed that the tubular population in chronic renal disease is very heterogeneous (Oliver 1939; Oliver et al. 1941). Some tubules were greatly enlarged in diameter, while others were atrophic. The same changes did not necessarily extend throughout the entire length of the nephron. Both large and small glomeruli were found connected to atrophic tubules. Aglomerular tubules of all sizes, from long hypertrophic and hyperplastic units to short small ones, were also described by Oliver (1939). Kramp et al. (1974) investigated rat kidneys 3–4 weeks after injection of potassium dichromate and mercuric chloride. Using microdissection they demonstrated that atrophy was found in some proximal tubules and hypertrophy and hyperplasia in others. A combination of these alterations was found in many of the proximal convolutions of individual nephrons. The single nephron glomerular filtration rate showed very heterogeneous values.

In 70 patients with various, mainly glomerular diseases a good correlation was found between the decreased glomerular filtration rate and changes in the tubules and interstitium, regardless of the basic disease in the kidneys, but there was a poor correlation between a score for glomerular disease and insulin clearance (Schainuck et al. 1970). This close relationship between tubulointerstitial changes and renal function has been demonstrated in many different renal diseases, such as minimal change disease, membranoproliferative glomerulonephritis, membranous glomerulonephritis, proliferative glomerulonephritis, IgA nephritis, and diabetic glomerulopathy (Bader et al. 1980; Fischbach et al. 1977; Jepsen and Mortensen 1979; Mackensen-Haen et al. 1988).

Also in experimental chronic nephropathy, interstitial fibrosis and tubular atrophy have been considered a major factor in the decreased renal function. In partially obstructed kidneys in pigs, electron microscopy revealed that the proximal tubules had a reduced volume of mitochondria per millimeter of tubular length and a reduction in the surface density of basolateral interdigitations (MØLLER 1986; MØLLER et al. 1986). At an early stage, no changes were seen in the relationship between tubules and peritubular capillaries and no interstitial fibrosis. When the hydronephrosis became more severe the proximal tubules became more simplified ultrastructurally, and an increasing separation of tubules and peritubular capillaries due to interposition of interstitial tissue was seen. In experimental pyelonephritis in the rat and the rabbit the tubular atrophy was pronounced, with loss of most proximal tubules, but in most areas normal-appearing glomeruli were present (HEPTINSTALL et al. 1960, 1963; HEPTINSTALL and STRYKER 1962; SHIMAMURA and HEPTINSTALL 1963). The interstitium contained chronic inflammatory cells and in the later stages was fibrotic.

The description of tubulitis in other chapters of this book as a significant factor in many renal diseases is relatively new. Tubulitis may lead to tubular destruction and to the formation of atubular glomeruli, but in acute interstitial nephritis lymphocytes are often present between normal-appearing tubular epithelial cells, and only later does destruction of the basement membrane take place (OLSEN et al. 1986). The grade of tubulitis seems mainly to depend mainly upon the interstitial infiltration, whereas the degree of fibrosis does not seem to contribute significantly to the severity of tubulitis (IVÁNYI et al. 1994).

In rabbits who were fed lithium for 12 months the glomerulosclerosis occurred later than the tubulointerstitial changes. In rats a significant reduction in renal function was found after lithium treatment for 8 or 16 weeks after birth. In these rats the volume and the length of proximal tubules were reduced by about 60% and the volume of interstitial tissue increased by up to ten times normal values (CHRISTENSEN et al. 1982; OTTOSEN et al. 1984).

Progressive renal changes were found after repeated doses of cisplatin, accompanied by reduction in volume and length of proximal tubules and an increase in fibrosis compared with controls (MARCUSSEN 1990; MARCUSSEN and JACOBSEN 1992) (Fig. 7). After termination of injections of cisplatin, the volume of interstitial fibrosis remained unchanged, whereas the volume of proximal tubules decreased, further indicating that the tubular changes may progress without a further increase in fibrosis.

The S_3 segment of the proximal tubule is particularly susceptible to ischemic injury (VENKATACHALAM et al. 1978). In renal artery stenosis the atrophy and disappearance of tubules seems to affect mostly the proximal tubules (MARCUSSEN 1991). This has been demonstrated by immunostaining for epithelial membrane antigen (EMA); the majority of the atrophic tubules were positive for EMA, indicating origin from distal convoluted or straight tubules or collecting ducts (Fig. 8).

Between atrophic tubules, clusters of hypertrophic nephrons with increased concentration of tubular and glomerular marker proteins can be seen in end-

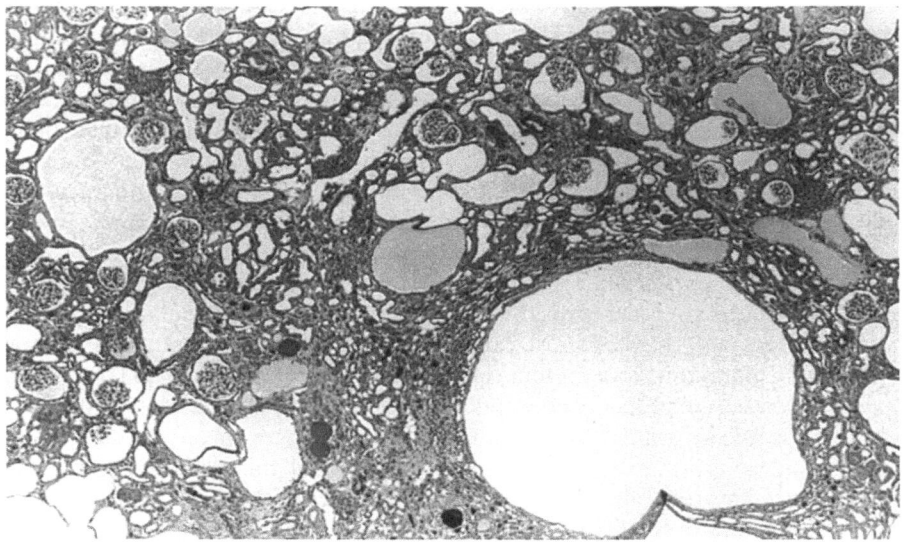

Fig. 7. Cisplatin nephropathy after 10 weeks of cisplatin treatment. Cysts, tubular dilation, atrophy of tubules, and increased interstitium are noted. PAS, × 60

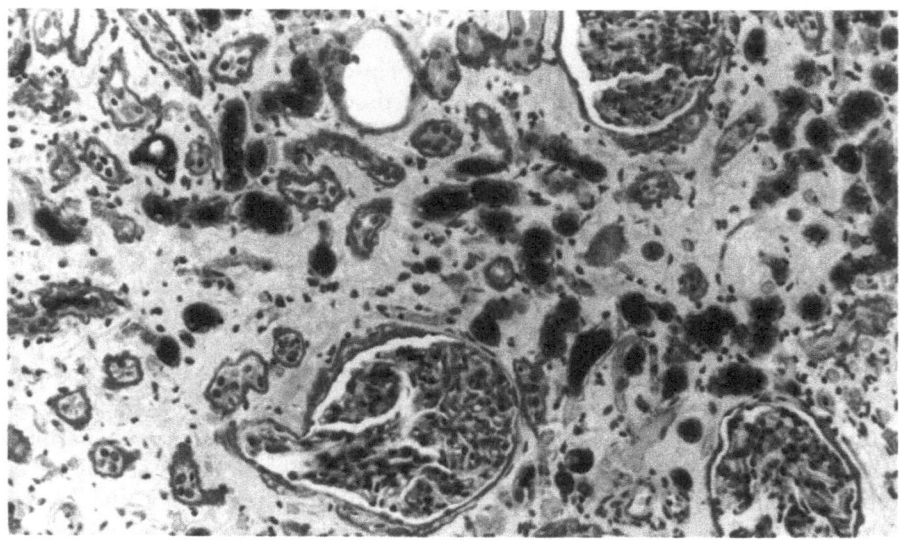

Fig. 8. Epithelial membrane antigen (EMA) staining of human kidney with stenosis of the renal artery. The tubules are atrophic and the majority stain wih EMA. This indicates that the atrophic tubules are of distal origin. PAS counterstain, × 300

stage renal disease. This indicates that the susceptibility of tubules and glomeruli to injury is variable, and some nephrons may escape destruction (SCHERBERICH et al. 1989).

6 The Importance of Atubular Glomeruli for Chronic Renal Failure

Atubular glomeruli cannot contribute to the formation of urine. A minute ultrafiltration could, however, be suggested as an explanation for the obvious dilation of Bowman's capsule in some atubular glomeruli in chronic nephropathies, such as renal artery stenosis and cisplatin-induced nephropathy in rats. The atubular glomerulus has open capillaries and may function as a vascular shunt, delivering blood to the intertubular capillary network. In this way the atubular glomeruli could contribute to the continuous function of the remaining intact nephrons.

Atubular glomeruli may provide an important explanation for the continuous decline in renal function in many chronic renal diseases. The presence of atubular glomeruli shows that factors other than glomerular sclerosis may explain the decline in kidney function. Atubular glomeruli also provide a good explanation for the correlation between the reduced volume and length of proximal tubules and the increased interstitial volume, on the one hand, and the reduced renal function on the other. The destruction and atrophy of proximal tubules lead to formation of atubular glomeruli. A relationship may then exist between atubular glomeruli and tubular atrophy if the glomerular alterations are only limited. Plasma urea correlated with the reduction in proximal tubules and with the increase in interstitial tissue (OTTOSEN et al. 1984). The percentage of glomeruli connected to normal proximal tubules was negatively correlated with the decrease in renal function measured by plasma urea or plasma creatinine (MARCUSSEN et al. 1989, 1991). However, the volume of interstitial fibrous tissue was also significantly related to the decrease in plasma creatinine when investigated using multiple regression analysis. The most significant correlations have been found between the percentage of glomeruli with normal proximal tubules and serum creatinine, and not between the proportion of atubular glomeruli and serum creatinine. This finding may be interpreted in the following way: Although a significant proportion of glomeruli are connected to atrophic tubules (Fig. 9), and thus theoretically may deliver some ultrafiltration, their contribution to the renal function is negligible and comparable to the function in atubular glomeruli (MARCUSSEN et al. 1991).

The atubular glomeruli may also explain the irreversibility of many chronic renal diseases. In renal artery stenosis their presence may have a special implication. In kidneys with stenosis of the renal artery, restoration of normal blood supply to the stenotic kidney is not always followed by improved renal function (BARAJAS et al. 1967; TEXTOR 1984). The irreversible cases are often seen when the renal changes are severe and may be explained by the presence of atubular glomeruli (MARCUSSEN 1991).

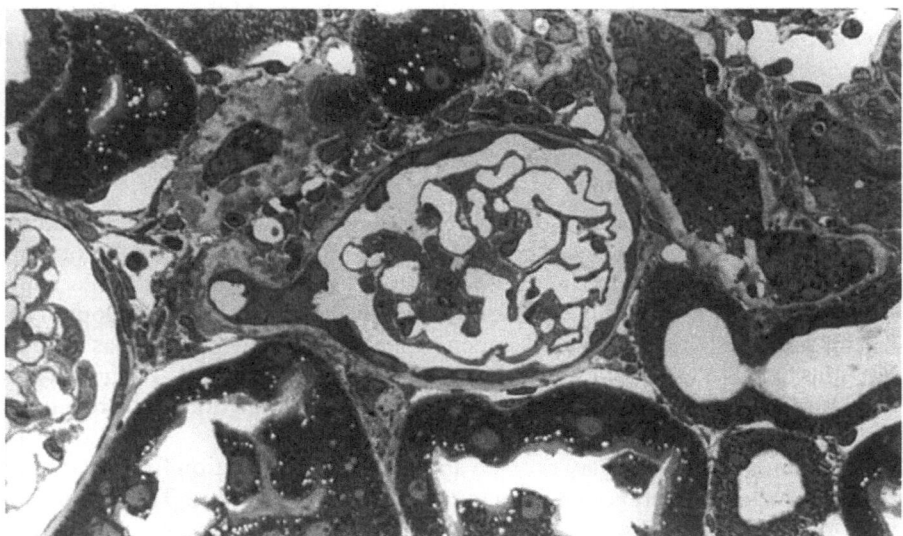

Fig. 9. Glomerulus connected to severely atrophic tubule in kidney from a rat treated with cisplatin for 10 weeks. Toluidine blue, × 750

It has not yet been proven that more atubular glomeruli are formed after termination of the initial disease process. If additional atubular glomeruli are formed, this may provide a direct explanation for the progression of chronic renal failure. It might, however, be difficult to demonstrate formation of extra atubular glomeruli, because many disease processes have an element of inflammatory reaction that does not stop when the initiating mechanism is removed. The present data show that when the disease is severe many atubular glomeruli are present. These findings have lead to the proposal of the following mechanisms to explain the progression of chronic renal failure (MARCUSSEN 1992): In primary glomerular diseases (glomerulonephritis, diabetic glomerulopathy), and perhaps also renal ablation and hypertension, the primary disease process or glomerular hyperfunction and hypertrophy are responsible for the progressive glomerulosclerosis, leading to continuous deterioration of renal function. An additional contribution to the progression of renal failure in these diseases may be tubulointerstitial changes. In nonglomerular diseases (pyelonephritis, toxic tubulointerstitial nephritis, and ischemic diseases) the primary disease process affects the tubules and interstitium with the formation of atubular glomeruli.

Some lines of evidence suggest that the atubular glomeruli continue to function as a shunt in the chronic diseased kidney and therefore are not eliminated. This conclusion is supported by the findings of atubular glomeruli in human renal diseases such as chronic pyelonephritis and renal artery stenosis. Rats treated with cisplatin for up to 12 weeks had nearly normal numbers of glomeruli and over one third of these were atubular; no sclerotic lesions were observed in the atubular glomeruli (MARCUSSEN 1990). In lithium-treated rats only minor ultrastructural changes were found; a fact that might indicate a continuous increase in the mesangium of the atubular glomeruli. Whether this mesangial increase leads to glomerulosclerosis is not known (MARCUSSEN et al. 1990). Elimination of atubular glomeruli could take place by continuous shrinkage of their volume with decreases in capillary size and number, ending in the collapse of capillaries.

7 The Significance of Atubular Glomeruli for Other Hypotheses of Chronic Renal Failure

Many hypotheses have been proposed to explain the progression and pathogenesis of chronic renal failure. They will be mentioned briefly here, because they may be of importance for the understanding of the disease process in chronic nephropathy and may play an additional role along with the atubular glomeruli and hyperfiltration theories.

7.1 The Intact Nephron Hypothesis

The intact nephron hypothesis was originally proposed by Bricker, who suggested that in chronic renal diseases the majority of nephrons that contribute to renal function behave as if they were normal, i.e., with preserved glomerulotubular balance (BRICKER 1969; BRICKER and FINE 1981). If structural damage impairs some glomerular or tubular functions in individual nephrons, there will be proportional changes in other functions of the same nephrons. MACKENSEN-HAEN et al. (1992) found that compensatory hypertrophy in man occurs only when more than 90% of the glomeruli are hyalinized. This is in contrast to the intact nephron hypothesis. However, in our own studies of atubular glomeruli in chronic pyelonephritis and renal artery stenosis, the glomeruli with normal proximal tubules were larger than atubular glomeruli and often had a larger volume than the normal glomeruli (MARCUSSEN 1992). The presence of atubular glomeruli and the distribution of the glomerular volumes in these chronic nephropathies gives some support to the hypothesis proposed by Bricker.

7.2 Tubulo-glomerular Feedback Mechanism

THURAU and SCHNERMANN (1965) demonstrated that an increased sodium chloride concentration at the macula densa results in a decrease in the filtration rate. The progressive interstitial fibrosis in chronic renal failure may lead to atrophy of the tubules, with disturbed function and impaired reabsorptive capacity for sodium chloride (Mackensen-Haen et al. 1981). Due to the tubulo-glomerular feedback, this would lead to a decrease in filtration. In a later study it was suggested that the mechanism most likely is active only when slight interstitial fibrosis and tubular atrophy are present (Bohle et al. 1987). It is possible that this mechanism is active along with the impairment of renal function due to the presence of atubular glomeruli.

7.3 Obliteration of Postglomerular Capillaries

Narrowing of the postglomerular capillaries in chronically diseased kidneys due to increased cortical interstitium may lead to a reduced blood flow in glomeruli and reduced glomerular filtration rate (Bohle et al. 1977, 1987). Bohle et al. (1987) have suggested that this mechanism is working when the interstitial fibrosis is severe and that it is an important factor in the decreased renal function of most glomerulopathies and tubulointerstitial diseases (Bohle et al. 1989b, 1990). However, morphometrical investigation of chronic obstructive nephropathy has shown that the relative volume of interstitial fibrosis was increased about three fold before any reduction in the length or surface area of the capillaries in the cortex was to be found (Møller 1986). The obliteration of postglomerular capillaries may or may not have an impact on the glomerular filtration. However, it could affect the tubules and their function by increasing the distance from the tubular cells to the blood supply.

7.4 Glomerular Hyperfiltration

The hypothesis that glomerular hyperfiltration is responsible for the progression of chronic renal failure is the one most discussed at the moment. It is based on altered function of the remaining glomeruli, and it suggests that the initial pathogenetic insults result in a reduced number of functioning glomeruli. The altered function, including hyperfiltration, and structural compensatory changes in the remnant glomeruli lead to glomerular damage and to segmental, and later global glomerulosclerosis (Brenner et al. 1982; Hostetter et al. 1981, 1982; Klahr et al. 1988; Olson et al. 1982).

The development of glomerulosclerosis after renal ablation has been proposed to be due to an increase in glomerular capillary pressure and flow, which results in an increased accumulation of macromolecules in the mesangium (Olson et al. 1982). Epithelial cell defects in the hypertrophic glomeruli may also play a role (Fries et al. 1989). Shea et al. (1978) suggested that glomerulosclerosis is a consequence of the glomerular hypertrophy. Others have shown, in rats, that glomerular damage became apparent only when elevated intracapillary pressure and increased glomerular volume were superimposed on hyperfiltration (TAPIA et al. 1990).

When many atubular glomeruli are present the remaining intact nephrons may hypertrophy, including the glomeruli. This may theoretically lead to secondary glomerulosclerosis of the glomeruli connected to normal tubules. This combination of lesions has not been described in lithium- or cisplatin-induced nephropathy in short-term studies in rats, but studies of longer duration may yield different results.

The hyperfiltration mechanism has been proposed to account for the pathogenesis of glomerulosclerosis in ageing, in renal ablation, and in intrinsic renal diseases (BRENNER et al. 1982). It should be noted that evidence for the role of glomerular hyperfiltration comes almost exclusively from studies in rats (WALSER 1988). The risk of developing significant deterioration of renal function after unilateral nephrectomy has been shown to be nil by some authors (ANDERSON et al. 1991), whereas others have found increased serum creatinine and mild proteinuria (OLSON and HEPTINSTALL 1988).

7.5 Tamm-Horsfall Protein

Tamm-Horsfall protein is normally present in the distal straight tubule and the first part of the distal convoluted tubule (KUMAR and MUCHMORE 1990). The protein may penetrate into the interstitium in different tubulointerstitial diseases, for example, infection caused by obstruction and vesicourethral reflux (HOSTETTER et al. 1988) and rejecting renal allografts (COHEN et al. 1984). It has been speculated that Tamm-Horsfall protein is liberated into the systemic circulation, thereby provoking antibody formation which could promote the progression of renal disease (HOSTETTER et al. 1988). Whether this mechanism is related to the presence of atubular glomeruli is unknown.

8 Morphometry in the Investigation of Atubular Glomeruli and Chronic Nephropathy

Morphometrical or stereological methods have gained importance in the investigation of chronic renal failure and of atubular glomeruli. These methods allow quantitation of the changes that take place in the chronically diseased kidney. These changes may then be compared with functional parameters, and important relationships may be detected. The use of morphometrical methods also provides us with some information that may not be detected in any other way (GUNDERSEN et al. 1988a,b). The atubular glomerulus can be identified only using serial sections, microdissection, or scanning electron microscopy. Determination of the exact volume of these glomeruli and, especially, of the distribution of the glomerular volumes requires unbiased stereological methods. Biased methods based on measurements of diameter or area of glomeruli may give results that are erroneous and may lead to wrong conclusions. Investigations of relationships between different renal structures may also require unbiased methods; an example might be the investigation of interactions between intertubular capillaries and the tubules. If stereological methods are not used it is impossible to estimate the number of glomeruli or nephrons in the kidney. In cases with glomerulosclerosis the counting of the number of glomeruli may prove to be very important.

9 Summary

The pathological changes in chronic renal failure are heterogeneous and may depend on the primary disease process. Renal function is better correlated with tubular and interstitial changes than with glomerular changes detectable in simple two-dimensional sections.

Atubular glomeruli have been demonstrated in many tubulointerstitial disorders. They constitute a significant portion of the glomerular population in some chronic renal diseases. The atubular glomeruli are generally small, but they have open capillaries and minor ultrastructural changes. The number of capillaries is decreased. Glomeruli connected to normal proximal tubules have volumes at the normal level or above. They have not been shown to be eliminated.

The presence of atubular glomeruli may explain the correlation between the volume of proximal tubules and the volume of interstitium, on the one hand, and altered renal function on the other. The presence of atubular glomeruli could explain the irreversibility of chronic renal diseases.

It is likely that interstitial fibrosis and tubular atrophy in themselves contribute to the decrease in renal function of both glomerular and nonglomerular renal diseases. In glomerular diseases, the glomerular lesion and hyperfiltration may play the major part in the pathogenesis of the deterioration of renal function. The available evidence points toward glomerulo-tubular disconnection as an important and common cause of progression and irreversibility of chronic renal diseases. It provides a simple explanation for the common observation of severely reduced kidney function and mostly normal-looking glomeruli—at least in two dimensions.

References

Anderson RG, Bueschen AJ, Lloyd LK, Dubovsky EV, Burns JR (1991) Short-term and long-term changes in renal function after donor nephrectomy. J Urol 145: 11–13
Bader R, Bader H, Grund KE, Mackensen-Haen S, Christ H, Bohle A (1980) Structure and function of the kidney in diabetic glomerulosclerosis. Correlations between morphological and functional parameters. Pathol Res Pract 167: 204–216

Barajas L, Lupu AN, Kaufman JJ, Latta H, Maxwell MH (1967) The value of the renal biopsy in unilateral renovascular hypertension. Nephron 4: 231–247

Baxter TJ (1965) Cysts arising in the renal corpuscle. A microdissection study. Arch Dis Child 40: 455–463

Biber TUL, Mylle M, Baines AD, Gottschalk CW, Oliver JR, MacDowell MC (1968) A study by micropuncture and microdissection of acute renal damage in rats. Am J Med 44: 664–705

Bidani AK, Mitchell KD, Schwartz MM, Navar LG, Lewis EJ (1990) Absence of glomerular injury or nephron loss in a normotensive rat remnant kidney model. Kidney Int 38: 28–38

Bohle A, Bader R, Grund KE, Mackensen S, Neunhoeffer J (1977) Serum creatinine concentration and renal interstitial volume. Analysis of correlations in endocapillary (acute) glomerulonephritis and in moderately severe mesangioproliferative glomerulonephritis. Virchows Arch [A] 375: 87–96

Bohle A, Mackensen-Haen S, von Gise H (1987) Significance of tubulointerstitial changes in the renal cortex for the excretory function and concentration ability of the kidney: a morphometric contribution. Am J Nephrol 7: 421–433

Bohle A, Gärtner H-V, Laberke H-G, Krück F (1989a) The kidney. Structure and function, 1st edn. Schattauer, Stuttgart, p 1

Bohle A, Kressel G, Müller CA, Müller GA (1989b) The pathogenesis of chronic renal failure. Pathol Res Pract 185: 421–440

Bohle A, Mackensen-Haen S, von Gise H, Grund K-E, Wehrmann M, Batz C, Bogenschütz O, Schmitt H, Nagy J, Muller C, Müller G (1990) The consequences of tubulo-interstitial changes for renal function in glomerulopathies. A morphometric and cytological analysis. Pathol Res Pract 186: 135–144

Brenner BM, Meyer TW, Hostetter TH (1982) Dietary protein intake and the progressive nature of kidney disease: the role of hemodynamically mediated glomerular injury in the pathogenesis of progressive glomerular sclerosis in aging, renal ablation, and intrinsic renal disease. N Engl J Med 307: 652–659

Bricker NS (1969) Editorial: On the meaning of the intact nephron hypothesis. Am J Med 46: 1–11

Bricker NS, Fine LG (1981) The renal response to progressive nephron loss. In: Brenner BM, Rector FC Jr (eds) The kidney. Saunders, Philadelphia, pp 1056–1096

Bricker NS, Morrin PAF, Kime SW (1960) The pathologic physiology of chronic Bright's disease. An exposition of the "intact nephron hypothesis." Am J Med 28: 77–98

Bright R (1827–1831) A report of medical cases, selected with a view to illustrating the symptoms and cure of diseases by a reference to morbid anatomy, vol 1. Longmans, Rees, Orme, Brown and Green, London

Burstone MS (1962) Enzyme histochemistry. Academic, New York

Christensen S, Ottosen PD, Olsen S (1982) Severe functional and structural changes caused by lithium in the developing rat kidney. Acta Pathol Microbiol Immunol Scand [A] 90: 257–267

Christensen S, Marcussen N, Petersen JS, Shalmi M (1992) Effects of uninephrectomy and high-protein feeding on lithium-induced chronic renal failure in rats. Renal Physiol Biochem 15: 141–149

Cohen AH, Border WA, Rajfer J, Dumke A, Glassock RJ (1984) Interstitial Tamm-Horsfall protein in rejecting renal allografts. Identification and morphologic pattern of injury. Lab Invest 50: 519–525

Couser WG, Stilmant MM (1975) Mesangial lesions and focal glomerular sclerosis in the aging rat. Lab Invest 33: 491–501

Damadian RV, Shwayri E, Bricker NS (1965) On the existence of non-urine-forming nephrons in the diseased kidney of the dog. J Lab Clin Med 65: 26–39

Evan AP, Tanner GA, Blomgren P, Knopp LC (1986) Proximal tubule morphology after single nephron obstruction in the rat kidney. Kidney Int 30: 818–827

Fischbach H, Mackensen S, Grund K-E, Kellner A, Bohle A (1977) Relationship between glomerular lesions, serum creatinine and interstitial volume in membrano-proliferative glomerulonephritis. Klin Wochenschr 55: 603–608

Franklin SS, Merrill JP (1960) The kidney in health; the nephron in disease. Am J Med 28: 1–7

Fries JWU, Sandstrom DJ, Meyer TW, Rennke HG (1989) Glomerular hypertrophy and epithelial cell injury modulate progressive glomerulosclerosis in the rat. Lab Invest 60: 205–218

Gibson IW, Downie I, Downie TT, Han SW, More IAR, Lindop GBM (1992) The parietal podocyte: a study of the vascular pole of the human glomerulus. Kidney Int 41: 211–214

Gibson IW, More IAR, Lindop GBM (1993) Acquired glomerulocystic change in human kidney: a scanning electron microscope study. EDTA/EDTNA congress, Glasgow, p 23 (abstract)

Grond J, Beukers JYB, Schilthuis MS, Weening JJ, Eleman JD (1986) Analysis of renal structural and functional features in two rat strains with a different susceptibility to glomerular sclerosis. Lab Invest 54: 77–83

Gundersen HJG, Bagger P, Bendtsen TF, Evans SM, Korbo L, Marcussen N, Møller A, Nielsen K, Nyengaard JR, Pakkenberg B, Sørensen FB, Vesterby A, West MJ (1988a) The new stereological tools: disector, fractionator, nucleator and point-sampled intercepts and their use in pathological research and diagnosis. APMIS 96: 857–881

Gundersen HJG, Bendtsen TF, Korbo L, Marcussen N, Møller A, Nielsen K, Nyengaard JR,Pakkenberg B, Sørensen FB, Vesterby A, West MJ (1988b) some new, simple and efficient stereological methods and their use in pathological research and diagnosis. APMIS 96: 379–394

Heptinstall RH (1983) Pathology of the kidney. Little, Brown, Boston Heptinstall RH, Gorrill RH (1955) Experimental pyelonephritis and its effect on the blood pressure. J Pathol Bacteriol 69: 191–198

Heptinstall RH, Stryker M (1962) Experimental pyelonephritis. A study of the susceptibility of the hypertensive kidney to infection in the rat. Bull Johns Hopkins Hosp 111: 292–306

Heptinstall RH, Michaels L, Brumfitt W (1960) Experimental pyelonephritis: the role of arterial narrowing in the production in the kidney of chronic pyelonephritis. J Pathol Bacteriol 80: 249–258

Heptinstall RH, Kissane JM, Still WJS (1963) Experimental pyelonephritis. Morphology and quantitative histochemistry of glomeruli in pyelonephritic scars in the rat. Bull Johns Hopkins Hosp 112: 299–311

Hoedemaeker PJ, Weening JJ (1989) Relevance of experimental models for human nephropathology. Kidney Int 35: 1015–1025

Hostetter TH, Olson JL, Rennke HG, Venkatachalam MA, Brenner BM (1981) Hyperfiltration in remnant nephrons: a potentially adverse response to renal ablation. Am J Physiol 241 (Renal Fluid Electrolyte Physiol 10): F85–F93

Hostetter TH, Rennke HG, Brenner BM (1982) Compensatory renal hemodynamic injury: a final common pathway of residual nephron destruction. Am J Kidney Dis I: 310–314

Hostetter TH, Meyer TW, Rennke HG, Brenner BM (1986) Chronic effects of dietary protein in the rat with intact and reduced renal mass. Kidney Int 30: 509–517

Hostetter TH, Nath KA, Hostetter MK (1988) Infection-related chronic interstitial nephropathy. Semin Nephrol 8: 11–16

Howie AJ, Gunson BK, Sparke J (1990) Morphometric correlates of renal exretory function. J Pathol 160: 245–253

Iványi B, Olsen TS (1991) Immunohistochemical identification of tubular segments in percutaneous renal biopsies. Histochemistry 95: 351–356

Iványi B, Olsen S, Marcussen N (1994) Tubulitis in primary vascular and glomerular renal disease. (submitted)

Jacobsen NO, Jørgensen F, Thomsen ÅC (1967) On the localization of some phosphatases in three different segments of the proximal tubules in the rat kidney. J Histochem Cytochem 15: 456–469

Jepsen FL, Mortensen PB (1979) Interstitial fibrosis of the renal cortex in minimal change lesion and its correlation with renal function. A quantitative study. Virchows Arch [A] 383: 265–270

Kaplan C, Pasternack B, Shah H, Gallo G (1975) Age-related incidence of sclerotic glomeruli in human kidneys. Am J Pathol 80: 227–234

Kappel B, Olsen S (1980) Cortical interstitial tissue and sclerosed glomeruli in the normal human kidney, related to age and sex. A quantitative study. Virchows Arch [A] 387: 271–277

Klahr S, Purkerson ML, Harris K (1988) Mechanisms of progressive renal failure in experimental animals and their applicability to man. In: Davison AM (ed) Nephrology, vol II. Proceedings of the 10th international congress on nephrology. Baillière Tindall, London, pp 1182–1191

Koletsky S, Goodsit AM (1960) Natural history and pathogenesis of renal ablation hypertension. Arch Pathol 69: 654–662

Kramp RA, MacDowell M, Gottschalk CW, Oliver JR (1974) A study by microdissection and micropuncture of the structure and the function of the kidneys and the nephrons of rats with chronic renal damage. Kidney Int 5: 147–176

Kumar S, Muchmore A (1990) Tamm-Horsfall protein—uromodulin (1950–1990). Kidney Int 37: 1395–1401

Lombet JR, Adler SG, Anderson PS, Nast CC, Olsen DR, Glassock RJ (1989) Sex vulnerability in the subtotal nephrectomy model of glomerulosclerosis in the rat. J Lab Clin Med 114: 66–74

Lubowitz H, Purkerson ML, Sugita M, Bricker NS (1969) GFR per nephron and per kidney in chronically diseased (pyelonephritic) kidney of the rat. Am J Physiol 217: 853–857

Mackensen-Haen S, Bader R, Grund KE, Bohle A (1981) Correlations between renal cortical interstitial fibrosis, atrophy of the proximal tubules and impairment of the glomerular filtration rat. Clin Nephrol 15: 167–171

Mackensen-Haen S, Eissele R, Bohle A (1988) Contribution on the correlation between morphometric parameters gained from the renal cortex and renal function in IgA nephritis. Lab Invest 59: 239–244

Mackensen-Haen S, Bohle A, Christensen J, Wehrmann M, Kendziorra H, Kokot F (1992) The consequences for renal function of widening of the interstitium and changes in the tubular epithelium of the renal cortex and outer medulla in various renal diseases. Clin Nephrol 37: 70–77

Malt RA (1983) Humoral factors in regulation of compensatory renal hypertrophy. Kidney Int 23: 611–615

Marcussen N (1990) Atubular glomeruli in cisplatin-induced chronic interstitial nephropathy. An experimental stereological investigation. APMIS 98: 1087–1097

Marcussen N (1991) Atubular glomeruli in renal artery stenosis. Lab Invest 65: 558–565

Marcussen N (1992) Atubular glomeruli and the structural basis for chronic renal failure. Lab Invest 66: 265–284

Marcussen N, Jacobsen NO (1992) The progression of cisplatin-induced tubulointerstitial nephropathy in rats. APMIS 100: 256–268

Marcussen N, Olsen TS (1990) Atubular glomeruli in patients with chronic pyelonephritis. Lab Invest 62: 467–473

Marcussen N, Ottosen PD, Christensen S, Olsen TS (1989) Atubular glomeruli in lithium-induced chronic nephropathy in rats. Lab Invest 61: 295–302

Marcussen N, Ottosen PD, Christensen S (1990) Ultrastructural quantitation of atubular and hypertrophic glomeruli in rats with lithium-induced chronic nephropathy. Virchows Arch [A] 417: 513–522

Marcussen N, Christensen S, Petersen JS, Shalmi M (1991) Atubular glomeruli, renal function and hypertrophic response in rats with chronic lithium nephropathy. Virchows Arch [A] 419: 281–289

Marcussen N, Nyengaard JR, Christensen S (1994) Compensatory growth of glomeruli is accomplished by an increased number of glomerular capillaries. Lab Invest 70: 868–874

Møller JC (1986) Dimensional changes of proximal tubules and cortical capillaries in chronic obstructive renal disease. A light-microscopic morphometric analysis. Virchows Arch [A] 410: 153–158

Møller JC, Jøgensen TM, Mortensen J (1986) Proximal tubular atrophy: qualitative and quantitative structural changes in chronic obstructive nephropathy in the pig. Cell Tissue Res 244: 479–491

Muehrcke RC, Kark RM, Pirani CL, Pollak UF (1957) Lupus nephritis: a clinical and pathologic study based on renal biopsies. Medicine (Baltimore) 36: 1–145

Nyengaard JR (1993) The quantitative development of glomerular capillaries in rats with special reference to unbiased stereological estimates of their number and sizes. Microvasc Res 45: 243–261

Nyengaard JR, Marcussen N (1993) The number of glomerular capillaries estimated by an unbiased and efficient stereological method. J Microsc 171: 27–37

Ogata K (1990) Clinicopathological study of kidneys from patients on chronic dialysis. Kidney Int 37: 1333–1340

Oliver J (1939) Architecture of the kidney in chronic Bright's disease. Hoeber, New York

Oliver J (1950) When is the kidney not a kidney? J Urol 63: 373–402

Oliver J (1953) Correlations of structure and function and mechanisms of recovery in acute tubular necrosis. Am J Med 15: 535–557

Oliver J, Bloom F, MacDowell M (1941) Structural and functional transformations in the tubular epithelium of the dog's kidney in chronic Bright's disease and their relation to mechanisms of renal compensation and failure. J Exp Med 73: 141–159

Olivetti G, Anversa P, Rigamonti W, Vitali-Mazza L, Loud AV (1977) Morphometry of the renal corpuscle during postnatal growth and compensatory hypertrophy. A light-microscope study. J Cell Biol 75: 573–585

Olsen TS, Wasssef NF, Olsen HS, Hansen HE (1986) Ultrastructure of the kidney in acute interstitial nephritis. Ultrastruct Pathol 10: 1–16

Olson JL, Heptinstall RH (1988) Nonimmunologic mechanisms of glomerular injury. Lab Invest 59: 564–578

Olson JL, Hostetter TH, Rennke HG, Brenner BM, Venkatachalam MA (1982) Altered glomerular permselectivity and progressive sclerosis following extreme ablation of renal mass. Kidney Int 22: 112–126

Ottosen PD, Sigh B, Kristensen J, Olsen S, Christensen S (1984) Lithium-induced interstitial nephropathy associated with chronic renal failure. Reversibility and correlation between functional and structural changes. Acta Pathol Microbiol Immunol Scand [A] 92: 447–454

Raaschou F (1948) Studies of chronic pyelonephritis with special reference to the kidney function. Munksgaard, Copenhagen

Remuzzi A, Pergolizzi R, Mauer MS, Bertani T (1990) Three-dimensional morphometric analysis of segmental glomerulosclerosis in the rat. Kidney Int 38: 851–856

Risdon RA, Sloper JC, de Wardener HE (1968) Relationship between renal function and histological changes found in renal-biopsy specimens from patients with persistent glomerular nephritis. Lancet 2: 363–366

Rosenbaum JL, Mikail M, Wiedmann F (1967) Further correlation of renal function with kidney biopsy in chronic renal disease. Am J Med Sci 254: 156–160

Schainuck LI, Striker GE, Cutler RE, Benditt EP (1970) Structural-functional correlations in renal disease, part II: the correlations. Hum Pathol 1: 631–641

Scherberich JE, Wolf G, Albers C, Nowark A, Stuckhardt C, Schoeppe W (1989) Glomerular and tubular membrane antigens reflecting cellular adaptation in human renal failure. Kidney Int 36 [Suppl 27]: S38–S51

Seyer-Hansen K, Hansen J, Gundersen HJG (1980) Renal hypertrophy in experimental diabetes. Diabetologia 18: 501–505

Seyer-Hansen K, Gundersen HJG, Østerby R (1985) Stereology of the rat kidney during compensatory renal hypertrophy. Acta Pathol Microbiol Immunol Scand [A] 93: 9–12

Shea SM, Raskova J, Morrison AB (1978) A stereologic study of glomerular hypertrophy in the subtotally nephrectomized rat. Am J Pathol 90: 201–210

Shimamura T, Heptinstall RH (1963) Experimental pyelonephritis. Nephron dissection of the kidney of experimental chronic pyelonephritis in the rabbit. J Pathol Bacteriol 85: 421–423

Shimamura T, Morrison AB (1975) A progressive glomerulosclerosis occurring in partial five-sixths nephrectomized rats. Am J Pathol 79: 95–101

Silva FG, Hogg RJ (1989) IgA nephropathy. In: Fischer CC, Brenner BM (eds) Renal pathology with clinical and functional correlations. Lippencott, Philadelphia, pp 434–493

Smith HW (1951) The kidney. Structure and function in health and disease. Oxford University Press, New York, pp 872–878

Smith SM, Hoy WE, Cobb L (1989) Low incidence of glomerulosclerosis in normal kidneys. Arch Pathol Lab Med 113: 1253–1255

Sterio DC (1984) The unbiased estimation of number and sizes of arbitrary particles using the disector. J Microsc 134: 127–136

Tanner GA, Evan AP, Summerlin DB, Knopp LC (1989) Glomerular and proximal tubular morphology after single nephron obstruction. Kidney Int 36: 1050–1060

Tapia E, Gabbai FB, Calleja C, Franco M, Cermeno JL, Bobadilla NA, Perez JM, Alvarado JA, Herrara-Acosta J (1990) Determinants of renal damage in rats with systemic hypertension and partial renal ablation. Kidney Int 38: 642–648

Textor SC (1984) Pathophysiology of renovascular hypertension. Urol Clin North Am 11: 373–381

Thurau K, Schnermann J (1965) Die Natriumkonzentration an den Macula densa-Zellen als regulierender Faktor für das Glomerulumfiltrat (Mikropunktionsversuche). Klin Wochenschr 43: 410–413

Tribe CR, Heptinstall RH (1964) The juxtaglomerular apparatus in scarred kidneys. An experimental study into the nature of the stimulus causing hyperplasia of the juxtaglomerular apparatus in rats. Br J Exp Pathol 46: 339–347

Venkatachalam MA, Bernard DB, Donohue JF, Levinsky NG (1978) Ischemic damage and repair in the rat proximal tubule: differences among the S1, S2 and S3 segments. Kidney Int 14: 31–41

Walser M (1988) Progression of renal failure. In: Davison AM (ed) Nephrology, vol II Proceedings of the 10th international congress on nephrology. Baillère Tindall, London, pp 1155–1181

Wehrmann M, Bohle A, Held H, Schumm G, Kendziorra H, Pressler H (1990) Long-term prognosis of focal sclerosing glomerulonephritis—an analysis of 250 cases with particular regard to tubulointerstitial changes. Clin Nephrol 33: 115–122

Wood JE Jr, Ethridge C (1933) Hypertension with arteriolar and glomerular changes in the albino rat following subtotal nephrectomy. Proc Soc Exp Biol Med 30: 1039–1041

Yoshida Y, Fogo A, Ichikawa I (1989) Glomerular hemodynamic changes vs. hypertrophy in experimental glomerular sclerosis. Kidney Int 35: 654–660

Yoshioka T, Shiraga H, Yoshida Y, Fogo A, Glick A, Deen WW, Hoyer J, Ichikawa I (1988) "Intact nephrons" as the primary origin of proteinuria in chronic renal disease. Study in the rat model of subtotal nephrectomy. J Clin Invest 82: 1641–1653

The Diabetic Renal Tubulointerstitium

F.N. ZIYADEH and S. GOLDFARB

1 Overview

Renal injury in diabetes mellitus is a major cause of morbidity and mortality. Approximately 30% of patients with type-I (insulin-dependent) diabetes mellitus (MOGENSEN 1982, 1990; BREYER 1992) and at least 10% of patients with type-II (non-insulin-dependent) diabetes mellitus (FABRE et al. 1982) will develop chronic renal failure requiring treatment in an end-stage renal disease program. Recent large-scale clinical trials have established that the best approach to the management of these patients is to detect the condition at an early stage and offer tight glycemic control (DCCT RESEARCH GROUP 1993) and to treat hypertension preferably with angiotension-converting enzyme inhibitors (LEWIS et al. 1993) in order to delay the progression of this life-threatening and costly complication of diabetes.

The stages of progression of diabetic nephropathy are best understood in the setting of type-I diabetes mellitus, although recent studies in the Pima Indian community, where type-II diabetes mellitus affects a relatively large fraction of the population, have shown stages of progression of nephropathy similar to those seen in type-I patients (MYERS et al. 1991). Diabetic nephropathy encompasses a host of structural alterations which are characterized by early hypertrophy of both glomerular and tubuloepithelial elements, thickening of the

Current Topics in Pathology
Volume 88, S.M. Dodd (Ed.)
© Springer-Verlag Berlin Heidelberg 1995

glomerular and tubular basement membranes (GBM and TBM, respectively), and progressive accumulation of extracellular matrix components, principally in the glomerular mesangium (HOSTETTER 1986; ZIYADEH et al. 1989; FIORETTO et al. 1992; ZIYADEH 1993a). There is no question that the glomerular lesions are of fundamental importance for the expression of the functional derangements which characterize the stage of overt diabetic nephropathy, namely frank proteinuria, hypertension, and the progressive decline in glomerular filtration rate (GFR) (HOSTETTER 1986; ZIYADEH et al. 1989; FIORETTO et al. 1992). However, progressive tubulointerstitial fibrosis and renal arteriosclerosis, less widely recognized lesions, are also important components of diabetic nephropathy because they give rise to important alterations in tubular as well as glomerular function, and they often contribute singnificantly to the development of ischemic or obliterative, global glomerulosclerosis and thus to the marked reduction in GFR (GELLMAN et al. 1959; DECKERT et al. 1986; ZIYADEH and GOLDFARB 1991; LANE et al. 1993). In fact, the degree of tubulointerstitial fibrosis in diabetic nephropathy closely correlates with the magnitude of mesangial matrix expansion (MAUER et al. 1984) and with the decline in GFR (BADER et al. 1980). Thus, as with many different renal glomerular diseases, the severity of the accompanying tubular atrophy and interstitial fibrosis is an excellent predictor of impaired kidney function, measured principally as a reduction in GFR (BOHLE et al. 1977a,b,c). Therefore, a full understanding of the mechanisms that culminate in irreversible kidney failure in diabetes mellitus requires a closer look at the status of the tubulointerstitium in this disease.

Another characteristic abnormality of the tubuloepithelial and interstitial compartments in the diabetic state in nephromegaly (SEYER-HANSEN 1983; RASCH 1984; KLEINMAN and FINE 1988; FLYVBJERG et al. 1992; ZIYADEH 1993). Nephromegaly is an early feature of the involvement of the kidney in this disease and is predominantly reflective of increased renal tubule mass, mostly as a consequence of cellular hypertrophy of the tubuloepithelium (SEYER-HANSEN et al. 1980; RASCH 1984). Much of the controversy in the literature on the pathogenesis of renal hypertrophy in type-I diabetes relates to whether an increase in GFR is a casual factor in the genesis of hypertrophy, or whether it is secondary to a primary increase in glomerular and kidney size (SCHWIEGER and FINE 1990). The importance of renal hypertrophy in the development of abnormalities in kidney function remains unsettled, but it can be speculated that tubular hypertrophy may contribute to the features of the disease, in a manner somewhat analogous to the more established relationship between glomerular hypertrophy and the eventual development of glomerulosclerosis (FOGO and ICHIKAWA 1989).

This review will first briefly summarize the functional disturbances that are thought to occur as a consequence of the tubular lesions in diabetic renal involvement (Table 1). We will propose the hypothesis that altered tubular transport and metabolic activity may contribute to the proteinuria in diabetes. We will explore in detail the structural disturbances of the tubulointerstitial compartment that characterize diabetic nephropathy, and provide evidence to

Table 1. Clinical manifestations of the diabetic kidney of nonglomerular origin

Tubular proteinuria
Fluid and electrolyte disorders
  Glycosuric osmotic diuresis
  Hypoaldosteronism
  Type-4 distal renal tubular acidosis
  Hypercalciuria
Obstructive nephropathy associated with neurogenic bladder dysfunction
Radiocontrast-induced nephrotoxic acute renal failure
Papillary necrosis
Pyelonephritis
  Bacterial
  Fungal
  Emphysematous
  Xanthogranulomatous

support the contention that interstitial fibrosis plays in important role in the ultimate expression of renal insufficiency in this disease.

2 Renal Tubular Functional Changes in Diabetes

2.1 Tubular Determinants of Microalbuminuria

Diabetic proteinuria is predominantly the result of increased glomerular filtration of protein. However, impairment of tubular reabsorption of filtered protein, as well as the excretion of proteins which originate from the tubular epithelium, may also variably contribute to the proteinuria (ABRASS 1984). Impaired tubular reabsorption not only leads to increased clearance of low-molecular-weight proteins, but may also be a contributory cause of the early abnormal urinary excretion of albumin (microalbuminuria) (ABRASS 1984; et al. 1993). This is because while the renal tubule can reabsorb significant amounts of filtered albumin via vesicular endocytosis, this capacity may eventually be exceeded. Thus, although microalbuminuria in early diabetes is generally taken to reflect the increased leakiness of the glomerular capillary to macromolecular traffic, recent experimental evidence (TUCKER et al. 1993) suggests that the increased glomerular filtration of albumin may not become detectable as increased urinary albumin excretion until the absolute proximal tubular reabsorption of albumin is decreased with progression of the diabetic state.

    Evidence of subtle damage to the renal tubule has been provided by the finding that the urinary excretion of N-acetyl-β-D-glucosaminidase is markedly increased in diabetes (MILTENYI et al. 1985; ROWE et al. 1987; GIBB et al. 1989). This lysosomal enzyme originating from the proximal tubule cell is not filtered by the glomerulus, but is liberated in the tubular fluid following proximal tubule injury. Moreover, careful morphological studies have recently demonstrated that proximal tubule brush-border height is significantly reduced after 2 months of diabetes in the streptozotocin-rat model, presumably indicative of decreased endocytic capacity that requires availability of apical membrane to form lysosomes, and this correlates with decreased absolute albumin reabsorption (TUCKER et al. 1993). Thus, while the microalbuminuria of early diabetes may represent an abnormality in glomerular barrier function and may herald or signify the presence of glomerular injury, which will inevitably lead to more substantial degrees of proteinuria and renal functional impairment, altered tubular handling of protein may also contribute to the development of proteinuria. The role of this abnormality in producing microalbuminuria has not been fully elucidated; however, such tubular changes could help to explain the finding that microalbuminuria may be dissociated from specific changes in glomerular structure in early clinical diabetes mellitus (CHAVERS et al. 1989). The clinical importance of alterations in the tubular component of protein handling for the prognostic and diagnostic value of microalbuminuria remains to be defined.

2.2 Sodium Transport

The induction of diabetes in the experimental animal brings about an adaptive change in the rates of transport of solutes and water, which maintains the volume and composition of the extracellular space at a new steady state. Glomerulotubular balance for sodium and glucose is maintained at a normal setting in the hypertrophied diabetic kidneys; i.e., a constant fraction of the filtered load of solute is reabsorbed by the renal tubules (VAAMONDE and PEREZ 1990).

During the first few days of experimental diabetes, excess natriuresis leads to a negative Na balance (CHRISTLIEB et al. 1979). Renal Na wasting results from hyperfiltration and the osmotic diuresis of glucose as well as from insulin deficiency, given the stimulatory effects of insulin treatment on Na reabsorption in the thick ascending limb (DEFRONZO et al. 1976; KIRCHNER 1988) and the proximal tubule (BAUM 1987). When significant ketoacidosis and ketonuria are present, cations (mainly Na^+, K^+, NH_4^+) are needed to accompany the large amounts of negatively charged ketone bodies excreted in the urine to maintain electrical neutrality. During this early stage, the contraction of the extracellular fluid volume stimulates mineralocorticoid secretion which in turn increases Na reabsorption in the collecting duct thereby serving to minimize Na wasting (CHRISTLIEB et al. 1979; WALD et al. 1986; KHADOURI et al. 1987). Additional renal and extrarenal effector mechanisms are also activated which maintain Na balance. In fact, as early as 3 weeks after the onset of experimental diabetes, the Na balance becomes positive and blood volume increases significantly (CHRISTLIEB et al. 1979; WALD et al. 1986; KHADOURI et al. 1987). Increased food intake, including Na, may also contribute to Na retention in the experimental animal. Furthermore, hyperglycemia induces an osmotic expansion of the extracellular fluid compartment, which partly explains the increase in circulating blood volume, renal blood flow, and GFR and could contribute to the deleterious increase in systemic blood pressure that is seen later in the disorder. Additionally, pathophysiologic responses in tubular transport function in diabetes that are linked to, or at least associated with, recognizable structural changes, including the induction of cellular hypertrophy, represent powerful renal adaptive mechanisms that contribute to the maintenance of a positive Na balance. In the proximal tubule, Na reabsorption increases proportionately to the increase in GFR, thus maintaining glomerular-tubular balance (MOGENSEN 1971; DITZEL and BROCHNER-MORTENSEN 1983; BROCHNER-MORTENSEN et al. 1984). The operation of peritubular Starling forces presumably favors a decrease in the back-leak of fluid via the paracellular route. Additionally, net transcellular Na reabsorption is also stimulated, as evidenced by a parallel increase in the activities of Na/H exchange in the luminal brush-border membrane (HARRIS et al. 1986) and the Na-K-ATPase in the basolateral membrane (WALD et al. 1986; KHADOURI et al. 1987). Intracellular Na concentration is also significantly increased, implying that the rate of luminal Na entry exceeds that of basolateral Na exit (KUMAR et al. 1988). Microvillus vesicle studies demonstrate that the activity of Na/H exchange is increased in both streptozotocin and autoimmune diabetic rats (HARRIS et al. 1986). Additionally, as $NaHCO_3$ treatment prevents this stimulation, it is concluded that the increase in net acid production and excretion in diabetes likely stimulates the activity of Na/H exchange (HARRIS et al. 1986). The stimulation of Na-K-ATPase in the proximal tubule occurs as early as the first 1–2 days following the induction of diabetes and precedes any detectable hyperfiltration (WALD et al. 1986; KHADOURI et al. 1987). It has been hypothesized that tubular hypertrophy may result from an activation in cellular Na transport, such as that due to an increase in Na/H exchange which is associated with cellular alkalinization (FINE et al. 1985), and/or from an increase in intracellular Na concentration (KUMAR et al. 1988). The increased filtered load of glucose stimulates the entry of glucose and Na into the renal cells, resulting in an increase in Na concentration. Although the mechanism is entirely conjectural at this time, it is suggested that the increase in intracellular Na may release stored Ca into the cytosol, increasing intracellular Ca and thus activating protein kinase C, which (in certain cell types) alkalinizes the cell via activation of the Na/H exchanger. These cellular events may result in the rapid expression of a set of protonocogenes that code for DNA-binding proteins, preparing the cell for DNA replication and hypertrophy (KUMAR et al. 1988; SCHWIEGER and FINE 1990). While this contention remains an attractive hypothesis, linking solute transport with the subsequent cellular events that lead to cell growth, experimental evidence is lacking at this time. In fact, in the models of NH_3-stimulated (GOLCHINI et al. 1989) or insulin-like growth factor 1-induced (MACKOVIC-BASIC et al. 1992) tubular hypertrophy in vitro, the increase in cell mass may persist even in the absence of stimulated Na/H exchange. In addition, treatment of mice with amiloride (an inhibitor of Na/H exchange) failed to prevent compensatory renal growth that follows uninephrectomy (GRANTHAM et al. 1989).

Stimulation of Na reabsorption in distal parts of the nephron also contributes to the maintenance of the Na balance in diabetes. The activity of Na-K-ATPase in the medullary (WALD et al. 1986; KHADOURI et al. 1987) and the cortical (WALD et al. 1986) thick ascending limb is stimulated, despite insulin deficiency, presumably due to the increase in the delivery of solute from the proximal nephron. The Na-K-ATPase activity is also stimulated in the collecting duct (WALD et al. 1986; KHADOURI et al. 1987). Here, the effect is most likely due to increased mineralocorticoid secretion, as evidenced by abrogation of stimulation in adrenalectomized diabetic rats (KHADOURI et al. 1987). It should be noted that the stimulation of Na-K-ATPase in the renal tubule of diabetic animals is segment specific. For instance, the activity of the enzyme in the distal convoluted tubule is not stimulated (WALD et al. 1986; KHADOURI et al. 1987). Moreover, in other tissues that may also become targets of diabetic complications the activity of Na-K-ATPase may actually be diminished, e.g., in glomeruli and in neural and vascular tissues (MACGREGOR and MATSCHINSKY 1986; GREENE et al. 1987; COHEN and KLEPSER 1988).

2.3 Potassium and Acid Transport

Defects in renal tubular potassium and hydrogen ion secretion related to the development of hypoaldosteronism (and/or tubular unresponsiveness to the action of aldosterone) are the main tubular abnormalities associated with mild to moderate diabetic nephropathy (DEFRONZO 1980). Because the transport of Na, K, and H in the distal tubule is under the influence of aldosterone, hypoaldosteronism is often associated with defects in K and H secretion. It is of interest that defects in Na conservation are rarely seen, and then only in cases in which tubular damage results in unresponsiveness to aldosterone. A form of distal renal tubular acidosis (also termed type 4) often develops in patients with pre-existing diabetic renal insufficiency. This entity may be recognized by the finding of hyperkalemia and/or hyperchloremic metabolic acidosis, which may be related to an underlying deficiency of renin and aldosterone production (VAAMONDE and PEREZ 1990). The two major factors responsible for the development of metabolic acidosis appear to be a reduction in renal hydrogen ion secretory capacity and ammonia production and/or diffusion into urine. The latter factor appears related both to mineralocorticoid deficiency and hyperkalemia. Patients with this form of distal renal tubular acidosis are at risk of developing severe hyperkalemia when they are hypovolemic or when medications affecting aldosterone production are introduced (e.g., angiotensin-converting enzyme inhibitors, heparin, nonsteroidal anti-inflammatory agents) (VAAMONDE and PEREZ 1990).

2.4 Glucose Transport

During uncontrolled hyperglycemia, the filtered load of glucose exceeds the renal threshold for its reabsorption. Under these conditions glucose, like any other nonreabsorbable solute (osmotic diuretic), prevents the reabsorption of water and sodium salts, leading to a progressive increase in urine flow. The osmotic diuresis of uncontrolled glycosuria is the major cause of salt and water losses in diabetic ketoacidosis.

Net renal glucose reabsorption is determined predominantly by the activity of Na^+-glucose co-transport in the luminal brush-border membrane and by the magnitude of paracellular back-leak of fluid from the peritubular region into the tubule lumen (VAAMONDE and PEREZ 1990). Net glucose reabsorption has been shown to increase proportionately with GFR and delivery rate (VAAMONDE and PEREZ 1990; ZIYZDEH and GOLDFARB 1991). Thus, with the development of hyperglycemia, combined with the hyperfiltration, the delivery of increased amounts of glucose in the filtrate is associated with a marked increase in the absolute rate of reabsorption of glucose in the proximal tubule, reflecting the maintenance of glomerular-tubular balance for glucose (MOGENSEN 1971; DITZEL and BROCHNER-MORTENSEN 1983). Presumably, the development of renal tubular hypertrophy implies an increased capacity for net glucose reabsorption mediated by an increase in the number of Na^+-glucose carriers (VAAMONDE and PEREZ 1990; ZIYADEH and GOLDFARB 1991). However, the intrinsic activity of the Na^+-glucose co-transporter measured in microvillus membrane vesicles is actually decreased in experimental models of diabetes (HARRIS et al. 1986). Thus, it is likely that the observed increase in net glucose transport in vivo may result from the marked increase in filtered glucose load, despite a decrease in intrinsic carrier-mediated transport (HARRIS et al. 1986).

It has been proposed that the increased tubular reabsorption of glucose may be the primary stimulus to renal hypertrophy; i.e., the kidney grows in response to the requirement for increased "work" necessary for glucose reabsorption (DITZEL and BROCHNER-MORTENSEN 1983). This hypothesis implies that GFR would rise secondarily and thus maintain glomerular-tubular balance.

In this context, it is important to indicate that high glucose concentrations in culture media exert direct effects in vitro on the structure and function of proximal tubule cells. For instance, HAZEN-MARTIN et al. (1989), employing a cell culture model of human proximal tubule cells, demonstrated that high glucose alters the ultrastructure of the cells, modifies the intercellular junctions, and reduces dome formation of confluent cell monolayers. These studies, along with our findings of the effects of glucose on proximal tubule growth and extracellular matrix biosynthesis (see below), emphasize the direct and potentially detrimental effects of ambient glucose on cellular structure and function.

2.5 Divalent Ions

A high prevalence of osteopenia has been demonstrated in diabetic patients, in part due to hypercalciuria (ZIYADEH and GOLDFARB 1991). The pathogenesis of hypercalciuria appears to be multifactorial. Hyperfiltration and osmotic diuresis, coupled with hyperphagia, increase urinary calcium excretion (GURUPRAKASH et al. 1988). Insulin treatment only partially corrects hypercalciuria (ZIYADEH and GOLDFARB 1991). In vivo microinjection studies (GURUPRAKASH et al. 1988) disclosed intrinsic defective tubular reabsorption of calcium in the loop of Henle (presumably in the thick ascending limb) and in the terminal regions of the nephron that were not attributable to a defect in parathyroid hormone secretion or action, or to an increased intake of calcium.

Patients with type-I (insulin-dependent) diabetes mellitus have a reversible dysfunction in the tubular handling of phosphate characterized by increased fasting urinary excretion of phosphate, related to a decrease in the maximal capacity of the renal tubular reabsorption of phsophate per unit filtrate (lowered TmPi/GFR) (DITZEL et al. 1982; VAAMONDE and PEREZ 1990). A modest decrease in fasting serum phosphate ensues.

These tubular abnormalities are also reversible and probably relate to suboptimal blood glucose control (DITZEL et al. 1982; VAAMONDE and PEREZ 1990). The phosphaturia in diabetes is not due to defects in parathyroid or growth hormone actions, as the levels of these hormones are reported to be not different from those in nondiabetic subjects (DITZEL et al. 1982; VAAMONDE and PEREZ 1990).

Despite hyperfiltration, proximal tubular reabsorption of phosphate is not concomitantly increased. This implies that for phosphate, in contrast to Na and glucose, glomerular-tubular balance is disrupted (DITZEL et al. 1982; DITZEL and BROCHNER-MORTENSEN 1983; VAAMONDE and PEREZ 1990). As both glucose and phosphate transport in the proximal tubules are coupled to active Na transport, it is likely that glucose reabsorption interferes with phosphate transport by inhibiting phosphate affinity at the tubular brush-border membrane. Glucose infusions sufficient to cause glycosuria result in a reduction in phosphate reabsorption. This response is not due to a nonspecific osmotic intraluminal effect, since mannitol infusion does not alter phosphate reabsorption (ZIYADEH and GOLDFARB 1991).

In the following discussion, we will detail the disturbances of the renal tubulointerstitial structure in diabetes and review several potential mechanisms for these abnormalities.

3 Early TBM Changes in Diabetes and the Relation to Tubular Cell Hypertrophy

The abnormalities of the TBM in diabetes may be conveniently divided into two stages: In the early phase of the disease there appears to be an acute increase in TBM mass, which accompanies the development of renal hypertrophy without discernible abnormalities in morphology; this is followed by the conspicuous thickening of the TBM which does not become apparent until a few years have elapsed. The early changes in TBM mass are best appreciated by considering the induction phase of experimental diabetes. SEYER-HANSEN et al. (1980) examined rat kidney growth in streptozotocin-induced diabetes by morphometric analysis of various anatomical structures at different intervals after the onset of the disease. After only 4 days, proximal tubule cell volume and epithelial cell height were significantly increased (by at least 20%). This was later accompanied by significant increases in tubule length and luminal diameter. Similar studies performed after 7–10 days of diabetes showed that proximal tubule length was increased by more than 30% while proximal tubule area was increased by approximately 50% (TUCKER et al. 1993). It would be reasonable to assume that TBM dimensions, particularly the surface area, were also increased as a necessary accompaniment to acute renal tubular hypertrophy. Moreover, it could be argued that, triggered by some of the anabolic events that are peculiarly restricted to the kidney, a substantial acceleration in TBM synthesis might have taken place, so as to augment TBM area (or volume). This argument is analogous to that previously made by OSTERBY and GUNDERSEN (1980) in their study on the fast accumulation of GBM material in experimental diabetes: An acute increase in the synthetic rate of GBM components accompanies acute glomerular hypertrophy, thus explaining the increase in GBM mass. At this early stage, alterations in the rate of degradation of membrane components play only a minor role, because even if total inhibition of degradation were to occur, this would not account for the acute changes, given the very slow rate of matrix degradation (COHEN and SURMA 1980; COHEN et al. 1982). However, considering the subsequent phases of diabetic nephropathy, it is likely that in addition to increased systhesis, decreased breakdown of BM components, particularly the collagens, may participate in the accumulation of extracellular matrix (STERNBERG et al. 1985).

Among the metabolic derangements that accompany the diabetic state, hyperglycemia is a necessary factor for the development of some of the renal manifestations of diabetes mellitus (MOGENSEN et al. 1978; CHRISTIANSEN et al. 1981; FELDT-RASMUSSEN et al. 1986; O'DONNEL et al. 1988; ZIYADEH et al. 1989; STACKHOUSE et al. 1990; PUGLIESE et al. 1991). LEVIN et al. (1975) hypothesized that elevated blood glucose levels (and high intrarenal concentrations) could be responsible for increased renal growth and basement membrane accumulation. Enzymes of the pentose-phosphate pathway show increased activity in the renal cortex of mature diabetic animals (BECKER 1976). Increases in the renal cortical pool of uridine triphosphate (UTP, essential for synthesis of RNA, glycogen, and glycoprotein through uridine diphosphoglucuronic enzymes) could be linked to increased pentose-phosphate activity and RNA content of hypertrophied kidneys. Unilateral nephrectomy further increases UTP pools and RNA content. These abnormalities are not corrected unless normoglycemia is achieved. There is also an early increase in de novo renal pyrimidine synthesis. Phosphoribosyl pyrophosphate (PRPP) serves as the substrate for the rate-limiting steps in the de novo synthesis of purines and pyrimidines in mammalian cells (SCHWIEGER and FINE 1990). There is a reciprocal relationship between kidney hypertrophy and whole kidney PRPP content in mature rats 2–3 days after creation of the diabetic state with either alloxan or streptozotocin. The increased synthesis of pyrimidines by the diabetic kidney facilitates the formation of uridine-diphospho-surgars and intermediates that are required for the synthesis of basement membrane collagen needed for growth (SCHWIEGER and FINE 1990).

To examine the isolated influence of elevated ambient glucose on renal cell metabolism, and to avoid the complicating roles of an altered metabolic milieu or the effects of renal hemodynamics on the process of diabetic renal hypertrophy, we previously developed a cell culture system in mouse proximal tubule epithelial cells where we were able to test the effects of elevated glucose concentration on cell growth and extracellular matrix biosynthesis (ZIYADEH et al. 1990; ZIYADEH and GOLDFARB 1991). Exposing the cells for 72 h to serum-free medium containing 25 mM (compared with 5.5 mM) D-glucose resulted in significant cellular hypertrophy, as defined by an increase in cell size (by cytofluorometry), increased total protein content, and stimulation of protein synthesis (ZIYADEH et al. 1990). This response was independent of changes in medium osmolality. Parallel studies also demonstrated that the high-glucose medium stimulated the secretion of collagen type IV by approximately twofold (ZIYADEH et al. 1990). There was also a concordant increase in steady-state levels of $\alpha 1(IV)$ mRNA and transcriptional activation of the gene encoding the $\alpha 1$ chain, providing evidence for increased collagen type-IV synthesis (ZIYADEH 1993b). Rates of collagen degradation were not measured in these short-term studies (ZIYADEH et al. 1990; ZIYADEH and GOLDFARB 1991; ZIYADEH 1993b).

Our in vitro studies on the effects of high levels of glucose concentration on collagen biosynthesis in proximal tubule appear to be relevant to the in vivo situation. In situ nucleic acid hybridization studies in rat kidney have demonstrated an early increase in collagen type-IV mRNA in hypertrophied proximal tubule cells in the streptozotocin-induced diabetic model (IHM et al. 1992). Moreover, increased synthesis of collagen type IV is also a feature of other models of renal hypertrophy, such as compensatory hypertrophy following partial kidney ablation (LEE et al. 1990) and angiotensin-II-induced proximal tubule cell hypertrophy (WOLF et al. 1991, 1993). In the latter in vitro model, we have demonstrated that the hypertrophogenic effect of angiotensin II required the presence of elevated ambient glucose concentration for its full expression (WOLF et al. 1991).

In summary, the developmental phase of renal tubular hypertrophy in diabetes mellitus is accompanied by an early increase in the mass of the normal constituents of the TBM. In vitro studies provide evidence that high glucose levels, independent of any hormonal factors, appear to be a major stimulus for the increased synthesis of collagen type IV by proximal tubule cells and for the induction of hypertrophy of these cells.

4 TBM Thickening in Diabetes

The renal TBM in diabetes mellitus, like the GBM and some other basement-membranes in other tissues, undergoes progressive thickening which develops slowly over several years (STEFFES et al. 1985). The increase in width of the TBM is almost uniform, although splitting and layered thickening may occur as in the GBM (FIORETTO et al. 1992; WALKER et al. 1992). There are virtually no detailed morphometric or ultrastructural studies devoted to the TBM in diabetes, in sharp contrast to the extensive studies on the GBM. Still lacking are large population surveys to derive data on mean and range of TBM width in normal adults similar to those generated for the GBM (STEFFES et al. 1983). Limited quantitative data have been obtained in a study of renal biopsies from seven pairs of identical twins who were discordant for insulin-dependent (type-I) diabetes (STEFFES et al. 1985). In each pair, the diabetic twin had a thicker TBM than the respective nondiabetic sibling; on average, the TBM of patients was 1100 nm, representing an almost 50% increase in thickness. When it was possible to differentiate between proximal and distal tubules, there were no consistent regional differences between the widths of their basement membranes. Similarly, GBM width in the diabetic twins (average width approximately 500 nm) exceeded that in the nondiabetic twins in each instance (approximately 330 nm). In this study (STEFFES et al. 1985), values for muscle capillary basement membrane width in the diabetic twins did not differ from those in their siblings. These results have demonstrated that the thickening of the TBM (and GBM) occurs relatively early, i.e., during the clinically silent course of the disease; moreover, this abnormality is predominantly a consequence of the metabolic perturbations of the diabetic state, rather than a generalized, hereditary disturbance affecting all basement membranes.

Several studies utilizing immunohistochemical techniques have revealed conspicuous linear binding of albumin and IgG along the length of the thickened TBM in kidneys from diabetic subjects (MICHAEL and BROWN 1981; MURRAH et al. 1984). The proteins were thought to have gained access to the TBM because of increased permeability of the peritubular capillaries. Thus, this phenomenon represents passive entrapment of circulating proteins rather than an active immune process, and it remains speculative whether this abnormality plays any role in the development of TBM thickening.

5 Glomerulosclerosis and the Relation to Nonglomerular Injury in Diabetic Nephropathy

It is widely held that the characteristic glomerular lesion of diabetic nephropathy, in particular the expansion of the mesangial matrix, is a primary abnormality arising in the glomerulus and largely responsible for the expression of the functional derangements which characterize the stage of overt dysfunction, namely frank proteinuria, hypertension, and renal failure (OSTERBY 1972, 1975; MOGENSEN and CHRISTENSEN 1984; BREYER 1992; FIORETTO et al. 1992). Histomorphometric analysis of kidney specimens from patients with a wide range of disease severity has established the close correlation between the expansion of the glomerular mesangial matrix and the declining surface area available for filtration (ELLIS et al. 1986; OSTERBY et al. 1988). Accordingly, the appearance of either diffuse or nodular glomerulosclerosis in moderately advanced stages of diabetic glomerulopathy has been thought to account, at least to a large extent, for the progressive decline in GFR (FIORETTO et al. 1992; WALKER et al. 1992). We will not dwell in this review on the established role of the glomerular lesions in the pathogenesis of the disease; rather, we will focus on the largely neglected role of the nonglomerular lesions, which are at least as important as the glomerular lesions in the expression of the functional derangements of diabetic nephropathy (Table 2).

Table 2. Nonglomerular structural lesions in diabetic nephropathy

Tubuloepithelial hypertrophy
Increased thickness of tubular basement membrane
Arteriolosclerosis (afferent and efferent)
Tubulointerstitial fibrosis
Armanni-Ebstein tubulopathy
Papillary necrosis

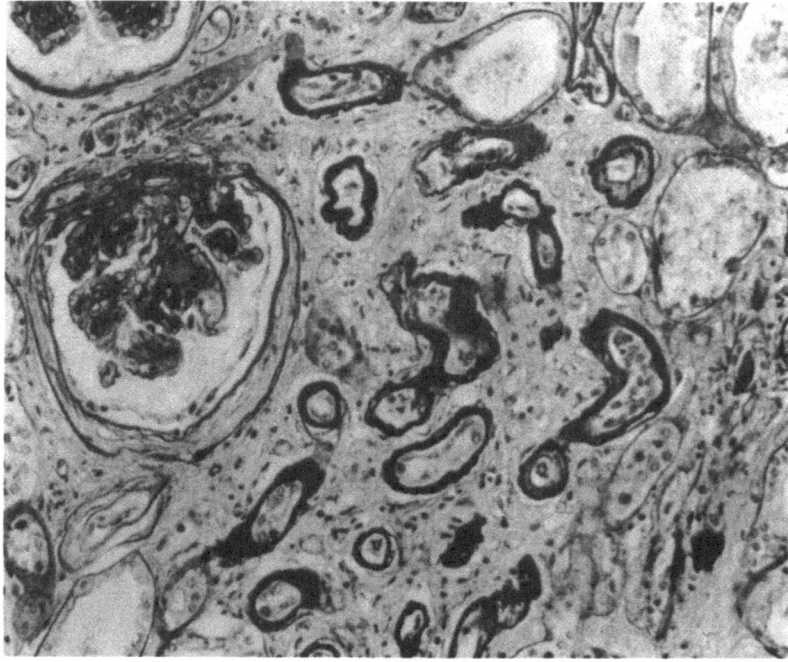

Fig. 1. Low-power view of kidney from patient with advanced diabetes showing tubular loss and thickening of tubular basement membranes and expanded area of interstitial fibrosis (*center*). The glomerulus (*upper left*) shows a variety of changes. PAS method, × 125. (Adapted with permission from Heptinstall 1983)

These nonglomerular lesions not only affect tubular function (DITZEL et al. 1982; ABRASS 1984; GURUPRAKASH et al. 1988; WALTON et al. 1988; GIBB et al. 1989) but may also exert potent secondary influences on the glomerular microcirculation, which eventually can culminate in obliterative or global glomerulosclerosis (Fig. 1).

6 Arteriosclerosis and Renal Injury in Diabetes

In a variety of tissues in patients with diabetes, a form of ischemic injury induced by exudative hyalinosis, which progressively obliterates small and medium sized arterioles, may be responsible for functional organ failure. In nerves, heart, and distal portions of the extremities, ischemic injury has been hypothesized. The potential role of such a vascular lesion in the kidney in advanced nephropathy seems likely (BADER et al. 1980; DECKERT et al. 1986).

As renal function deteriorates, progressive and global obliteration of glomeruli occurs, and this clearly plays an important role in reducing total kidney GFR (HORLYCK et al. 1986). OSTERBY and co-workers (1988) have suggested that this pathological entity occurs in a peculiar columnar-like pattern of distribution within all levels of the renal cortex (HORLYCK et al. 1986). This, in turn, suggested a vascular component to the phenomenon of glomerular occlusion, as these "columns" corresponded to the distribution of large renal interlobular vessels. Vascular occlusion in medium-sized renal vessels could predispose to glomerular occlusion and nephron destruction characterized by afferent arteriolar exudative hyalinosis. Examining biopsies of 44 patients with various stages of diabetic nephropathy DECKERT and colleagues (1986) also found that an arteriopathy is an important characteristic of the kidney in advanced diabetic nephropathy.

The role of arteriolar lesions in inducing diabetic changes has been inferred from several observations. First, in biopsies from patients with diabetic nephropathy BADER et al. (1980) found a clear correlation between the degree of diabetic glomerulosclerosis and a quantitative index of arteriolar hyalinization and occlusion. It was clear from these observations that the degree of vessel obstruction and obliteration was inversely correlated with the level of renal function and directly correlated with the greater severity of both diabetic glomerular sclerosis and interstitial fibrosis. Similarly, DECKERT et al. (1986) found that arteriolar hyalinosis tended to be more severe in patients with overt nephropathy and increased interstitial tissue volume, but this abnormality was also found in patients with milder forms of nephropathy and therefore could not be used to distinguish those individuals with more severe lesions. However, the fact that 20% of glomeruli were totally occluded in patients with overt nephropathy, whereas less than 10% of glomeruli were occluded in the less severely affected group, suggests that vascular occlusion could represent an important mechanism of the loss of glomeruli in the more severely affected individuals.

In summary, direct arteriolar obliteration could play an important role in the progressive renal failure of diabetic nephropathy by producing glomerular occlusion or by producing chronic tubulointerstitial ischemia and thereby stimulating interstitial fibrosis. As noted below, the latter may also be a primary event related to the direct biochemical effects of sustained hyperglycemia.

7 Tubulointerstitial Fibrosis in Diabetic Nephropathy

Interstitial fibrosis could also originate from nonvascular injury, thus comprising a primary abnormality in diabetic nephropathy. BOHLE and colleagues (1977a,b,c) suggested that changes in the renal interstitium may represent the crucial parameter that produces renal failure in a variety of renal diseases as well as in diabetes. This hypothesis derives from a histomorphometric study of biopsies of 105 patients with various degrees of diabetic nephropathy. In this study, there was a striking correlation between the percent of kidney volume occupied by the renal interstitium and the decline in GFR as measured by serum creatinine level (BADER et al. 1980). It should be noted that this relationship exists over a wide range of serum creatinine values.

Additionally, there is a strong direct correlation between interstitial expansion and the progression of glomerular sclerosis. This could suggest a parallel process damaging the glomeruli and tubulointerstitial structures, or the changes in the interstitium could be initiating a secondary glomerular process, as will be discussed below. FRØKJÆR THOMSEN et al. (1984) examined autopsy specimens from 34 long-term type-I diabetic patients and found that interstitial and mesangial lesions both correlated with serum creatinine and the presence of clinical nephropathy. MAUER and colleagues (1984) also observed similar relationships. In their study of the histomorphometry of renal biopsies from 45 patients with diabetes mellitus, interstitial fibrosis was evident even at the earliest stages of diabetic nephropathy, although it was subtle and required careful examination for its detection (Fig. 2). As glomerular filtration fell, the interstitial fibrosis became much more prominent (MAUER et al. 1984).

BADER and colleagues (1980) proposed that the interstitial fibrosis of diabetes might be directly responsible for producing the decline in glomerular filtration as well as contribute to the structural glomerulopathy through a number of possible mechanisms. First, progressive expansion of the renal interstitium could lead to a progressive obliteration of vascular elements and thus induce an ischemic nephropathy. This could also contribute to the process of the glomerular occlusion that characterizes the later phases of diabetic nephropathy. In addition, the increased interstitial fibrosis could not only lead to increased resistance or at least reduced compliance in the pre- and postglomerular vessels, but also potentiate the transmission of systemic hypertension of glomerular structures by imparing vascular autoregulation. Such changes could contribute to glomerular hypertension obsersed in experimental animals with diabetes.

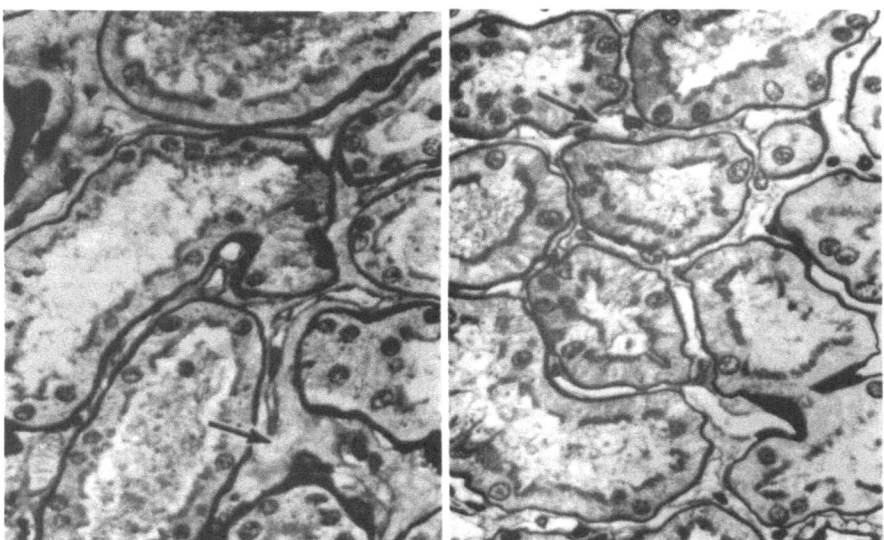

Fig. 2. *Left panel*: representative cortical area from a kidney biopsy obtained from an insulin-dependent diabetic patient with subtle interstitial fibrosis (*arrow*); the mean index of interstitial fibrosis was only 0.25. The index of interstitial fibrosis was determined as a semiquantitative estimate of the space occupied by fibrous tissue separating cortical tubules; 0 was used as normal, 1.0 as twice normal thickness, 2.0 as three times normal thickness, etc., in each 500 × field. *Right panel*: representative cortical area from a kidney biopsy in another insulin-dependent diabetic patient with more extensive interstitial fibrosis (*arrow*) in cortical area; the mean index of interstitial fibrosis was 2.75 PAS, × 350. (Adapted with permission from Mauer et al. 1984)

Also, to the extent that tubular obstruction could result from interstitial fibrosis, increased intratubular pressure could lead to progressive glomerular injury. Finally, if tubular dropout occurs, GFR would be eliminated in an affected nephron, thereby contributing to a decline in total number of functioning nephrons.

While all of these studies have shown relationships between interstitial lesion and various measures of renal function, none have simultaneously quantitated glomerular lesions, interstitial expansion, and renal function (BADER et al. 1980; FRØKJAER THOMSEN et al. 1984; Mauer et al. 1984). Furthermore, each study demonstrated or suggested a correlation between mesangial and interstitial expansion. However, in a recent study LANE and co-workers (1993) attempted to explore further the relationship between interstitial and glomerular lesions in type-I diabetic patients, especially mesangial expansion, arteriolar hyalinosis, and global glomerulosclerosis, as well as the relationship of these structural parameters to renal function and urinary albumin excretion. In this study, 84 patients with type-I diabetes mellitus of varying severity underwent studies of renal function and quantitative renal morphometry, including mesangial volume fraction, index of arteriolar hyalinosis, percentage of globally sclerosed glomeruli, and interstitial volume fraction per total renal cortex (Fig. 3). There

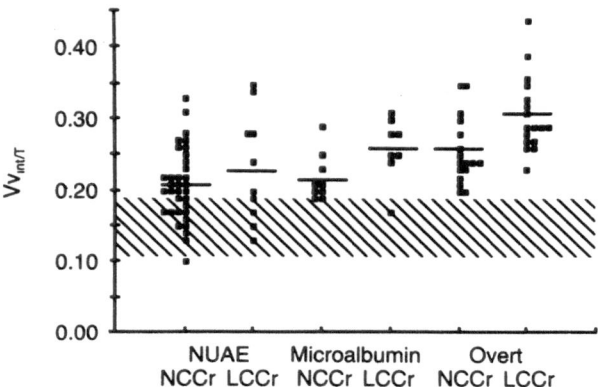

Fig. 3. Tubulointerstitial lesions in six groups of insulin-dependent diabetic patients with a wide range of disease severity. Abbreviations: $V_{Vint/T}$, interstitial volume fraction for total renal cortex (i.e., the proportion of the renal cortex made up of the expanded interstitial tissue, containing areas of atrophic tubules and thickening or wrinkling of tubular basement membranes as assessed by semiquantitative histomorphometry on specimens obtained by percutaneous kidney biopsy); *NUAE*, normal urinary albumin excretion; *Microalbumin*, microalbuminuria (45–200 mg/24 h); *Overt*, overt proteinuria (> 200 mg/24 h); NC_{Cr}, normal (90–120 ml/min/1.73 m²) or elevated (> 120 ml/min/ 1.73 m²) creatinine clearance; LC_{Cr}, low creatinine clearance (< 90 ml/min/1.73 m²). The range of values (mean ± 2 SD) seen in age- and sex-matched nondiabetic kidney donors is *shaded.* A correlation can be seen between the grade of tubulointerstitial lesion and the severity of clinical disease, as assessed by urinary albumin excretion and glomerular filtration rate (creatinine clearance). $p < 0.001$ by ANOVA for the six insulin-dependent diabetic groups compared with the nondiabetic group. The interstitial volume fraction for total renal cortex in all the diabetic groups was greater than in the nondiabetic group (by Dunnett's *t*-test, $p < 0.05$ for NUAE/LC$_{Cr}$ vs. Overt/LC$_{Cr}$ vs. nondiabetic group; $p < 0.01$ for other comparisons). ANOVA remained significant when the nondiabetic group was excluded ($p < 0.001$). Among the diabetic groups, the following comparisons had $p < 0.005$ by Scheffé F-test: NUAE/NC$_{Cr}$, and micro/NC$_{Cr}$ vs. Overt/LC$_{Cr}$. (From Lane et al. 1993, with permission)

was significant correlation among the four structural parameters. Moreover, all four parameters correlated with GFR and the log of urinary albumin excretion.

Abnormalities in renal tubulointerstitial structures have also been observed in experimental diabetes in animals. WEIL et al. (1976) showed that after 4 months of experimental diabetes induced by streptozotocin infusion in rats, there was a progressive tubulopathy characterized by the accumulation of myeloid-like bodies in the proximal tubular cells with progressive tubular disruption. RASCH (1984) also studied the pathology of short-term streptozotocin diabetic rats in order to investigate the site and mechanism of the Armanni-Ebstein lesion, the most specific tubular morphological abnormality of diabetes mellitus. With hematoxylin-eosin staining, cells appear clear and completely empty (vacuolization); glycogen can be demonstrated with periodic acid-Schiff (PAS) staining, predominantly in distal nephron and ascending limb cells. However, the pathophysiological importance of myeloid bodies or glycogen accumulation in both the cytoplasm and the nuclei of these epithelial cells remains to be determined. Proximal tubular morphological alterations which are associated with heavy proteinuria are also recognized and include enhanced lipid deposition (fatty vacuolization) and increased number of protein-containing lysosomes. The functional significance of these alterations is not known.

We have investigated the long-term changes in the renal interstitium in diabetes and have discovered tubulointerstitial changes which occur after 6–9 months of sustained hyperglycemia in streptozotocin-treated rats (ZIYADEH and GOLDFARB 1991). Assaying for the presence of interstitial fibrosis, tubular cell atrophy, interstitial inflammatory infiltrates, or tubular dilation, we found that 11 of 14 long-term diabetic rats demonstrated mild interstitial lesions whereas only three of 16 age-matched control animals on a normal diet manifested similar changes. Thus, it appears that tubular interstitial changes seen in the diabetic patients have their experimental conterpart in rats rendered diabetic with streptozotocin.

In summary, while it is unquestioned that changes in the glomerular mesangium and glomerular capillary basement membrane in diabetes contribute to the structural changes of progressive, diffuse diabetic glomerulosclerosis, the contribution of tubulointerstitial changes to the progressive decline in GFR seems equally likely. This hypothesis may be particularly relevant in explaining how the kidneys ultimately fail in diabetic nephropathy, rather than how the glomerular morphological changes develop. The progression from a normal or a modestly reduced GFR to a level requiring renal replacement therapy may be critically determined by these changes described in the tubulointerstitium and vascular compartments.

8 Tubulointerstitial Infection and Papillary Necrosis

Pyelonephritis and papillary necrosis are occasionally observed in patients with diabetes mellitus. While these lesions may be important in any given patient, they are not a common agent of progressive renal decline. Papillary necrosis is occasionally seen in patients with diabetes, and in fact diabetes mellitus is probably the most common co-morbid condition with papillary necrosis reported in the literature. For example, in an autopsy series from Johns Hopkins Hospital (HEPTINSTALL 1983), diabetes was found in 44% of 25 cases of papillary necrosis. The mechanism leading to this lesion is not clear, but several possibilities have been forwarded. First, vascular obstruction could lead to a reduction of blood flow to the oxygen-deficient renal papilla. This could accelerate an ischemic injury and induce areas of necrosis in the inner medulla. In addition, infection may occur more frequently in patients with diabetes because of glycosuria and diabetic cystopathy. In this circumstance, the combination of ischemia induced by vasculopathy and infection could act in concert to induce papillary necrosis. Other possibilities include an exaggerated degree of interstitial fibrosis in the inner medulla, which could further compromise blood flow to the inner portions of the medullary and papillary regions.

The speculation that "pyelonephritis" in diabetic patients is attributable to infection is not supported by clinicopathological analyses (VEJLSGAARD 1966). Several studies have indicated a rather modest degree of urinary tract infection or chronic bacteriuria in patients with diabetes. It has been suggested that bacteriuria is relatively uncommon and occurs in less than 10% of patients with diabetes (RENGARTS 1959). In addition, studies of patients with bacteriuria suggest that renal function does not necessarily deteriorate in these individuals (BATALLA et al. 1971). Thus, it is unlikely that the tendency to demonstrate interstitial fibrosis and inflammation in patients with diabetes is a secondary manifestation of chronic infection.

9 Mediators of Diabetic Renal Injury

Although capillary hypertension (MOGENSEN et al. 1978; HOSTETTER 1986; ZATZ et al. 1986; BREYER 1992), an abnormal metabolic environment (ZIYADEH et al. 1989; MOGENSEN 1990), and/or genetic predisposition (BORCH-JOHNSEN et al. 1992; KROLEWSKI et al. 1992) may all participate in the pathogenesis of diabetic nephropathy, the details of the cell-signaling mechanisms and the putative molecular mediators remain to be firmly established. A detailed account of these mediators is beyond the scope of this review, and only a brief exposition will be attempted of the mechanisms which are linked to the deleterious consequences of the hyperglycemic milieu (Table 3).

Nonenzymatic glycation reactions resulting in both the early ketoamine linkages (Amadori products) (COHEN 1989; ZIYADEH et al. 1989) and the later-

Table 3. Cellular mediators of diabetic renal involvement

Altered intrarenal hemodynamics
'Direct' effects of hyperglycemia on renal growth and extracellular matrix production
Nonenzymatic glycation of circulating or structural proteins
    Amadori glucose adducts
    Advanced glycosylation end-products ('AGE')
Humoral imbalance
    Insulin deficiency
    Activation of intrarenal hormones or cytokines
        Angiotensin II
        Transforming growth factor-β
        Thromboxane
        Insulin-like growth factor I
        Platelet-derived growth factor
Activation of pathyways of glucose metabolism
    Polyol pathway (increased sorbitol)
    Pentose-phosphate shunt (increased UDP glucose)
    De novo synthesis of diacylglycerol and stimulation of protein kinase C
    Disordered *myo*-inositol metabolism
    Altered cellular redox state (increased $NADPH/NADP^+$, $NADH/NAD^+$)
    Altered glycosphingolipid metabolism (increased glucosylceramide and ganglioside GM3)
Genetic predisposition

---

developing advanced glycosylation end-products (AGE) (BROWNLEE 1984, 1988; BROWNLEE 1991) often affect long-lived matrix constituents and may contribute in a significant way to the aberrations in the structure or function of basement membranes, the impaired susceptibility of the GBM to degradation (COHEN et al. 1980; STERNBERG et al. 1985; COHEN 1989; ZIYADEH et al. 1989; BROWNLEE 1991), and the increased production of mesangial matrix (SOULIS-LIPAROTA et al. 1991; DOI et al. 1992). Additionally, our recent studies on mesangial cells indicate that Amadori glucose adducts in glycated serum proteins (e.g., albumin), when added to the culture media, inhibit mesangial cell proleferation, stimulate collagen type-IV gene expression, and increase collagen production (ZIYADEH and COHEN 1993; COHEN and ZIYADEH 1994).

Increased flux through insulin-independent pathways for intracellular glucose utilization, particularly the polyol pathway, has been advanced as a factor mediating the early functional changes in certain diabetic target organs (MAUER et al. 1989; PEDERSON et al. 1991; TILTON et al. 1992). Increased oxidation of sorbitol to fructose is coupled to reduction of NAD^+ to NADH (TILTON et al. 1992), and a higher cytosolic ratio of $NADH/NAD^+$ may result in abnormalities in hormone responsiveness and signal-transduction pathways which eventually lead to cellular dysfunction. These disorders may also relate to alterations in cellular *myo*-inositol metabolism; *myo*-inositol supplementation may correct some of the disturbances that are attributed to increased activity of the polyol pathway (GREENE et al. 1987; WINEGRAD 1987; GOLDFARB et al. 1991). Evidence in favor of an involvement of the polyol pathway in some of the renal manifestations of diabetes has been provided by our recent demonstration that the early glomerular hyperfiltration in streptozotocin-induced diabetic rats can be ameliorated by a diet supplemented with *myo*-inositol (1%), or by the administration of sorbinil, an aldose reductase inhibitor (ARI) which blocks the rate-limiting step in the polyol pathway (the conversion of glucose to sorbitol) (GOLFARB et al. 1991). These effects were not associated with changes in blood glucose levels or blood pressure, and they were specific, in that the hyperfiltration induced by increased protein feeding was not modulated by these maneuvers. In a recent study on a small number of diabetic patients, the hyperfiltration was also favorably decreased by ARI therapy (PEDERSON et al. 1991).

It is less clear whether increased activity of the polyol pathway is crucial in the genesis of the altered metabolism of renal extracellular matrix. COHEN et al. (1988) were not able to reverse the undersulfation of GBM proteoglycan by ARI administration to diabetic rats. Moreover, treatment with statil, another ARI, did not reduce the increased levels of laminin B1 mRNA in rat kidneys (POULSOM et al. 1988). However, a significant reduction in GBM thickness was demonstrated in diabetic rats after several months of sorbinil therapy (MAUER et al. 1989). Furthermore, a favorable reduction of the microalbuminuria in diabetic rats has been reported with sorbinil treatment (BEYER-MEARS et al. 1984).

In our in vitro studies on the effects of elevated ambient glucose on proximal tubule cell growth and matrix production we found that the stimulation by high glucose of collagen type-IV secretion and α1(IV) mRNA level was abolished when the cells were treated with 0.1 mM sorbinil (BLEYER et al. 1994) or when the high-glucose medium was supplemented with 800 µM myo-inositol (ZIYADEH et al. 1991b). In contrast, the induction of cellular hypertrophy by high glucose was not modified by ARI treatment or myo-inositol treatment, suggesting that only particular actions of high-glucose media are directly linked to the polyol pathway or to disturbances in myo-inositol metabolism.

An intriguing pathogenetic link between the products of the polyol pathway (and other pathways of glucose metabolism) and the reactions of nonenzymatic glycation has been proposed (SUAREZ et al. 1988; PETERSEN et al. 1990; SZWERGOLD et al. 1990). This is based on the observation that these glycation reactions can also involve metabolites of glucose which are the products of the polyol pathway (e.g., fructose) (SUAREZ et al. 1988) and which can be further phosphorylated via novel pathways of glucose metabolism that are activated in diabetes mellitus (PETERSEN et al. 1990; SZWERGOLD et al. 1990). Sorbitol-3-phosphate, fructose-3-phosphate (PETERSEN et al. 1990), 3-deoxyglucosone (B.S. Szwergold, personal communication), and other metabolites are increased in erythrocytes of diabetic subjects and could participate in protein glycation and cross-linking.

The intracellular signaling pathways which mediate some of the effects of elevated ambient glucose levels may involve activation of protein kinase C (PKC) as a consequence of stimulation of de novo synthesis of the endogenous PKC activator diacylglycerol (CRAVEN et al. 1990; AYO et al. 1991; STUDER et al. 1993). Stimulation of de novo synthesis of diacylglycerol may also result from the glucose-induced increase in the ratio of NADH/NAD$^+$ (TILTON et al. 1992). Increased activity of PKC in glomerular mesangial cells may lead to an increase in extracellular matrix expression, such as fibronectin, laminin, and type-IV collagen (SUAREZ et al. 1988; AYO et al. 1991). It has also been suggested that an increased NADPH/NADP$^+$ ratio resulting from activation of the pentose-phosphate shunt pathway (STEER et al. 1982) and the increased accumulation of glycosphingolipids (e.g., glucosylceramide and ganglioside GM3) in the kidney may mediate the renal hypertrophy in streptozotocin- induced diabetes in the rat (ZADOR et al. 1993).

Several of the manifestations of diabetic nephropathy may also be a consequence of altered production of local or circulating growth factors and/or modulation in the response to these factors, for example, TGF-β, IGF-1, prostanoids (e.g., thromboxane), angiotensin II, and platelet-derived growth factor (LEE et al. 1989; LEDBETTER et al. 1990; AYO et al. 1991; BLAZER-YOST et al. 1991; ROCCO and ZIYADEH 1991; WOLF et al. 1991; BLAZER-YOST et al. 1992; DOI et al. 1992; ROCCO et al. 1992; SHARMA and ZIYADEH 1993; STUDER et al. 1993). A discussion of the role of each of these mediators will not be given here. However, TGF-β deserves special consideration because it is produced by several cell types including renal cells, and it has a central role in promoting the synthesis and accumulation of different extracellular matrix moieties (ROBERTS et al. 1991; ROCCO and ZIYADEH 1991; SHARMA and ZIYADEH 1993). In recent studies, we gathered evidence that the effects of elevated ambient glucose in cultured mesangial or renal tubular cells are mediated by autocrine activation of TGF-β (ZIYADEH et al. 1991a; ROCCO et al. 1992). Neutralizing anti-TGF-β antibodies reverse the stimulation by high glucose of collagen biosynthesis in cultured mesangial cells (ZIYADEH et al. 1994). Moreover, the hypertrophy of the tubuloepithelium induced by elevated ambient glucose appears to be mediated largely by autocrine activation of endogenous TGF-β, since the neutralizing anti-TGF-β antibodies also prevent the high-glucose-induced hypertrophy. Whether a similar phenomenon is operative in vivo remains to be established, but it is interesting to note that in two rodent models of spontaneous insulin-dependent diabetes (NOD mouse and BB rat) we have recently demonstrated an increase in the expression of TFG-β1 in the kidney within a few days of the appearance of hyperglycemia (SHARMA and ZIYADEH 1994).

10 Concluding Remarks

Tubulointerstitial fibrosis in diabetes is an important pathological feature of diabetic nephropathy, particular in patients with associated renal insufficiency. There is a clear correlation between the degree of interstitial fibrosis and the development of a reduced GFR. The mechanism of this relationship could be an alteration in blood flow through the fibrosed interstitium, or altered hemodynamics induced by affected vascular structures passing through the fibrotic tissue. In addition, the direct effects on tubular function and on tubuloglomerular feedback could be important contributing features. One likely mediator of these effects could be the non-enzymatic glycation of various matrix proteins which alters their structure and function and prevents normal degradation of collagen. In addition, recent evidence suggests that high levels of glucose directly promote collagen biosynthesis by stimulating collagen gene expression, thus raising the possibility that the actions of diabetes in producing renal insufficiency could be due in part to direct effects of glucose on tubular epithelial cell matrix synthesis. A role for various growth factors, especially transforming growth factor-β, in producing renal tubular growth and hypertrophy also seems likely. New therapeutic strategies aimed at reducing collagen synthesis in the kidney, or at preventing the formation of early Amadori glucose adducts as well as of long-standing cross-links of advanced glycation end-products in various extracellular matrix proteins, provide the possibility of altering the natural history of diabetic nephropathy through strategies that complement the well-described benefits of antihypertensive therapy (PARVING et al. 1983; MOGENSEN 1985), especilly cinvertin enzyme inhibitors (LEWIS et al. 1993), strict glycemic control (DCCT RESEARCH GROUP 1993; REICHARD et al. 1993), and perhaps reduced dietary protein intake (WALKER et al. 1989; ZELLER et al. 1991).

Acknowledgments. The studies conducted in the authors' laboratories were supported by the Juvenile Diabetes Foundation, the American Diabetes Association, and the National Institutes of Health, Grants DK07006, DK39565, DK45191, and DK44513.

References

Abrass CK (1984) Diabetic proteinuria. Glomerular or tubular origin? Am J Nephrol 4: 337–346

Ayo SH, Radnik R, Garoni JA, Kreisberg J (1991) High glucose increases diacylglycerol mass and activates protein kinase C in mesangial cell culture. Am J Physiol 261: F571–F577

Bader R, Bader H, Grund K, Markensen-Haen S, Christ H, Bohle A (1980) Structure and function of the kidney in diabetic glomerulosclerosis: correlations between morphologic and functional parameters. Pathol Res Pract 167: 204–216

Batalla MA, Balodimos MC, Bradley RF (1971) Bacteriuria in diabetes mellitus. Diabetologia 7: 297–305

Baum M (1987) Insulin stimulates volume absorption in the rabbit proximal convoluted tubule. J Clin Invest 79: 1104–1109

Becker MA (1976) Patterns of phosphoribosylpyrophosphate and ribose-5-phosphate concentration and generation in fibroblasts. J Clin Invest 57: 308–318

Beyer-Mears A, Ku L Cohen MP (1984) Glomerular polyol accumulation in diabetes and its prevention by oral sorbinil. Diabetes 33: 604–607

Blazer-Yost BL, Goldfarb S, Ziyadeh FN (1991) Insulin, insulin-like growth factors and the kidney. In: Goldfarb S, Ziyadeh FN (eds) Contemporary issues in nephrology: hormones, autacoids, and the kidney. Churchill Livingstone, New York, pp 339–363

Blazer-Yost BL, Watanabe M, Haverty TP, Ziyadeh FN (1992) Role of insulin and IGF1 receptors in proliferation of cultured renal proximal tubule cells. Biochim Biophys Acta 1133: 329–335

Bleyer A, Fumo P, Snipes ER, Goldfarb S, Simmons DA, Ziyadeh FN (1994) Polyol pathway mediates high-glucose-induced collagen synthesis in proximal tubule. Kidney Int 42: 659–666

Bohle A, Bader R, Grund KE, Mackensen S, Neunhoffer J (1977a) Correlations between relative interstitial volume of the renal cortex and serum creatinine concentrations in minimal changes with nephrotic syndrome and in focal sclerosing glomeruloneohritis. Virchows Arch [A] 376: 221–232

Bohle A, Bader R, Grund KE, Mackensen S, Tolon M, Neunhoffer J (1977b) Serum creatinine concentration and renal interstitial volume. Analysis of correlations in endocapillary (acute) glomerulonephritis and in moderately severe mesangio-proliferative glomerulonephritis. Virchows Arch [A] 375: 87–96

Bohle A, Bader R, Grund KE, Makensen S, Tolon M (1977c) Correlations between renal interstitium and level of serum creatinine. Morphometric investigations of biopsies in perimembranous glomerulonephritis. Virchows Arch [A] 373: 15–22

Borch-Johnsen K, Norgaard K, Hommel E, Mathiesen ER, Jensen JS, Deckert T, Parving HH (1992) Is diabetic nephropathy an inherited complication? Kidney Int 41: 719–722

Breyer JA (1992) Diabetic nephropathy in insulin-dependent patients. Am J Kidney Dis 20: 533–547

Brochner-Mortensen J, Stockel M, Sorensen PJ, Nielson AH, Ditzel J (1984) Proximal glomerular tubular balance in patients with type-1 (insulin-dependent) diabetes mellitus. Diabetologia 27: 189–192

Brownlee M (1991) Glycosylation products as toxic mediators of diabetic complications. Annu Rev Med 42: 159–166

Brownlee M, Vassara H, Cerami A (1984) Nonenzymatic glycosylation and the pathogenesis of diabetes complications. Ann Intern Med 101: 527–537

Brownlee M, Cerami A, Vlassara H (1988) Advanced glycosylation end products in tissue and the biochemical basis of diabetic complications. N Engl J Med 318: 1315–1321

Chavers BM, Bilous RW, Ellis EN, Steffes M, Mauer SM (1989) Glomerular lesions and urinary albumin excretion in type-I diabetes without overt proteinuria. N Engl J Med 320: 966–970

Christiansen JS, Franden M, Parving HH (1981) Effect of intravenous glucose infusion on renal function in normal man and in insulin-dependent diabetes. Diabetologia 27: 368–373

Christlieb AR, Long R, Underwood RH (1979) Renin-angiotensin-aldosterone system, electrolyte homeostasis and blood pressure in alloxan diabetes. Am J Med Sci 277: 295–303

Cohen MP (1989) Nonenzymatic glycation and enhanced polyol pathway activity in the pathogenesis of diabetic nephropathy. In: Heidland A, Koch KM, Heidbreder E (eds) Diabetes and the kidney: contributions to nephrology. Karger, Basel, pp 59–72

Cohen MP, Klepser H (1988) Glomerular Na/K-ATPase activity in acute and chronic diabetes and with aldose reductase inhibition. Diabetes 37: 558–562

Cohen MP, Klepser H, Wu VY (1988) Heparan sulfate of glomerular basement membrane is undersulfated in experimental diabetes and is not corrected with aldose reductase inhibition. Diabetes 37: 1324–1327

Cohen MP, Surma ML (1980) Renal glomerular basement membrane. In vivo biosynthesis and turnover in normal rats. J Biol Chem 225: 1767–1770

Cohen MP, Surma ML, Wu VY (1982) In vivo biosynthsis and turnover of glomerular basement membrane in diabetic rats. Am J Physiol 242: F385–F389

Cohen MP, Urdanivia E, Surma M, Wu VY (1980) Increased glycosylation of glomerular basement membrane collagen in diabetes. Biochem Biophys Res Commun 95: 765–769

Cohen MP, Ziyadeh FN (1994) Amadori glucose adducts modulate mesangial cell growth and collagen gene expression. Kidney Int 45: 475–484

Craven P, Davidson C DeRubertis F (1990) Increase in diacylglycerol mass in isolated glomeruli by glucose from de novo synthesis of glycerolipids. Diabetes 39: 667–674

Deckert T, Parving HH, Thomsen OF, Jorgensen HE, Brun C, Thomsen AC (1986) Renel structure and function in type-I (insulin-dependent) diabetic patients. Diabetic Nephropathy 4: 163–168

DeFronzo RA (1980) Hyperkalemia and hyporeninemic hypoaldosteronism (clinical conference). Kidney Int 17: 118–134

DeFronzo RA, Goldberg M, Agus ZS (1976) The effects of glucose and insulin on renal electrolyte transport. J Clin Invest 58: 83–90

Diabetes Control and Complications Trial Group (1993) The effects of intensive insulin treatment of diabetes on the development and progression of long-term complications in insulin-dependent diabetes mellitus. N Engl J Med 329: 977–986

Ditzel J, Brochner-Mortensen J (1983) Tubular reabsorption rates as related to elevated glomerular filtration in diabetic children. Diabetes 32: 28–33

Ditzel J, Brochner-Mortensen J, Kawahara R (1982) Dysfunction of tubular phosphate reabsorption related to glomerular filtration and blood glucose in diabetic children. Diabetologia 23: 406–410

Doi TT, Vlassara H, Kirstein M, Yamada Y, Striker GE, Striker L (1992) Receptor-specific increase in extracellular matrix production in mouse mesangial cells by advanced glycosylation end products is mediated via platelet-derived growth factor. Proc Natl Acad Sci USA 89: 2873–2877

Ellis EN, Steffes MW, Goetz FC, Sutherland DE, Mauer SM (1986) Glomerular filtration surface in type-I diabetes mellitus. Kidney Int 29: 889–894

Fabre J, Balant LP, Dayer PG, Fox HM, Vernet AT (1982) The kidney in maturity-onset diabetes mellitus: a clinical study of 510 patients. Kidney Int 21: 730–738

Feldt-Rasmussen B, Mathiesen ER, Deckert T (1986) Effect of two years of strict metabolic control on progression of incipient nephropathy in insulin-dependent diabetes. Lancet 2: 1300

Fine LG, Badie-Dezfooly B, Lowe AG, Hamzeh A, Wells J, Salehmoghaddam S (1985) Stimulation of Na^+-H^+ antiport is an early event in hypertrophy of renal proximal tubular cells. Proc Natl Acad Sci USA 82: 1736–1740

Fioretto P, Steffes MW, Brown DM, Mauer SM (1992) An overview of renal pathology in insulin-dependent diabetes mellitus in relationship to altered glomerular hemodynamics. Am J Kidney Dis 20: 549–558

Flyvbjerg A, Marshall SM, Frystyk J, Hansen KW, Harris AG, Orskov H (1992) Octreotide adminstration in diabetic rats: effect on renal hypertrophy and urinary albumin excretion. Kidney Int 41: 805–812

Fogo A, Ichikawa I (1989) Evidence for the central role of glomerular growth promoters in the development of sclerosis. Semin Nephrol 9: 329–342

Frokjaer Thomsen O, Andersen A, Christiansen JS, Deckert T (1984) Renal changes in long-term type-1 (insulin-dependent) diabetic patients with and without clinical nephropathy: a light microscopic, morphometric study of autopsy material. Diabetologia 26: 361–365

Gellman DD, Pirani CL, Soothill JF, Muehrcke RC, Kark RM (1959) Diabetic nephropathy: a clinical and pathologic study based on renal biopsies. Medicine (Baltimore) 38: 321–367

Gibb DM, Tomlinson PA, Dalton NR, Turner C, Shah V, Barratt TM (1989) Renal tubular proteinuria and microalbuminuria in diabetic patients. Arch Dis Child 64: 129–134

Golchini K, Norman J, Boham R, Kurtz I (1989) Induction of hypertrophy in cultured proximal tubule cells by extracellular NH_4Cl. J Clin Invest 84: 1767–1779

Golfarb S, Ziyadeh FN, Kern EFO, Simmons DA (1991) Effects of polyol-pathway inhibition and dietary *myo*-inositol on glomerular hemodynamic function in experimental diabetes mellitus in rats. Diabetes 40: 465–471

Grantham JJ, Grantham JA, Donoo VS, Cragoe EJ (1989) Effect of amiloride on the compensatory renal growth that follows uninephrectomy in mice. J Lab Clin Med 114: 129–134

Greene DA, Lattimer SA, Sima AAF (1987) Sorbitol, phosphoinositides and the sodium-potassium ATPase in the pathogenesis of diabetic complications. N Engl J Med 316: 599–606

Guruprakash GH, Krothapalli RK, Rouse D, Babino H, Suki WN (1988) The mechanism of hypercalciuria in streptozotocin-induced diabetic rats. Metabolism 37: 306–311

Harris RC, Brenner BM, Seifter JL (1986) Sodium-hydrogen exchange and glucose transport in renal microvillus membrane vesicles from rats with diabetes mellitus. J Clin Invest 77: 724–733

Hazen-Martin DJ, Sens MA, Detrisac CJ, Blackburn JG, Sens DA (1989) Elevated glucose alters paracellular transport of cultured human proximal tubule cells. Kidney Int 35: 31–39

Heptinstall RH (1983) Diabetes mellitus and gout. In: Heptinstall RH (ed) Pathology of the kidney. Little-Brown, Boston, p 1426

Horlyck A, Gunderson HJG, Osterby R (1986) The cortical distribution pattern of diabetic glomerulopathy. Diabetologia 29: 146–150

Hostetter T (1986) Pathogenesis of diabetic nephropathy. In: Mitch W (ed) The progressive nature of renal disease: contemporary issues in nephrology. Chruchill Livingstone, New York, pp 149–166

Ihm C, Lee G, Nast C, Artishevsky A, Guillermo R, Levin R, Glassock R, Adler S (1992) Early increased procollagen α1(IV) mRNA levels in streptozotocin-induced diabetes. Kidney Int 41: 768–777

Khadouri C, Barlet-Bas C, Doucet A (1987) Mechanism of increased tubular Na-K-ATPase during stretozotocin-induced diabetes. Pflugers Arch 409: 296–301

Kirchner KA (1988) Insulin increases loop segment chloride reabsorption in the euglycemic rat. Am J Physiol 255: F1206–F1213

Kleinman KS, Fine LG (1988) Prognostic implications of renal hypertrophy in diabetes mellitus. Diabetes Metab Rev 4: 179–189

Krolewski AS, Warram JH, Laffel LMB (1992) Genetic susceptibility to diabetic nephropathy. Adv Nephrol 21: 69–81

Kumar AM, Gupta RK, Spitzer A (1988) Intracellular sodium in proximal tubules of diabetic rats. Role of glucose. Kidney Int 33: 792–797

Lane PH, Steffes MW, Fioretto P, Mauer SM (1993) Renal interstitial expansion in insulin-dependent diabetes mellitus. Kidney Int 43: 661–667

Ledbetter S, Copeland EJ, Noonan D, Vogeli G, Hassell JR (1990) Altered steady-state mRNA levels of basement membrane proteins in diabetic mouse kidneys and thromboxane synthase inhibition. Diabetes 39: 196–203

Lee GCL, Nast OC, Ihm CG, Guillermo R, Levin PS, Glassock RJ, Adler G (1990) Renal hypertrophy preceded elevated procollagen α1 (IV) mRNA levels after $1\frac{2}{3}$ nephrectomy. J Am Soc Nephrol 1: 635 (abstract)

Lee TS, Saltsman KA, Ohashi H, King GL (1989) Activation of protein kinase C by elevation of glucose concentration. Proposal for a mechanism in the development of diabetic vascular complications. Proc Natl Acad Sci USA 86: 5141–5145

Levin NW, Silveira E, Cortes P (1975) Relation of renal growth to diabetic glomerulosclerosis. Lancet 1: 1120–1121

Lewis EJ, Hunsicker LG, Bain RP, Rohde RD (1993) The effect of angiotensin-converting-enzyme inhibition on diabetic nephropathy. N Engl J Med 329: 1456–1462

MacGregor LC, Matschinsky FM (1986) Altered retinal metabolism in diabetes. II. Measurement of (Na,K)-ATPase and total sodium and potassium in individual retinal layers. J Biol Chem 261: 4052–4058

Mackovic-Basic M, Fine LG, Norman JT, Cragoe EJ, Kurtz I (1992) Stimulation of Na^+/H^+ exchange is not required for induction of hypertrophy of renal cells in vitro. J Am Soc Nephrol 3: 1124–1130

Mauer SM, Steffes MW, Azar S, Brown DM (1989) Effects of sorbinil on glomerular structure and function in long-term diabetic rats. Diabetes 38: 839–846

Mauer SM, Steffes MW, Ellis EN, Sutherland DER, Brown DM, Goetz FC (1984) Structural-functional relationships in diabetic nephropathy. J Clin Invest 74: 1143–1155

Michael AF, Brown DM (1981) Increased concentration of albumin in kidney basement membranes in diabetes mellitus. Diabetes 30: 843–846

Miltenyi M, Korner A, Tulassay T, Szabo A (1985) Tubular dysfunction in type-I diabetes mellitus. Arch Dis Child 60: 929–931

Mogensen C (1990) Prevention and treatment of renal disease in insulin-dependent diabetes mellitus. Semin Nephrol 10: 260–273

Mogensen CF (1971) Maximum tubular reabsorption capacity of glucose and renal hemodynamics during rapid hypertonic glucose infusion in normal and diabetic man. Scand J Clin Lab Invest 28: 101–109

Mogensen CE (1982) Diabetes mellitus and the kidney. Kidney Int 21: 673–675

Mogensen CE (1985) Long-term antihypertensive treatment inhibiting progression of diabetic nephropathy. Br Med J 285: 685–688

Mogensen CE, Christensen CK (1984) Predicting diabetic nephropathy in insulin-dependent patients. N Engl J Med 311: 89–93

Mogensen CE, Christensen NJ, Gunderson HJG (1978) The acute effect of insulin on renal hemodynamics and protein excretion in diabetes. Diabetologia 15: 153–157

Murrah V, Crosson J, Sauk J (1984) Abnormal binding of negatively charged serum proteins to diabetic basement membranes is largely a systemic phenomenon. Virchows Arch [A] 405: 141–154

Myers BD, Nelson RG, Williams GW, Bennett PH, Hardy SA, Berg RL, Loon L, Knowler WC, Mitch WE (1991) Glomerular function in Pima Indians with noninsulin-dependent diabetes mellitus to recent onset. J Clin Invest 88: 524–530

O'Donnel MP, Kaseske BL, Keane WF (1988) Glomerular hemodynamic and structural alterations in experimental diabetes mellitus. FASEB J 2: 2339–2347

Osterby R (1972) The number of glomerular cells and substructures in early juvenile diabetes. Acta Pathol Microbiol Scand [A] 80: 785–800

Osterby R (1975) Early phases in the development of diabetic glomerulopathy. A quantitative electron-microscopic study. Acta Med Scan 574 [Suppl]: 1–82

Osterby R, Gunderson HJG (1980) Fast accumulation of basement membrane material and the rate of morphological changes in acute experimental diabetic glomerular hypertrophy. Diabetologia 18: 493–500

Osterby R, Parving H, Nyberg G, Jorgensen H, Lokkegaard H, Svalander C (1988) A strong correlation between glomerular filtration rate and suface in diabetic nephropathy. Diabetologia 31: 265–270

Parving HH, Andersen AR, Smidt UM, Svendsen PAA (1983) Early aggressive anti-hypertensive treatment reduces rate of decline in kidney function in diabetic nephropathy. Lancet 2: 1175–1179

Pederson MM, Christiansen JS, Mogensen CE (1991) Reduction of glomerular hyperfiltration in normoalbuminuric IDDM patients by 6 months of aldose reductase inhibition. Diabetes 40: 527–531

Petersen A, Szwergold BS, Kappler F, Weingarten M, Brown TR (1990) Identification of sorbitol 3-phosphate and fructose 3-phosphate in normal and diabetic human erythrocytes. J Biol Chem 265: 17424–17427

Poulsom R, Kurkinen M, Prockop DJ, Boot-Hanford RP (1988) Increased steady-state levels of laminin B1 mRNA in kidneys of long-term streptozotocin-diabetic rats. No effect of aldose reductase inhibitor. J Biol Chem 263: 10072–10076

Pugliese G, Tilton RG, Williamson JR (1991) Glucose-induced metabolic imbalances in the pathogenesis of diabetic vascular disease. Diabetes Metab Rev 7: 35–59

Rasch R (1984) Tubular lesions in streptozotocin diabetic rats. Diabetologia 27: 32–37

Reichard P, Nilsson B, Rosenqvist U (1993) The effect of long-term intensified insulin treatment on the development of microvascular complications of diabetes mellitus. N Engl J Med 329: 304–309

Rengarts RT (1959) Asymptomatic bacilluria in 68 diabetic patients. Am J Med Sci 239: 159–171

Roberts AB, Kim SJ, Sporn MB (1991) Is there a common pathway mediating growth inhibition by TGF-β and the retinoblastoma gene product? Cancer Cells 3: 19–21

Rocco MV, Chen Y, Goldfarb S, Ziyadeh FN (1992) Elevated glucose stimulates TGF-β gene expression and bioactivity in proximal tubule. Kidney Int 41: 107–114

Rocco MV, Ziyadeh FN (1991) Transforming growth factor-beta: an update on systemic and renal actions. In: Goldfarbs, Ziyadeh FN (eds) Hormones, autacoids and the kidney: contemporary issues in nephrology. Chruchill Livingstone, New York, pp 391–410

Rowe DJF, Anthony F, Polak A, Shaw K, Ward CD, Watts GF (1987) Retinol binding protein as a small molecular weight marker of renal tubular function in diabetes mellitus. Ann Clin Biochem 24: 477–482

Schwieger J, Fine LG (1990) Renal hypertrophy, growth factors, and nephropathy in diabetes mellitus. Semin Nephrol 10: 242–253

Seyer-Hansen K (1983) Renal hypertrophy in experimental diabetes mellitus. Kidney Int 23: 643–646

Seyer-Hansen K, Hansen J, Gunderson HJG (1980) Renal hypertrophy in experimental diabetes. A morphometric study. Diabetologia 18: 501–505

Sharma K, Ziyadeh FN (1993) The transforming growth factor-β system and the kidney. Semin Nephrol 13: 116–128

Sharma K, Ziyadeh FN (1994) Renal hypertrophy is associated with upregulation of TGF-β1 gene expression in diabetic BB rat and NOD mouse. Am J Physiol 267: F1094–F1101

Soulis-Liparota T, Cooper M, Papazoglou D, Clarke B, Jerums G (1991) Retardation by aminoguanidine of development of albuminuria, mesangial expansion, and tissue fluorescence in streptozotocin-induced diabetic rat. Diabetes 40: 1328–1334

Stackhouse S, Miller PL, Park SK, Meyer TE (1990) Reversal of glomerular hyperfiltration and renal hypertrophy by blood glucose normalization in diabetic rats. Diabetes 39: 989–995

Steer KA, Sochor M, Gonzalez A-M, Mclean P (1982) Regulation of pathways of glucose metabolism in kidneys. Specific linking of pentose-phosphate pathway activity with kidney growth in experimental diabetes and unilateral nephrectomy. FEBS Lett 150: 494–498

Steffes M, Sutherland D, Goetz F, Rich S, Mauer S (1985) Studies of kidney and muscle biopsy specimens from identical twins discondant for type-I diabetes mellitus. N Engl J Med 312: 1282–1287

Steffes MW, Barbosa J, Basgen JM, Sutherland DER, Najarian JS, Mauer SM (1983) Quantitative glomerular morphology of the normal human kidney. Lab Invest 49: 82–86

Sternberg M, Cohen-Fortere L, Peyroux J (1985) Connective tissue in diabetes mellitus: biochemical alterations of the intercellular matrix with special reference to proteoglycans, collegens and basement membranes. Diabete Metab 11: 27–50

Studer RK, Craven PA DeRubertis FR (1993) Role of protein kinase C in the mediation of increased fibronectin accumulation by mesangial cells grown in high-glucose medium. Diabetes 42: 118–126

Suarez G, Rajaram R, Bhuyan KC, Oronsky AL, Goidi JA (1988) Administration of an aldose reductase inhibitor induces a decrease of collagen fluorescence in diabetic rats. J Clin Invest 82: 624–627

Szwergold BS, Kappler F, Brown TR (1990) Identification of fructose 3-phosphate in the lens of diabetic rats. Science 247: 451–454

Tilton RG, Baier LD, Harlow JE, Smith SR, Ostrow E, Williamson JR (1992) Diabetes-induced glomerular dysfunction: links to a more reduced cytosolic ratio of NADH/NAD$^+$. Kidney Int 41: 778–788

Tucker BJ, Rasch R, Blantz RC (1993) Glomerular filtration and tubular reabsorption of albumin in preproteinuric and proteinuric diabetic rats. J Clin Invest 92: 686–694

Vaamonde CA, Perez GO (1990) Tubular function in diabetes mellitus. Semin Nephrol 10: 203–218

Vejlsgaard R (1966) Studies on urinary infection in diabetes. II. Significant bacteriuria in relation to long-term diabetic manifestations. Acta Med Scand 179: 183–195

Wald H, Scherzer P, Popovtzer MM (1986) Enhanced renal tubular ouabain-sensitive ATPase in streptozotocin diabetes mellitus. Am J Physiol 251: F164–F170

Walker JD, Close CF, Jones SL, Rafftery M, Keen H, Viberti GC, Osterby R (1992) Glomerular structure in type-I (insulin-dependent) diabetic patients with normo- and microalbuminuria. Kidney Int 41: 741–748

Walker JD, Dodds RA, Murrells TJ, Bending JJ, Mattock MB, Keen H, Viberti GC (1989) Restricition of dietary protein and progression of renal failure in diabetic nephropathy. Lancet 2: 1411–1415

Walton C, Bodansky HJ, Wales JK, Forbes MA, Cooper EH (1988) Tubular dysfunction and microalbuminuria in insulin-dependent diabetes. Arch Dis Child 63: 244–249

Weil R, Nozawa M, Koss M, Reemtsma K, McIntosh R (1976) The kidney in streptozotocin diabetic rats. Morphological ultrastructural and functional studies. Arch Pathol Lab Med 100: 37–49

Winegrad A (1987) Banting Lecture 1986: Does a common mechanism induce the diverse complications of diabetes? Diabetes 36: 396–406

Wolf G, Neilson EG, Goldfarb S, Ziyadeh FN (1991) The influence of glucose concentration on angiotensin-II-induced hypertrophy of proximal tubular cells in culture. Biochem Biophys Res Commun 176: 902–909

Wolf G, Mueller E, Stahl RAK, Ziyadeh FN (1993) Angiotensin-II-induced hypertrophy of cultured murine proximal tubular cell is mediated by endogenous TGF-β. J Clin Invest 92: 1366–1373

Zador IZ, Deshmukh GD, Kunkel R, Johnson K, Radin NS, Shayman JA (1993) A role for glycosphingolipid accumulation in the renal hypertrophy of streptozotocin-induced diabetes mellitus. J Clin Invest 91: 797–803

Zatz R, Dunn BR, Meyer TW, Anderson S, Rennke HG, Brenner BM (1986) Prevention of diabetic glomerulopathy by pharmacological amelioration of glomerular capillary hypertension. J Clin Invest 77: 1925–1930

Zeller K, Whittaker E, Sullivan L, Raskin P, Jacobson HR (1991) Effect of restricting dietary protein on the progression of renal failure in patients with diabetes mellitus. N Engl J Med 324: 78–84

Ziyadeh FN (1993a) The extracellular matrix in diabetic nephropathy. Am J Kidney Diss 22: 736–744

Ziyadeh FN (1993b) Renal tubular basement membrane and collagen type IV in diabetes mellitus. Kidney Int 43: 114–120

Ziyadeh FN, Cohen MP (1993) Effects of glycated albumin on mesangial cells: evidence for a role in diabetic nephropathy. Mol Cell Biochem 125: 19–25

Ziyadeh FN, Goldfarb S (1991) The renal tubulointerstitium in diabetes mellitus. Kidney Int 39: 464–475

Ziyadeh FN, Goldfarb S, Kern EFO (1989) Diabetic nephropathy: metabolic and biochemical mechanisms. In: Brenner BM, Stein JH (eds) The kidney in diabetes mellitus. Churchill Livingstone, New York, pp 87–113

Ziyadeh FN, Snipes ER, Watanabe M, Alvarez RJ, Goldfarb S, Haverty TP (1990) High glucose induces cell hypertrophy and stimulates collagen gene transcription in proximal tubule. Am J Physiol 259: F704–F714

Ziyadeh FN, Chen Y, Davila A, Goldfarb S, Wolf G (1991a) Self-limited stimulation of mesangial cell growth in high glucose: autocrine activation of TGF-β reduces proliferation but increases mesangial matrix. J Am Soc Nephrol 2: 304 (abstract)

Ziyadeh FN, Simmons DA, Snipes ER, Goldfarb S (1991b) Effect of *myo*-inositol on cell proliferation and collagen transcription and secretion in proximal tubule cells cultured in elevated glucose. J Am Soc Nephrol 1: 1220–1229

Ziyadeh FN, Sharma K, Ericksen M, Wolf G (1994) Stimulation of collagen gene expression and protein synthesis in murine mesangial cells by high glucose is mediated by activation of transforming growth factor-β. J Clin Invest 93: 536–542

Selected Experimental Models of Renal Tubular Atrophy and of Cystic Tubular Cell Hyperplasia

H.-J. Gröne

Abbreviations: AI, angiotensin I; AII, angiotensin II; ATP, adenosine triphosphate; BSA, bovine serum albumin; C, casein diet; CF, casein fat diet; D, daunomycin; FF, filtration fraction; GFR, glomerular filtration rate; HPF, high power field (objective × 40 ocular × 10); i.p., intraperitoneal; i.v., intravenous; NAD, nicotinamide adenine dinucleotide; P, regular pelleted rat chow; PAN, puromycinaminonucleoside; PRA, plasma renin activity; RAS, renin angiotensin system; RBF, renal blood flow; RPF, renal plasma flow; RRA, renal renin activity; RVR, renal vascular resistance.

Current Topics in Pathology
Volume 88, S.M. Dodd (Ed.)
© Springer-Verlag Berlin Heidelberg 1995

1 Introduction

1.1 Clinical-Pathologic Relevance of Renal Tubular Lesions

The nephron constitutes the smallest functional unit of the kidney. It consists of glomerulus, proximal tubule, Henle's loop, and distal tubule. The relative volume of the tubuli exceeds that of any other renal structure. About 85% of the total volume of the renal cortex is taken up by tubules (PEDERSON et al. 1980). The different tubular segments have been characterized structurally and functionally in detail (BOYLAN et al. 1970; CHRISTENSEN and MAUNSBACH 1980; MAACK et al. 1985; MAUNSBACH 1966; VON MÖLLENDORF 1930; TRUMP et al. 1985). Tubular lesions exert a major influence on the extent and course of renal and glomerular diseases. Patients with severe proliferative extracapillary glomerulonephritis may have normal excretory renal function if lesions of tubuli do not occur. On the other hand, a glomerulonephritis with slight glomerular alterations but with severe tubulointerstitial reactive lesions may be accompanied by a significant reduction in renal function (BOHLE et al. 1986).

Two modes of renal tubular alterations can be observed in chronic renal disease:

1. Atrophic epithelia without segmental differentiation, which can be found in ectatic and collapsed tubuli.
2. Hypertrophic and hyperplastic epithelia. A proliferation of epithelia in differentiated and in regressively altered tubular segments is a frequent phenomenon in cystic kidney disease (GARDNER and EVAN 1984).

1.2 General Aim of the Study

In order to study pathogenetic factors that are relevant to renal tubular atrophy and renal tubular hyperplasia, new experimental models of atrophy and hyperplasia of renal tubular epithelia were developed. These animal models enabled us to compare the functional and morphological characteristics of these tubular alterations and to demonstrate common and contrasting features. A major criterion for the establishment of a given model was its clinical relevance.

1.3 Clinical and Pathophysiologic Basis and Hypothesis of the Model of Tubular Atrophy

1.3.1 Clinical Basis

Arterial hypertension is a frequent disease in industralized nations. Epidemiologic studies prove the efficiency of antihypertensive therapy, which reduces the deleterious consequences of arterial hypertension, such as cerebral ischemia and chronic renal insufficiency (GRÖNE and DUNN 1985; SCHELER and GRÖNE 1982).

Unwanted effects of a reduction of arterial pressure on renal function have been published in case reports but not examined systematically (SCHELER and GRÖNE 1982). The development and clinical application of antihypertensives that inhibit the renin-angiotensin system (RAS) have instigated studies on the renal effects of these substances, since a decrease in renal function was sometimes observed during RAS inhibition and since the RAS seems to have and blood pressure reduction, an important physiologic role in the regulation of renal hemodynamics (GROSS et al. 1991; NAVAR and ROSIVALL 1984; SWEET et al. 1981).

1.3.2 Pathophysiologic Basis

Renin is synthesized in the epithelioid cells of the juxtaglomerular apparatus; it catalyzes the conversion of angiotensionogen into angiotensin I (AI). The decapeptide AI is converted to the octapeptide angiotensin II (AII) by angiotensin-converting enzyme (ACE). AII in plasma is rapidly degraded by angiotensinases (CUSHMAN et al. 1980). AII binds specifically to receptors with different affinities in structures such as the adrenal gland, arterial vessels, and renal tubules (DOUGLAS 1987; GRÖNE et al. 1992). It increases the synthesis of aldosterone in the adrenal cortex; vessels are constricted by nanogram concentrations of AII. AII effects on renal tubular epithelia are concentration dependent: low concentrations increase the reabsorption of sodium; high AII concentrations lead to natriuresis (HARRIS and NAVAR 1985). AII also has hyperplastic and hypertrophic effects on the renal tubular epithelium (NORMAN et al. 1987).

Animal experiments and investigations of patients with arterial hypertension have demonstrated the pathogenetic role of the RAS in different forms of arterial hypertension, especially hypertension due to renal artery stenosis (HELMCHEN and KNEISSLER 1976; SCHWIETZER 1980). After construction of the renal artery, baroreceptors of afferent arterioles activate the secretion of renin and the RAS. The increased AII synthesis leads to systemic arterial hypertension and to arterial normotension in the kidney distal to the renal artery stenosis.

Inhibition of the AII receptors by AII antagonists, inhibition of ACE or of the enzymatic activity of renin can lower the increased systemic arterial pressure (HELMCHEN and KNEISSLER 1976; LEVENSON and DZAU 1987; SPERTINI et al. 1981). Antihypertensive therapy with ACE inhibitors thus seems reasonable in renovascular hypertension. This therapeutic approach is advantageous for the systemic circulation, but not necessarily for the stenosed kidney. During arterial hypotension AII differentially affects the resistance of renal arterial and arteriolar vessels to ascertain a relative constancy of the effective glomerular filtration pressure and glomerular filtration rate (GFR) (STEINHAUSEN 1987).

ANDERSON et al. (1979) demonstrated that in acute constriction of the renal artery of the dog the blockade of AII dramatically increased the effective resistance of the renal artery clip. AII thus reduced the fall in arterial pressure on the renal artery clip and increased the intrarenal perfusion pressure to maintain glomerular filtration.

1.3.3 Hypotheses

Our studies were designed to test the hypotheses that

1. Blockade of the RAS leads to a decrease in renal excretory function in a kidney distal to a stenosis.
2. Chronic RAS inhibition leads to renal tubular damage and a decrease in tubular function due to the inhibition of the hemodynamic and direct tubular effects of AII.

Since a "clipped" kidney does not constitute an immunologic glomerular disease or an inflammatory lesion of the tubulointerstitial compartment, and does not have hypertensive lesions, (a) the effect of a disturbed hemodynamic situation on renal tubular function and (b) the chronic effect of a suspected tubular lesion on renal function without interference by other factors seemed to be testable.

Clinical observations by our group and case reports of other clinical groups on a significant reduction of renal function during ACE inhibition in patients with bilateral renal artery stenosis supported the clinical relevance of the experimental studies (Gröne et al. 1982; Kindler et al. 1981; Levenson and Dzau 1987).

A further aim of our experiments was to test whether the expected tubular atrophy was reversible after discontinuing RAS inhibition.

1.4 Clinical and Pathophysiologic Basis and Hypothesis
of the Model of Cystic Hyperplasia of Renal Tubules

1.4.1 Clinical Basis

Cystic renal diseases are genetic or acquired alterations of the kidney (Garner 1976). The incidence of autosomal dominant polycystic kidney disease is 1–5%, according to autopsy series (Torres et al. 1985). The prevalence of the gene of polycystic kidneys has been estimated to be 2.5% (Dalgaard 1957; Iglesias et al. 1983; Torres et al. 1985). Almost 500 000 persons in the U.S.A. and about 150 000 patients in West Germany carry the polycystic kidney disease gene. Autosomal dominant polycystic kidney disease is therefore not a rare genetic disease (Schimke 1985).

Prior to peritoneal and hemodialysis, 50–60 of patients with autosomal dominant polycystic kidney disease died of uremia. Today, about 8% of all dialysis patients have polycystic kidneys (Kramer et al. 1982).

Twenty-seven to 47% of chronic dialysis patients have cysts in their kidneys. These cystic kidneys are known as acquired polycystic kidneys and may be either shrunken or enlarged (DUNNILL et al. 1977; DUNNILL 1985; ELLIOTT et al. 1977; FEINER et al. 1981; HUGHSON et al. 1986; THOMPSON et al. 1986). In patients with chronic renal disease but without dialysis therapy, acquired polycystic kidneys have also been described (FAVEMI and ALI 1980; GRANTHAM 1985; KREMPIEN and RIETZ 1980). Restrospective analysis has confirmed that acquired polycystic kidneys increase the risk of developing a renal tubular cell tumor. Papillary epithelial proliferations in cysts as well as renal cell carcinomas were described (CHUNG-PARK et al. 1983; FARROW and WILKINSON 1979; GARDNER 1984; ISHIKAWA et al. 1980). The incidence of renal cell carcinomas in acquired polycystic kidney disease is 5–6% almost eightfold higher than in the normal population (HUGHSON et al. 1980, 1986; HUGHSON 1985; MATAS et al. 1975). Although a tubular cell proliferation can also be documented in autosomal dominant polycystic kidneys, the risk of developing renal cell carcinoma does not seem to be increased in this patient group as compared with the normal population (ZEIER et al. 1987).

In addition, the clinical relevance of genetic or acquired polycystic kidney disease is based on the fact that hemorrhages and bacterial infections can occur in renal cysts (BENNETT 1985; NARASIMHA et al. 1986; SWEET and KEANE 1979).

1.4.2 Pathophysiologic Basis

Cystic kidneys show numerous light-microscopically, ultrastructurally and functionally *divergent* aspects. Atrophic tubules and, in relation to the total number of nephrons, relatively few cystic tubular segments can be observed beside normal tubules. Tubular cysts can show pores to neighboring tubules or have no communication to nephron (GRANTHAM et al. 1987). Cystic epithelia either show normal segmental differentiation by light microscopy and electron microscopy or consist only of dedifferentiated, flat epithelia. Tubular basement membranes and the interstitial extracellular matrix may not be increased or significantly thickened (COHEN and HOYER 1986; WINSTON and SAFIRSTEIN 1985). The intraluminal cystic pressure may be elevated, comparable to the normal tubular pressure, or diminished (GRANTHAM 1983). The absorptive and secretory activity of cystic epithelia varies enormously. In contrast to solitary renal cysts, those in cystic kidneys may still constitute parts of a functionally active nephron and, depending on their topography as proximal or distal tubular segments, may reabsorb sodium or secrete potassium and hydrogen ions (BRICKER and PATTON 1955; CUPPAGE et al. 1980; GARDNER 1969; GARDNER et al. 1976; MILUTINOVIC et al. 1980). The total excretory renal function can be normal or significantly decreased in renal cystic disease (MARTINEZ-MALDONADO 1985; PREUSS et al. 1979; REUBI 1985).

Within the context of our experiments on tubular cystogenesis, it did not seem sensible to take the aforementioned heterogeneous characteristics of cystic kidneys as the basis of this study. Rather, we tried to characterize a constant feature of cystic kidneys. In experimental and human cystic kidneys, a proliferation of epithelia that cover a dilated tubule or the tubular cyst can always be found (BERNSTEIN et al. 1987; McKINLEY 1920; STRUM 1875). Independent of biochemical and cell biological investigations, this epithelial hyperplasia can be deduced from the geometry of renal cysts (GRANTHAM 1983). A normal human kidney tubule has a diameter of 40 μm; the epithelium has a height of almost 7.5 μm. If after tubular dilatation the tubular diameter is 5 or 10 mm, epithelial height without epithelial proliferation will be 48.8 or 24.4 nm. These epithelial heights are no longer visible with the light microscope. However, cystic epithelium in human cystic kidneys can be seen by light microscopy quite easily. In human and experimentally induced cystic kidneys, morphometric investigations have frequently shown epithelial heights comparable to that of normal tubular epithelium. By scanning electron microscopy, polypoid epithelial proliferations were often found (BERNSTEIN et al. 1987; EVAN and GARDNER 1976, 1979).

The exogeneous and endogenous features that can initiate a proliferation of tubular epithelia are shown in Fig. 1 (BERNSTEIN et al. 1987; CROCKER et al. 1987; HAY 1983; WILSON and SHERWOOD 1991). Epithelial hyperplasia would be a secondary phenomenon if increased mitotic activity occurred after dilatation of the tubules due to an enhanced compliance of the basement membrane. Cells in culture can be induced to synthesize new DNA by simple stretching (BRUNETTE 1984). The remaining factors for epithelial proliferative activity shown in Fig. 1 can primarily change the proliferative kinetics of tubular epithelia. "Primary" epithelial hyperplasia could contribute to cystogenesis in different modes.

The proliferated epithelium partially or totally obstructs the tubular lumen with consecutive dilatation of the proximal tubular segments during conserved

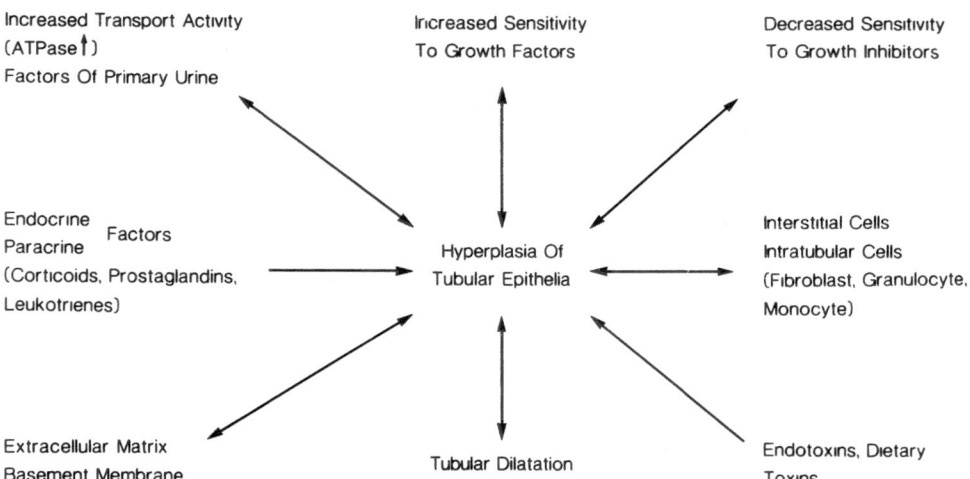

Fig. 1. Possible hyperplastic factors of renal tubular epithelia. →unidirectional action; ↔ interaction

glomerular filtration. Changed structure and compliance of the tubular basement membrane and hyperplasia of the tubular epithelium may contribute to cystogenesis. A proliferating epithelium could produce abnormal basement membrane components and thus change the compliance of the tubular membrane. The multitude of factors that can potentially stimulate tubular epithelium suggests that hyperplasia of the tubular epithelium does not constitute an epiphenomenon, but rather the primary feature of cystogenesis.

A controlled investigation of the role of epithelial hyperplasia in the genesis of cystic kidneys does not seen feasible in humans. Functional, biochemical, and morphological investigations cannot be performed continuously, but only at the time of an operation or at the end stage of a disease. The dynamics of the disease process thus have not been elucidated. Experiments on the characteristics of proliferation of tubular epithelium and its role in cystogenesis therefore demand an experimental approach.

Several experimental models of cystic kidneys have been described (CROCKER et al. 1972; DOBYAN et al. 1981; RESNICK et al. 1976; SAFOUH et al. 1970). (GRANTHAM et al. 1987; AVNER et al. 1988; COWLEY et al. 1993; RAHILLY et al. 1992; TAKAHASHI et al. 1991). Besides genetically determined cystic kidney disease models, antioxidants, antimycotics, and antihelmintics have been applied as so-called cystogenic substances (BAXTER 1960; EVAN et al. 1978; GARDNER and EVAN 1983; GOODMAN et al. 1970; McGEOCH and DARMADY 1973). Some of these substances have been found in foods and could also be effective in human renal cystogenesis (GARDNER and EVAN 1984). Nevertheless, one has to consider that only a small percentage of people who consume these dietary cystogenic substances indeed develop renal cysts or cystic kidneys. Endogenous influences thus seem to be of importance in the pathogenesis of acquired cystic kidneys.

1.4.3 Hypothesis

In our own experiments on the development of renovascular hypertension in rats, glomerular lesions and the consecutive proteinuria were followed by hyperplasia of the tubular epithelium and dilated tubules. In rats with nephrotic syndrome, cystic tubular alterations were described (ANDREWS 1977; BERTANI et al. 1986; GIROUX et al. 1984).

Reports on renal biopsy results in related infants with so-called infantile Finnish-type nephrosis suggested that the typical tubular cysts of this renal disease occurred after loss of the glomerular permselectivity and with glomerular proteinuria (AUTIO-HARMAINEN et al. 1981; HUTTUNEN 1976; RISDON and TURNER 1980).

Kidneys with excretory impairment due to chronic vascular, glomerular, or interstitial disease and end-stage kidneys of dialysis patients with some residual renal function are prone to develop renal cysts and quite often have glomerular proteinuria of the functioning nephrons.

The following experiments therefore tested the hypothesis that proteinuria may induce tubular epithelial hyperplasia and lead to tubular cysts. It was the aim of this study to investigate etiologically different models of proteinuria in the rat to determine the general importance of proteinuria for tubular dilatation and cytogenesis. Besides induction of glomerular proteinuria by administration of heterologous bovine serume albumin (BSA), nephrotic syndromes were induced by the chemotherapeutic substances daunomycin (D) and puromycinaminonuc-leoside (PAN). Experiments in the rat indicated that the growth of the kidney may be fostered by so-called synthetic protein diets and a high fat content of the diet. We therefore additionally tested whether diets with varying protein and fat contents could perhaps enhance the suspected tubular effect of glomerular proteinuria.

2 Experimental Design

2.1 Model of Tubular Atrophy

The experiment was done using rats with renovascular hypertension with two-kidney, one-clip hypertension. A silver clip with an internal diameter of 0.2 mm was placed on the left renal artery of anesthetized male Wistar rats with a body weight of 160–180 g (WILSON et al. 1986). Four weeks later, those rats with a systolic arterial pressure exceeding 150 mmHg received a sodium-deficient diet (13 mM Na/kg diet; diet no. 1036, Altromin GmbH, D-4910 Lage, FRG.) and distilled water ad libitum. After a week of sodium-deficient diet, the animals were treated with the ACE inhibitor MK 421 or with the vasodilator dihyd-ralazine (KOCH-WESER 1976; SPERTINI et al. 1981; SWEET et al. 1981). Control animals were fed a sodium-deficient diet only. The reversibility of the tubular alterations was tested under four different conditions:

Group 1: After 14 days of antihypertensive therapy, the left renal artery was unclipped and the right contralateral kidney was excised. The animals were then observed for a period of 2–7 days, equivalent to a total experiment time of 16–21 days.

Group 2: Only the silver clip on the left renal artery was removed after 14 days of MK 421 therapy. Observation time after therapy and surgery was 7–21 days, corresponding to a total experiment time of 21–35 days.

Group 3: After discontinuing ACE inhibition after 14 days of treatment and without surgery, the rats were observed for 10, 28, and 49 days, corresponding to a total experiment time of 24, 42, and 63 days.

Group 4: Rats with renovascular hypertension were treated with MK 421 for 14, 31, and 51 days.

2.2 Models of Cystic Hyperplasia of Renal Tubules

Male Wistar rats with a body weight of 180–220 g were nephrectomized on the left side. After 3 weeks the animals received heterologous BSA or D or PAN.

Group 1 (heterologous albuminuria): The rats were injected intraperitoneally (i.p.) with 1.5 g BSA/4 ml H_2O/24 h for 4, 7, 28, and 56 days. Controls received a solution containing the same electrolyte content as the albumin solution in equal volumes.

Group 2 (uninephrectomized rats with daunomycin nephrosis): D leads to a nephrosis with pronounced glomerular proteinuria in rats (SHIRAIWA et al. 1986; STERNBERG 1970). D was injected once in a dose of 5 mg/kg body wt. into the tail vein. The experiment time varied from 9 to 56 days.

Group 3 (puromycinaminonucleoside nephrosis): PAN, like D, increases the permeability of the glomerular basement membrane (HAASE et al. 1965; HOCH-LIGETI 1960). PAN was injected three times in a dosage of 35 mg/kg body wt. i.p. at 7-day intervals. Experiment time after the last PAN injection was 49 days. Rats of the three groups received different diets. They contained similar amounts of total protein but varied in the quality of the protein. P was conventional rat chow with a mixture of different proteins; C contained only casein; CF was a casein- and fat-rich diet with a total fat content of 39% and a cholesterol content of 5%. The respective diet was started in the first group 1 week before and in groups 2 and 3 1 day after administration of the drug to adapt the animals to the diet at the start of the glomerular proteinuria.

3 Results

3.1 Model of Tubular Atrophy

Animals with renal vascular hypertension (two-kidney, one clip model) received long-term treatment with two antihypertensives: (a) the nonspecific vasodilator dihydralazine and (b) the specific angiotensin-converting-enzyme (ACE) blocker MK 421 (Fig. 2).

MK 421 inhibited plasma ACE activity until the end of therapy (MK 421 $n = 13$: 72 ± 13 versus hypertensive controls $n = 19$: 293 ± 12 nmol/l/min). Renal cortical renin activity was significantly increased in the clipped left kidney as compared with the right normal kidney (MK 421 $n = 13$, left kidney 1.77 ± 0.39, right kidney 0.65 ± 0.05 ng/mg/h).

Plasma creatinine and urea concentrations were in the normal range after 2 weeks of dihydralazine or MK 421 therapy (POPPER et al. 1937). In contrast, significant differences in glomerular filtration rate (GFR) were measured within and between groups when split renal function measurements were done (Fig. 2b).

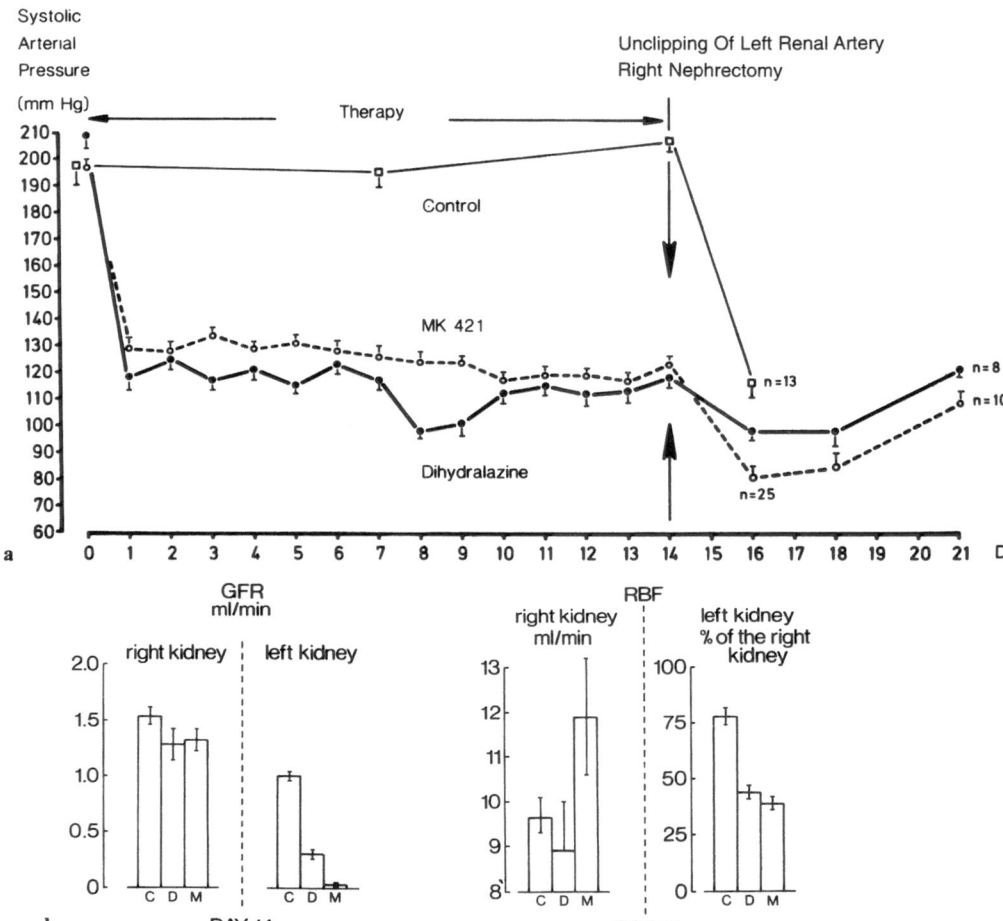

Fig. 2. a Systolic arterial pressure in sodium-depleted rats with two-kidney, one-clip hypertension (PFEFFER et al. 1971). Two-week treatment period was followed by contralateral nephrectomy and unclipping of the left renal artery. **b, c** Split renal function, glomerular filtration rate (GFR), and renal blood flow (RBF) in sodium-depleted rats with two-kidney, one-clip hypertension after 14 days of antihypertensive therapy with dihydralazine (*D*) or with the angiotensin-converting enzyme inhibitor MK 421 (*M*). **b** Mean GFR of the clipped kidneys of hypertensive control rats (*C*) was only about 66% of mean GFR of the contralateral right kidneys but 3.7-fold higher than the GFR of clipped kidneys of dihydralazine-treated rats, and 34-fold higher than GFR of clipped kidneys of MK 421-treated rats. **c** Mean RBF of the left clipped kidneys of control rats was significantly higher than that of clipped kidneys of both treatment groups. Mean RBF of the clipped kidney of dihydralazine-treated rats did not differ significantly from that of clipped kidneys of MK 421-treated animals

In hypertensive controls, the left GFR was 33% less than the GFR of the right kidney (1.03 ± 0.03 versus 1.55 ± 0.08 ml/min). In dihydralazine-treated animals, the mean GFR of the left clipped kidney was only 22% of the GFR of the right kidney and only 27% of the left GFR of control hypertensive animals.

In ACE inhibitor MK 421-treated rats, glomerular filtration was drastically reduced in the clipped left kidney. The GFR was only 0.03 ± 0.01 ml/min and thus only 2–3% of the GFR of the contralateral kidney, and only 10% of the GFR of the clipped kidneys of animals treated with the nonspecific vasodilator dihydralazine. In animals with RAS blockade, urine flow stopped when systemic mean arterial pressure was less than 90–59 mmHg. In contrast, urine flow stopped with systemic mean arterial pressures of 75–70 mmHg or lower in dihydralazine-treated rats. The GFR of the right kidney was comparable in both treatment groups and control hypertensive animals.

Renal plasma flow (RPF) of clipped kidneys was not significantly different in the two treatment groups (Fig. 2c). The left renal blood flow (RBF) of treated animals was nevertheless significantly lower than in left kidneys of control hypertensive rats. Animals that were treated with ACE inhibitor showed a significantly higher RBF in unmanipulated right kidneys as compared with control hypertensive and dihydralazine-treated rats. Filtration fraction (FF) of right kidneys in MK 421-treated rats had decreased to 23% and was significantly lower than in the control and dihydralazine groups. The left clipped kidneys of animals treated with RAS blockade had significantly lower weights after 14 days of therapy than kidneys distal to renal artery stenosis in the control hypertensive and dihydralazine groups. Kidney weights decreased further with continued therapy (80% loss of kidney weight as compared with clipped kidneys of control hypertensive rats after 51 treatment days) (Figs. 3 and 4f).

The main light-microscopic alterations in the shrunken, clipped kidneys could be seen within the tubules. Glomeruli showed only slight changes. Glomerular diameters were smaller in animals with RAS blockade than in those with untreated clipped kidneys. The visceral epithelial cells appeared to have lost the fine interdigitated foot processes, as seen by scanning electron microscopy (Fig. 6d). Essentially, two tubular alterations were seen in the shrunken clipped kidneys of animals treated by ACE inhibition (MK 421):

1. Atrophic proximal tubules with small or no lumina
2. Proximal tubules with flattened segment-dedifferentiated epithelia and seemingly widened lumina. In either case, segments of the atrophic, collapsed, proximal tubules were lined by epithelia with clear cytoplasm. Ultrastructurally, the number of mitochondria had decreased significantly; the brush border had flattened (Figs. 5, 6a–c).

According to this ultrastructural finding, villin as a specific structural protein of the brush border was only focally observed in MK 421-treated animals after 14 days of therapy and was not documented in animals with severe tubular epithelial atrophy (51 treatment days with MK 421). The atrophic epithelia did not show a basal labyrinth; tubular basement membranes appeared convoluted and slightly thickened due to the collapse of the tubular lumina. The interstitium was not enlarged. In atrophic kidneys with dilated tubules, a slight interstitial fibrosis and thickening of the tubular basement membrane was observed with continued therapy (more than 14 treatment days). The epithelia of the dilated tubules were

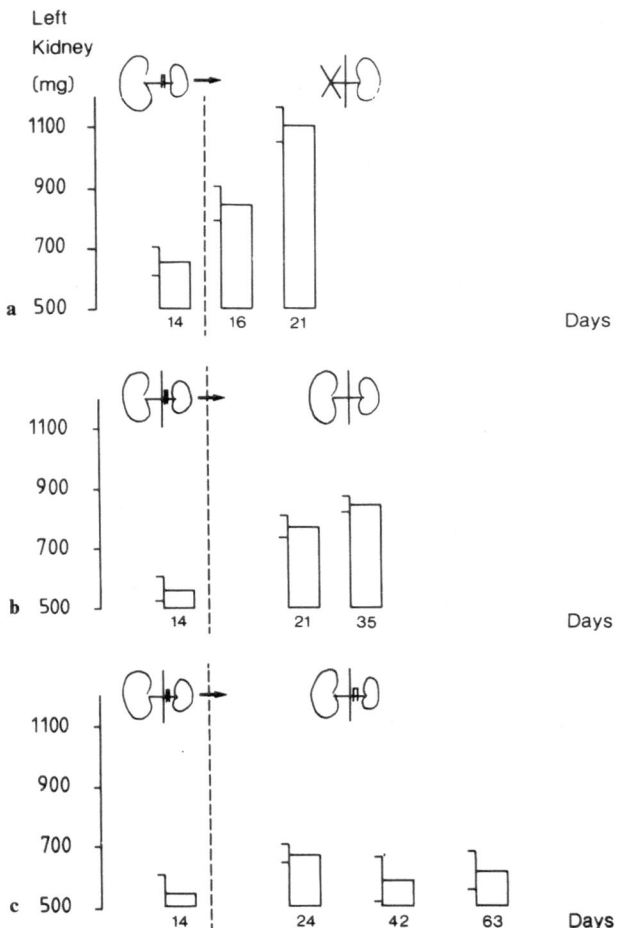

Fig. 3a–c. Development of mean weights of left clipped kidneys of MK 421-treated rats with two-kidney, one-clip hypertension after a 14-day treatment phase. **a** After unclipping and contralateral nephrectomy, the mean weight of clipped kidneys increased by about 170% within 7 days. **b** After unclipping and cessation of MK 421 therapy, mean weight of clipped kidneys increased by about 150% within 21 days. **c** After cessation of therapy but without contralateral nephrectomy and without unclipping, the mean weight of clipped kidneys did not change significantly within the 7-week post-therapeutic observation period

flattened and did not possess a brush border. Necrosis or mitosis of epithelia were only seldom observed.

The atrophic epithelia of collapsed tubules often showed a structureless cytoplasm without a prominent expression of filaments. Nevertheless, in a few epithelia and groups of tubules that were dilated, the co-expression of the intermediate filaments keratin and vimentin was observed (Fig. 13e, f). Normal tubular epithelia of adult rat kidneys were negative for the intermediate filament vimentin and exclusively expressed the intermediate filament-type keratin, as did other epithelial cells. The co-expression of vimentin and keratin in atrophic, clear, and didifferentiated flat epithelia was observed in MK 421-treated animals independent of the extent of tubular atrophy. As will be shown for the model of cystic kidney disease, tubular epithelia in hyperplastic and hypertrophic tubules can show a co-expression of the intermediate filaments keratin and vimentin. Distal tubules did not demonstrate major alterations. The epithelium appeared only slightly lower in height than normal. The arrangement of cytoplasmic organelles, especially of mitochondria, was only slightly disturbed in comparison to distal tubules of clipped kidneys of hypertensive control animals.

The atrophy of the proximal tubules in clipped kidneys of animals with RAS blockade was shown morphometrically. The cross-sectional areas of tubules in MK 421 rats were only 45% of those of control animals (Fig. 4).

The activity of two key enzymes of cellular metabolism of proximal tubular epithelia was determined to characterize the function of the described atrophic proximal tubules. Na-K-ATPase is a major enzyme for energy-dependent, transepithelial transport processes (ROSSIER et al. 1987). Cathepsins are lysosomal enzymes that degrade proteins reabsorbed from primary urine in proximal tubular epithelia; they also catalyze the degradation of cell proteins.

In dissected proximal tubular segments S1 Na-K-ATPase activity was significantly lowered in MK 421-treated animals. This difference was seen in comparison to the contralateral kidney of the same animal and also in comparison to the clipped kidneys of hypertensive control rats (GARG et al. 1981). Cathepsin B and L activities were decreased in dissected proximal tubular segments S1 of kidneys behind the renal artery stenosis in rats with ACE inhibition in comparison to contralateral kidneys of the same rats and in comparison to clipped kidneys of hypertensive control rats.

If ACE inhibition continued for 5 and 7 weeks, tubular atrophy progressed. Brush borders disappeared; the tubular lumina were filled with autofluorescent material. Proximal and distal tubules in cortex and medulla were eventually completely destroyed. The interstitium was infiltrated with a few mononuclear cells and was only slightly expanded considering the extensive atrophy of the clipped kidney.

Clipped kidneys of animals treated with the vasodilator dihydralazine demonstrated a barely discernible atrophy of proximal tubules that was convincingly shown only by morphometry (Fig. 4a vs. b). Especially in animals with temporary drastic reduction of arterial pressure, the stenosed kidneys showed small foci of ectatic tubules with flattened dedifferentiated epithelia. Clear tubular atrophy was only rarely observed. The mean cross-sectional area of proximal tubules was nevertheless 25% less than in clipped kidneys of hypertensive control rats. The left clipped kidneys of untreated hypertensive rats generally showed a regular morphology. The kidneys were protected from the systemically increased arterial pressure by the renal artery clip. Only very small foci of atrophic tubules with seemingly thickened basement membranes and a very slight fibrosis of the surrounding interstitium were visible.

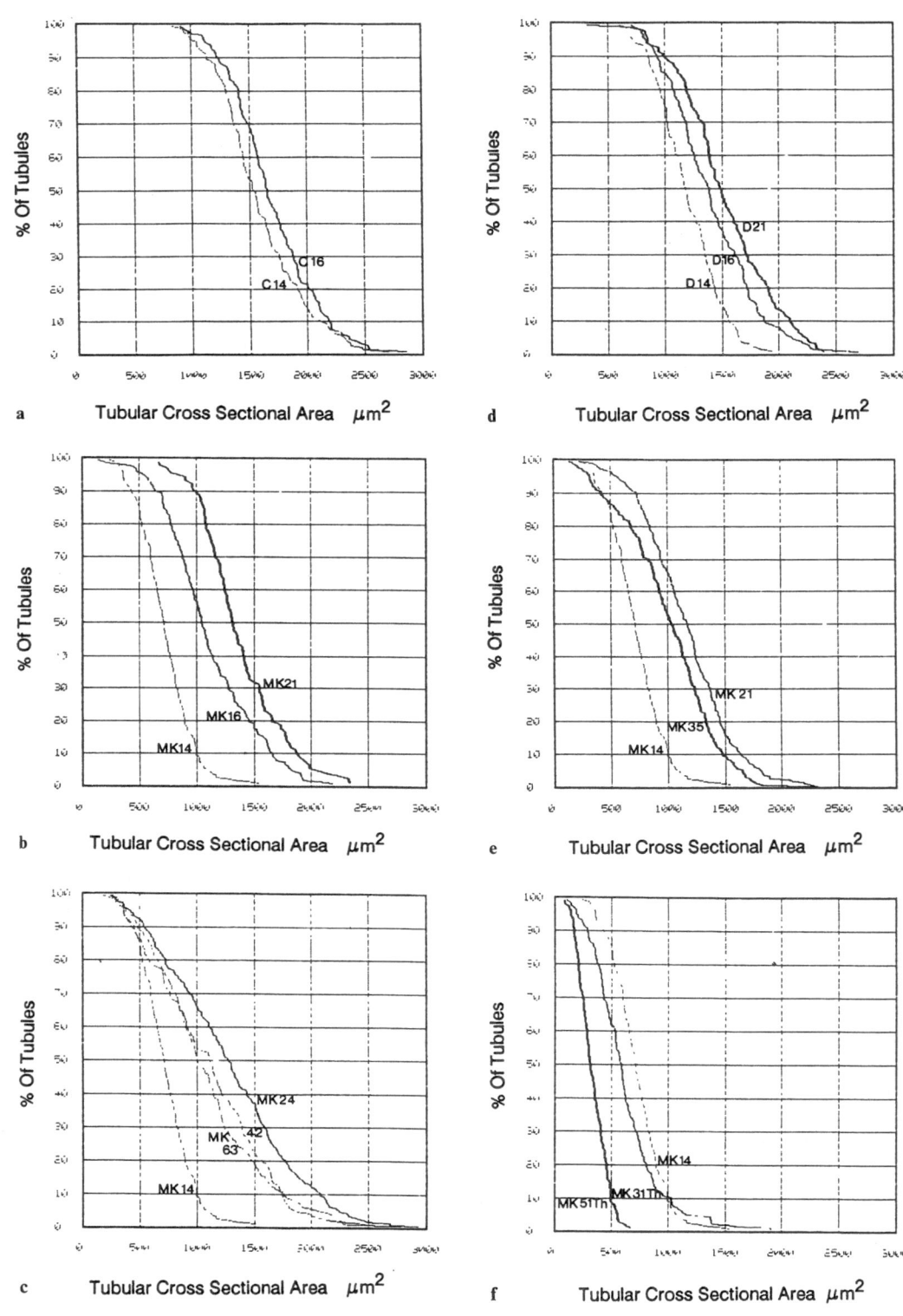

3.2 Reversibility of Tubular Atrophy

The reversibility of tubular atrophy was investigated under three different conditions:

1. Antihypertensive therapy was stopped after 14 days and the left-sided renal artery stenosis was corrected; after unclipping, a contralateral nephrectomy was performed.
2. Following cessation of the ACE inhibition by MK 421 after 14 days, only the renal artery stenosis of the left kidney was corrected.
3. ACE inhibition was stopped after 14 days but the renal artery clip was left in place.

3.2.1   In hypertensive, nontreated control rats, the arterial pressure decreased to normal values. In both treatment groups arterial pressure sank even lower than during antihypertensive therapy. In formerly MK 421-treated rats, 2 days after cessation of therapy a mean systolic pressure of 80 mmHg was measured.

Plasma creatinine concentration of the control group increased slightly from 0.7 ± 0.07 mg% to 1.0 ± 0.09 mg% after contralateral nephrectomy; in the dihydralazine group, plasma creatinine concentration increased from 0.69 ± 0.03 mg% to 1.12 ± 0.18 mg%. In animals with 14-day RAS blockade and atrophic single kidneys, excretory renal insufficiency developed. Two days after therapy was stopped, the plasma creatinine concentration was fourfold higher than during therapy.

GFR, RPF, RBF, and RVR were determined in both treatment groups 1 week after cessation of antihypertensive treatment. The hemodynamic parameters, especially GFR, were again similar in both groups and in the normal range (GFR: MK 421 1.25 ± 0.008, D: 1.38 ± 0.13 ml/min; FF: MK 421 27 ± 2, D: 27 ± 2; RPF: MK 421 4.75 ± 0.37, D: 5.26 ± 0.30 ml/min, MK 421 $n = 7$, $Dn = 6$). Accordingly, formerly atrophic kidneys of MK 421-treated rats showed almost regular tubular structures by light microscopy 7 days after the end of therapy; focally, small groups of dilated tubules with flattened epithelium were seen. Ultrastructurally, mitochondria were again arranged in a normal pattern at

----

Fig. 4a–f. Cumulative frequency curves of cross-sectional areas of proximal tubules in the outer cortex of clipped kidneys in: **a** Hypertensive control animals (*C*) after 14 (C14) and 16 (C16) days; **b** dihydralazine-treated rats (*D*) after 14 therapy days (D14) and 2 and 7 days after therapy end, unclipping of the left renal artery, and right nephrectomy (D16, D21); **c** MK 421-treated rats (*MK*) after 14 treatment days (Mk14) and 2 and 7 days after end of therapy, unclipping of the left renal, and right nephrectomy (MK16, MK21); **d** MK 421-treated rats (MK) after 14 treatment days (MK 14) and 7 and 21 days after cessation of therapy and unclipping of the left renal artery (MK21, MK35); **e** MK 421-treated rats (MK) after 14 treatment days (Mk14) and 10, 28, and 49 days (MK24, MK42, MK63) after end of therapy without unclipping and without nephrectomy. In rats with MK 421 therapy (c), cross-sectional surface areas of proximal tubules only reached those observed in dihydralazine-treated rats in b. In d and e an decrease in cross-sectional surface areas was noted with increased post-therapeutic observation time (MK21 vs MK35 and MK24 vs MK63); **f** MK 421-treated rats after 14 (MK14), 31 MKTH31) and 51 (MKTH51) treatment days. A significant decrease of cross-sectional surface areas was observed during therapy

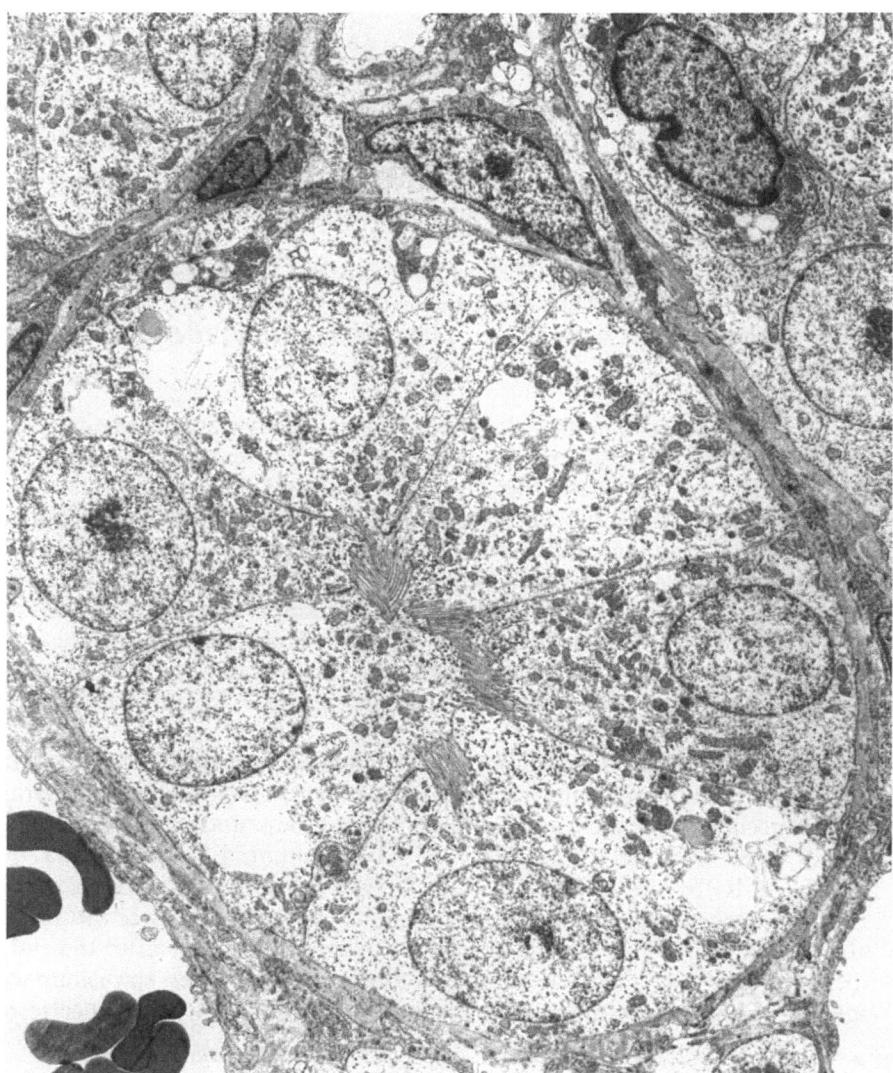

Fig. 5. Transmission electron microscopy. Ultrastructure of atrophic proximal tubular epithelia of a clipped kidney after 14 days of RAS blockade with MK 421. A tubule without lumen is seen; atrophic epithelia had only a few mitochondria and no basolateral plasma membrane invaginations. The brush border was lower then normal. × 3570

right angles to the tubular basement membrane in proximal tubules; the basal labyrinth was normally differentiated. The cross-sectional areas of proximal tubules had increased compared with those values during therapy. For the partes rectae of proximal tubules, the values even reached those of the control group. In dissected segments of proximal tubules, the activities of Na-K-ATPase and

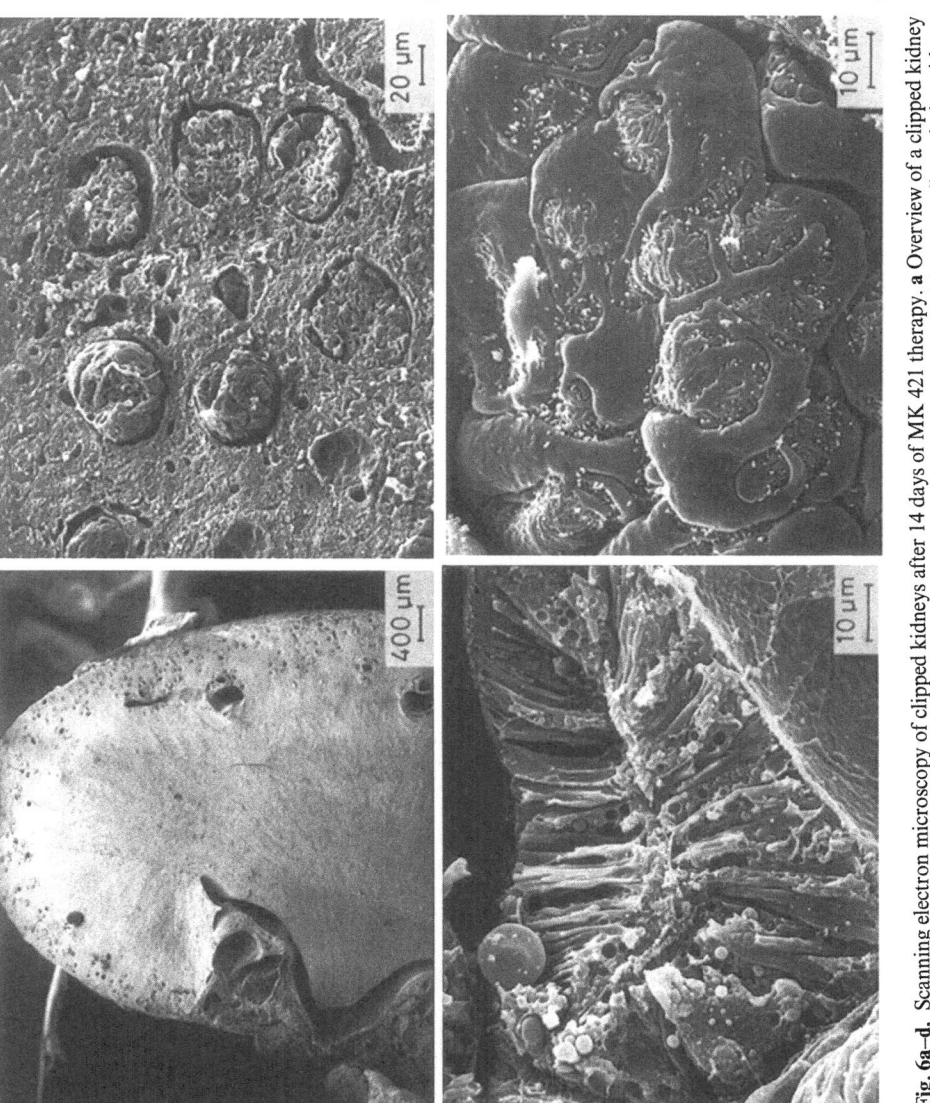

Fig. 6a–d. Scanning electron microscopy of clipped kidneys after 14 days of MK 421 therapy. **a** Overview of a clipped kidney with thin cortex with densely packed glomeruli. **b** Glomeruli arranged in a clockwise fashion with surrounding tubules without lumina. **c** A collapsed proximal tubule with a decreased number of cytoplasmic globules. **d** Glomerulus with visceral epithelial cells that show relatively broad interdigitations

cathepsins B and L did not differ significantly from those of nontreated clipped kidneys.

3.2.2   Normalization of blood pressure also occurred when ACE inhibition was stopped after 14 days and the stenosis of the left renal artery was eliminated. The GFR of the formerly clipped kidney rose in comparison to the value during treatment but even after 15 days did not attain those values measured in animals that were also contralaterally nephrectomized. The mean weight of the atrophic kidneys increased by about 50% until 3 weeks after discontinuing therapy.

In almost 40% of the animals, variably large foci of atrophic and ectatic tubules were still seen 21 days after the end of therapy, although tubular atrophy and generally regressed qualitatively and also morphometrically. Despite the further increase in kidney weight from day 21 to day 35 after therapy was stopped, the extent of atrophic tubules also increased (Fig. 4). These atrophic tubules were surrounded by a fibrosed interstitium with a slight mononuclear cell infiltrate.

3.2.3   Renal atrophy after RAS blockade was only partially reversible if anti-hypertensive treatment was discontinued but the renal artery stenosis left in place. Within a 7-week observation period after discontinuation of the anti-hypertensive drug, the fresh weight of the atrophic kidneys did not increase significantly (Fig. 3c). The mean cross-sectional areas of proximal tubules re-mained significantly decreased in comparison to the values of hypertensive controls (Fig. 4e). The majority of tubules were smaller than normal but were lined by normally differentiated epithelium with a regular brush border. In some cortical areas, atrophic tubules with only slight surrounding interstitial fibrosis were seen. As in animals in whom only the artery clip had been removed after MK 421 therapy, the number of atrophic tubules and interstitial fibrosis in-creased with continued post-therapy observation time.

3.3 Models of Cystic Tubular Cell Hyperplasia

3.3.1 Acute and Chronic Heterologous Albuminuria

The hemodynamic and morphological renal effects of daily intrapertioneal administration of heterologous bovine serum albumin (BSA) with consecutive proteinuria were studied over a period of up to 8 weeks. Other experiments related to the effects of heterologous albuminuria covered relatively short periods of up to 7 days and included functional and morphological alterations of glomeruli only (LAWRENCE and BREWER 1981, 1982, 1984).

The intraperitoneal administration of bovine albumin led to a massive increase of urinary protein excretion within 24 h; proteinuria persisted with chronic injection of heterologous albumin. Microdisc electrophoresis showed that besides albumin, rat plasma proteins with a molecular weight higher than 60 000 and proteins with a molecular weight lower than that of rat albumin were excreted in the urine. Animals fed a casein and fat-enriched diet had significantly higher proteinuria than animals fed normal rat chow. The bovine albumin did not influence GFR even though it was administered in high doses (1.5 g/24 h). Exclusively in animals on regular rat chow, renal plasma flow rose slightly but significantly. Arterial pressures did not differ between albumin- and placebo-injected rats.

Fresh renal weight of albuminuric rats was significantly higher than that of control animals starting after 7 days of BSA injection (Fig. 7). The increase in weight was preceded by a higher than normal mitotic activity and ^{3}H-thymidine

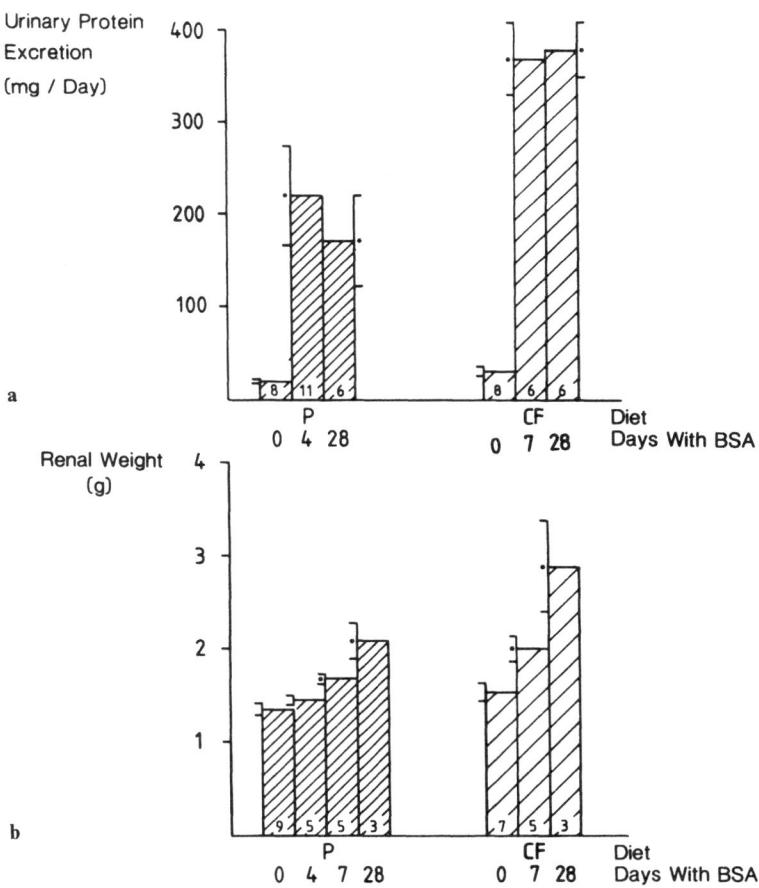

Fig. 7a, b. Urinary protein excretaion (**a**) and kidney weight (**b**) of uninephrectomized rats before and during chronic administration of heterologous bovine serum albumin (*BSA*). *P*, regular pelleted rat chow; *CF*, fat- and cholesterol-rich diet; *, significant difference to value on day 0 within one diet group. (From WEBER et al. 1986)

DNA incorporation of tubular epithelium. In animals with casein-, fat- and cholesterol-rich diets, the mitotic index remained high in comparison to control animals with regular rat chow (Fig. 8). The number of dilated and cystic tubules rose in parallel to the elevated proliferation of tubular epithelia in animals with heterologous proteinuria and was most pronounced in animals with the casein- and fat-rich diets.

Animals with fat-rich diets already had a threefold higher ^{3}H-thymidine DNA incorporation than animals with regular rat chow before injection of bovine albumin. Cystic or dilated tubules were not observed, however, in these control rats, with fat-rich diets.

After 4 weeks of BSA administration the increase in kidney weight leveled off and the number of tubular dilations no longer increased. The injection of

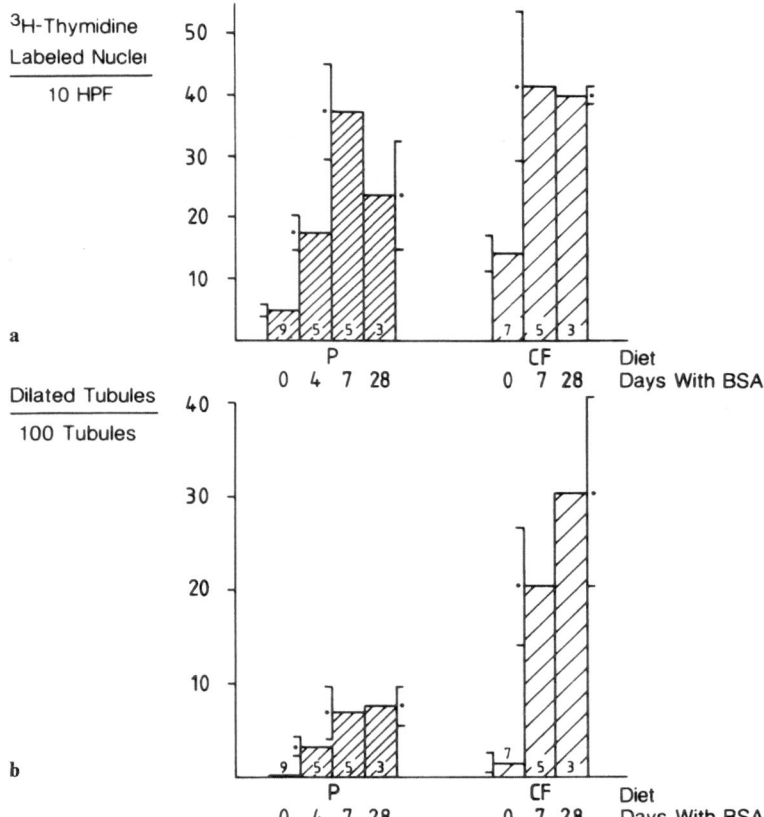

Fig. 8a, b. Extent of tubular epithelial proliferation. **a** and number of dilated tubules. **b** during chronic administration of bovine serum albumin (*BSA*). An increase of the number of dilated and cystic tubules was observed concurrent with an increase in DNA synthesis of tubular epithelia. The CF diet had a permissive effect on cystogenesis, independent of the proliferative activity of the epithelia. *, Significant difference to value on day 0 within one diet group

heterologous albumin led to a segmental and focal glomerular sclerosis. After 4 weeks, 16% of the glomeruli of animals with regular rat chow and 31% of glomerular areas in animals with fat-rich diet showed partial sclerosis (Fig. 9). The glomerular sclerosis occurred after the start of tubular epithelial proliferation and after dilation of tubules. This was especially evident in animals with a fat-rich diet. The incidence of atrophic tubules with small lumina, dedifferentiated epithelia, and thickened basement membranes increased with the number of partially sclerosed glomeruli (Fig. 9).

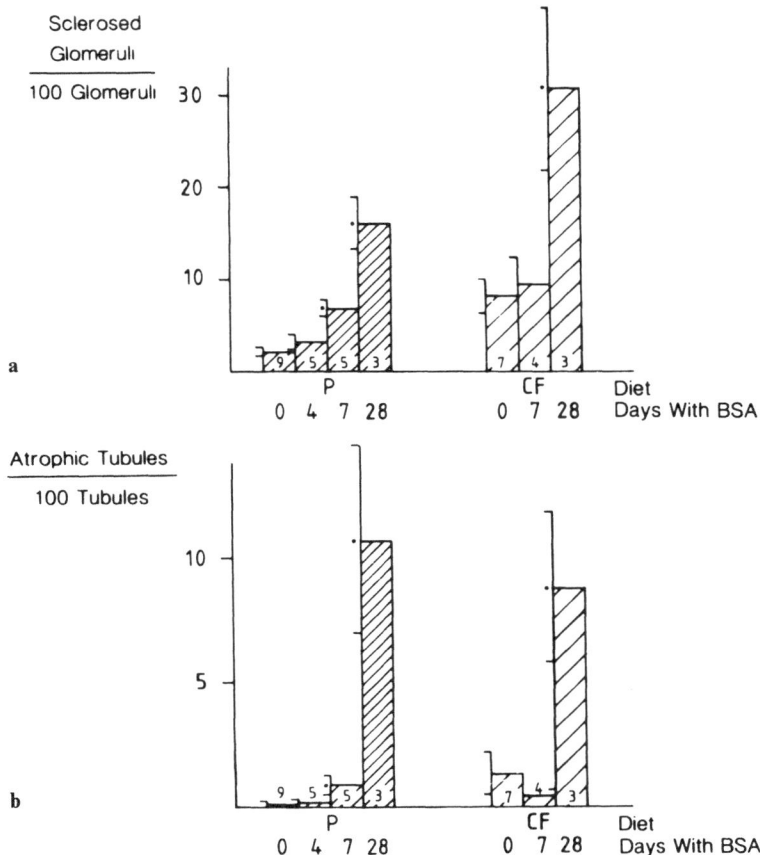

Fig. 9a, b. Number of partially or totally sclerosed glomeruli. **a** and number of atrophic tubules. **b** during chronic heterologous proteinuria induced by intraperitoneal injection of bovine serum albumin (*BSA*). A relevant increase in glomerular sclerosis occurred only after a significant increase of tubular dilatation (Fig. 8b). *, Significant difference to the value on day 0 within the respective diet group

3.3.2 Homologous Proteinuria

Intravenous injection of D and repeated administration of PAN induced a nephrotic syndrome. The studies can be divided into two groups:

1. D nephrosis in unilaterally nephrectomized animals
2. PAN nephrosis in unilaterally nephrectomized animals

3.3.2.1 D Nephrosis in Unilaterally Nephrectomized Rats

Almost a week after intravenous injection of D (5 mg/kg body wt.) a significant glomerular proteinuria was noted that increased slightly up to the fourth week after injection. By microdisc electrophoresis of urine, an increased excretion of proteins was observed. Scanning electron microscopy showed the typical loss of foot processes of the podocytes of glomeruli in nephrotic rats. On the other hand, the podocytes had multiple microvilli-like structures protruding into Bowman's space. Kidney size increased 18 days after daunomycin injection. Kidneys were larger in rats with a casein-rich diet than in rats with regular rat chow.

A fat- and cholesterol-rich diet in addition to the casein diet (CF) led to a further increase in kidney weight. Eight weeks after daunomycin injection, the kidneys of groups CF were 2.6-fold heavier than those of control rats. Numerous cysts with light yellow fluid were seen on the surface of decapsulated large kidneys. The increase in kidney size leveled off 37 days after D injection.

During the development of acquired cystic kidney disease, GFR decreased significantly to values 10–15% of controls on day 55, independent of the respective diet. RBF decreased by 33% (diet P) and 43% casein diet (C and CF) of control values. Arterial pressure remained constant and in the normal range during the whole study period.

The number of dilated tubules in D-treated rats increased steadily after the nephrotic syndrome was manifest with hypoproteinuria, hypercholesterolemia, and hypertriglyceridemia. About one third of all tubules in the cortex were dilated 37 days after D injection in rats with the casein diet (C); in rats with regular rat chow (P) the number of dilated tubules was only one third of that in groups C and CF.

Dilated proximal tubules outnumbered dilated and cystic distal tubules. Tubules in the inner stripe of the outer medulla and the inner medulla were rarely dilated. The dilated tubules often had constrictions and the appearance of a colon-like structure (Fig. 11a–d). The tubular epithelium was flattened without segment differentiation on light and electron microscopy; partly a residual or clearly visible brush border of proximal tubular epithelia was observed. In many sections a multilayered epithelium was seen that grew in a polypoid arrangement (Fig. 10a, b). Complete observation of the tubular lumen by proliferated epithelium was not observed.

The proliferative activity of tubular epithelium was noted with the occurrence of glomerular proteinuria. The mitotic rate was 6- to 16-fold higher in

D-rats than in control rats 3 weeks after D injection. The mitotic rate remained elevated until the end of the study. An increase in tubular atrophy was also observed in parallel to the dilation of tubules and cystogenesis. Five weeks after D injection, almost 13% of all tubular cross-sectional areas showed atrophy in the cortex and outer stripe of the outer medulla in the three daunomycin groups with diets P, C, and CF. The interstitium was fibrosed to a moderate extent and infiltrated by mononuclear cells. Some mononuclear cells infiltrated atrophic and hyperplastic tubular segments that had thickened basement membranes.

The co-expression of keratin and vimentin was observed by immunohistology in numerous tubular epithelia (Fig. 12a–d). Epithelia that were regularly differentiated, as judged by light microscopy, solely synthesized the intermediate filament keratin that is typical for epithelial cells. The intermediate filament vimentin was only expressed in altered, either hyperplastic or atrophic, epithelia. There was a positive correlation between the extent of tubular dilatation and the extent and intensity of intermediate coexpression.

3.3.2.2 PAN Nephrosis of Uninephrectomized Rats

To eliminate a possible specific cystogenic influence of D, homologous proteinuria was induced in unilaterally nephrectomized rats by a substance that shows no structural similarity to D (PAN). PAN was injected three times intraperitoneally in a dose of 35 mg/kg body wt. PAN-injected animals had significantly higher proteinuria until the end of the experiments, 49 days after PAN injection, than control rats. The nephrotic syndrome, however, was less severe than that observed in D nephrosis, as glomerular proteinuria was only two thirds of that in D nephrosis. Hypercholesterolemia and hypertriglyceridemia were moderately severe.

After 7 weeks, dilated proximal tubules and numerous tubular cysts were observed in the cortex and outer strip of the outer medulla in rats with PAN-induced homologous proteinuria. Renal weight had increased in rats with casein diet and in rats with casein- and fat-rich diets. Rats with the fat-rich diet CF had a slightly but not significantly higher kidney weight than animals with casein diet without cholesterol enrichment.

4 Discussion

4.1 Model of Tubular Atrophy

4.1.1 Pathogenesis of Tubular Atrophy

In rats with chronic renovascular hypertension, arterial pressure distal to a fixed renal artery stenosis had been found to be in the normal range (ANDERSON et al.

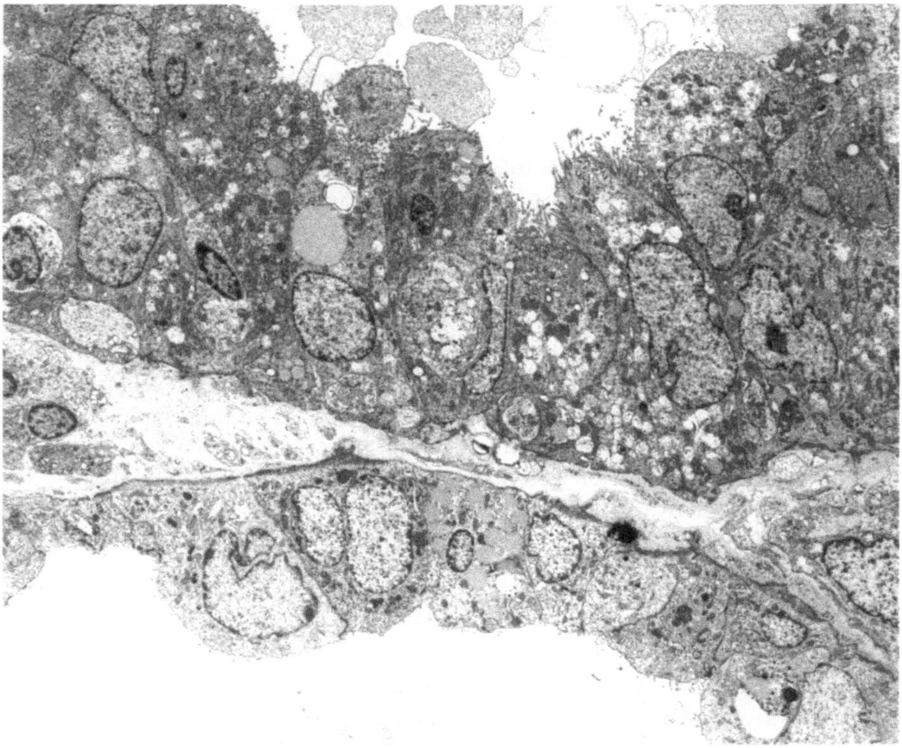

a

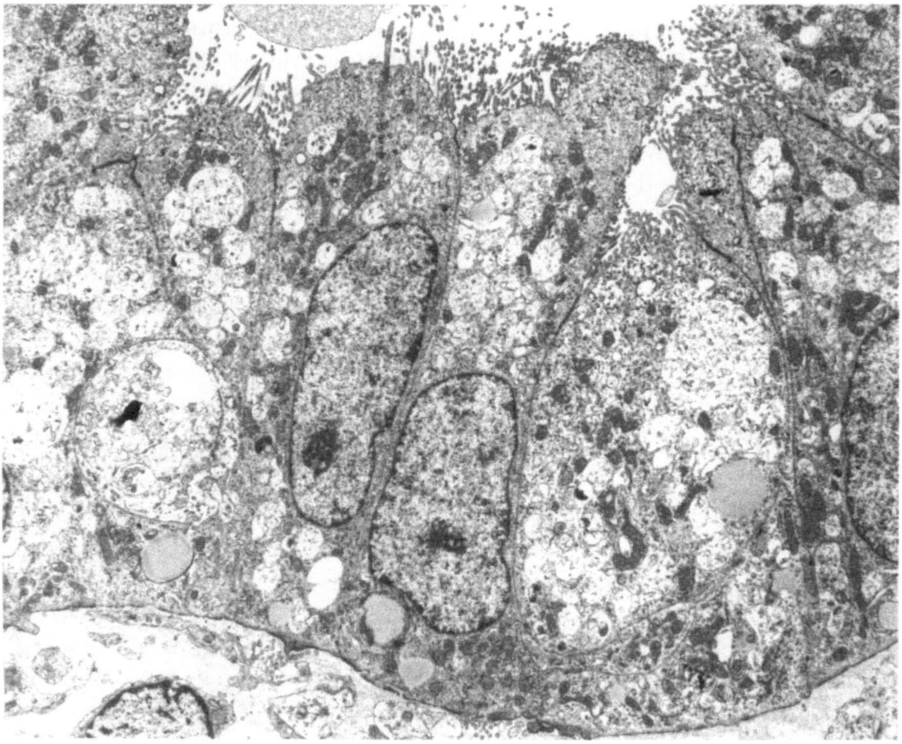

b

1981; HELMCHEN and KNEISSLER 1976). From a teleological viewpoint, the purpose of the systemic arterial hypertension in renal artery stenosis is to achieve normal arterial pressure distal to the stenosis and thereby a sufficient filtration of the clipped kidney (HELMCHEN and KNEISSLER 1976).

Prolonged antihypertensive therapy led to a persistent decrease of systemic arterial pressure and to a decrease in excretory function of the kidney distal to a renal artery stenosis. The extent of renal insufficiency and tubular alterations was dependent on the antihypertensive mechanism of the respective drug. Dihydralazine dilates arterial and arteriolar vessels and stimulates neural and hormonal mechanisms which antagonize the reduction of arterial pressure (KOCH-WESER 1976). During the 2-week treatment it was necessary to increase the dose of dihydralazine five to six fold to keep systolic arterial pressure in the normotensive range. The GFR of the clipped kidney decreased by about 75% with regard to the clipped kidney of the hypertensive control rats; renal blood flow sank by about 50%. The low perfusion pressure distal to the fixed renal artery stenosis seemed to be the main factor for this pronounced derangement of renal hemodynamics and excretory renal function.

Blood flow and glomerular filtration were nevertheless sufficient during dihydralazine treatment to maintain a cortical and medullary renal structure that by light and electron microscopy did not show major differences from the structures in control animals. Glomerular filtration stopped exclusively in animals with subnormal systemic mean arterial pressures of less than 75 mmHg. In kidneys of these animals, tubules with flattened dedifferentiated epithelia and wide lumina were observed. Intrarenal compensatory mechanisms were apparently ineffective with these low arterial pressures during dihydralazine therapy. In animals in whom the arterial pressure reduction was achieved by blockade of the renin angiotensin system (MK 421), a decrease of systemic arterial pressure to 95–90 mmHg stopped urine flow. Total GFR was nominally zero (Fig. 2b).

This functional finding was supported by the light-microscopic and electron-microscopic appearance of glomeruli and proximal tubules. Glomerular diameters were smaller than normal (Fig. 6b). The proximal tubules showed only focally small lumina. In contrast to the acute collapse of tubules after a sudden stop of renal blood flow, the proximal tubular changes in these experiments with ACE blockade were evidence for atrophy of the tubules after a stop of urine flow. The clear epithelia showed relatively small brush borders that often touched each other (Fig. 5a). Only in animals in whom the RAS was chronically inhibited was this drastic reduction of renal function and atrophy of the clipped kidney observed. It could be excluded that the effects of the MK 421 therapy were caused by a substance-specific effect that was independent of ACE inhibition.

◄―――

Fig. 10a, b. Transmission electron microscopy: Hyperplastic tubular epithelia in solitary kidney of a rat with daunomycin nephrosis and casein- and cholesterol-rich diet (CF) 37 days after daunomycin injection. Only rudimentary brush borders are seen. Several epithelia have formed blebs into the tubular lumina. The cytoplasm showed disarranged mitochondria, numerous liposomes, and autophagosomes. Tubular basement membranes were broadened. **a** × 2808; **b** × 5535

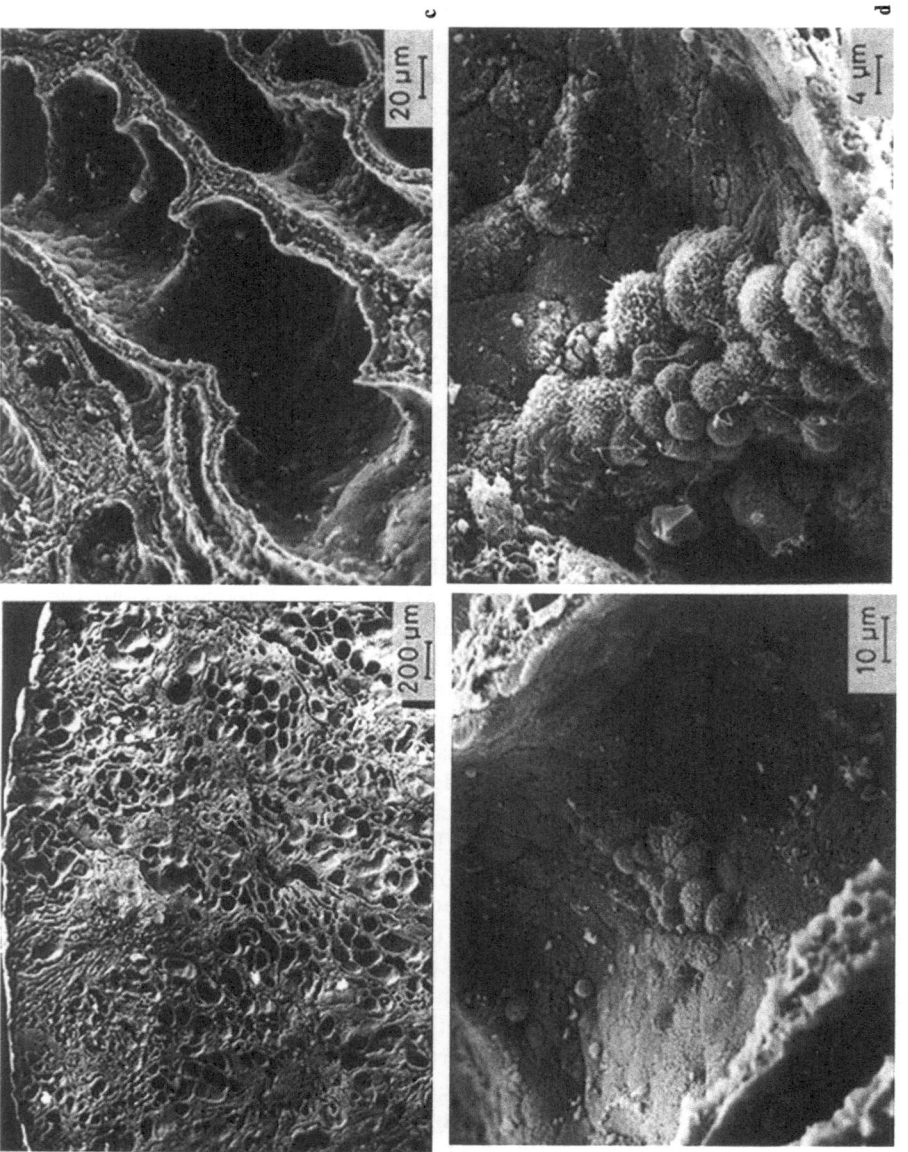

Fig. 11a–d. Scanning electron microsocopy of a cystically transformed solitary kidney of a rat with daunomycin nephrosis and casein- and cholesterol-rich diet (CF) 37 days after daunomycin injection. **a** Cortex and outer stripe of outer medulla with numerous dilated and cystic tubules. **b** A dilated tubule with a colon-like structure. **c, d** Polypous epithelial proliferations of different degree in dilated proximal tubules. Epithelia had partly flattened brush borders, partly showed no tubular segmental differentiation

Captopril, an ACE inhibitor with a structure chemically different from MK 421, had similar effects on the clipped kidney after systemic blood pressure reduction in rats with two-kidney, one-clip hypertension and in rats with one-kidney, one-clip hypertension (unpublished data). Sarisoleucine, a peptide antagonist of AII, led to a normalization of systemic blood pressure in rats with bilateral renal artery stenosis and to acute renal insufficiency (GRÖNE and HELMCHEN 1982; HELMCHEN et al. 1982).

The functional and structural alterations of the clipped kidney after chronic reduction of systemic blood pressure by MK 421 can thus be regarded as a specific effect of the blockade of AII. The pathogenesis of this renal insufficiency can be understood in more detail if one considers our functional data and findings on the AII effects on renal vessels.

The autoregulation of the kidney, e.g., the perfusion pressure-dependent regulation of renovascular resistance, assures optimal conditions for glomerular filtration. STEINHAUSEN (1987) found that in rats preglomerular vessels, with the exception of the glomerular pole of the vas afferens, dilated increasingly when renal perfusion pressure sank; the vas efferens did not exhibit this dilatory capacity with a decrease in renal perfusion pressure (STEINHAUSEN 1987). OSSWALD et al. (1979) reported that in dogs a fall of renal arterial pressure from 121 mmHg to 65 mmHg was coupled with a significant increase in vascular resistance of postglomerular vessels.

In micropuncture experiments in the rat kidney, the resistance of the efferent arteriole increased during low renal perfusion pressure. The result was an almost constant effective transcapillary hydrostatic pressure gradient of the glomeruli. In these experiments of DEEN et al. (1972), no definitive statement could be made with regard to the mechanism of this preferential constriction of the efferent arteriole.

The renin angiotensin system has the essential function of preserving glomerular hemodynamics and filtration during hypotonic conditions. The data from our own experiments and the results of other groups support this assumption.

STEINHAUSEN et al. (1983, 1986; STEINHAUSEN 1987) determined the reactivity of preglomerular arteries and arterioles of the glomerulus and of the vas efferens to AII using the model of the hydronephrotic kidney. AII constricted pre- and postglomerular vascular segments in a dose-dependent manner. A decrease of renal perfusion pressure caused by an aortic clip during systemic AII infusion was followed by a significant decrease in vasoconstriction in all preglomerular vessels, with the exception of the immediate preglomerular part of the vas afferens. The constriction of the vas efferens even increased under these experimental conditions. ANDERSON et al. (1979, 1981) investigated the renal hemodynamic effects of the RAS after acute stenosis of the renal artery. During inhibition of ACE by teprotide, the effective resistance of the renal artery stenosis increased dramatically. The renal blood flow remained constant, but the preglomerular arterial pressure decreased.

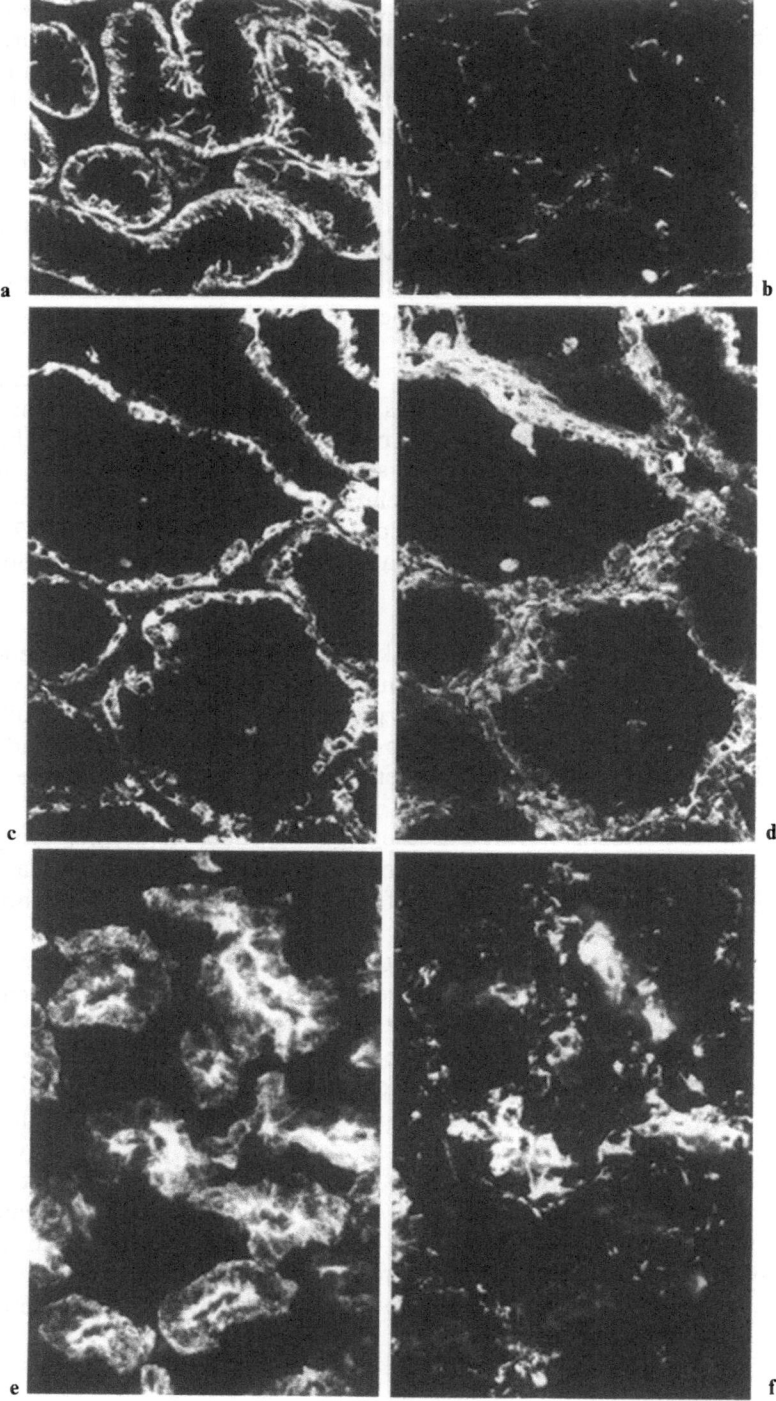

In several experimental series, Hall et al. documented convincingly that AII is important for the preservation of filtration during low renal perfusion pressures. In dogs with chronic renin depletion by deoxycorticosteronacetate administration and salt-enriched diet, a decoupling of autoregulation of RBF and GFR was achieved by low renal perfusion pressures (70–100 mmHg). Though RBF decreased moderately (maximally 15%), GFR and FF were reduced markedly, up to 60%. In dogs with sodium depletion and significantly, stimulated RAS, autoregulation of GFR was eliminated by the AII antagonist SAR^1, Ile^8-AII during low renal perfusion pressure. As RBF sank by only 10% with a renal perfusion pressure of 70 mmHg, GFR and FF decreased by about 60%. In animals with a regular sodium diet, normal sodium balance, and regular activity of the RAS, GFR decreased only slightly when renal perfusion pressure was lowered and the RAS inhibited; renal blood flow even increased by about 20%. Calculations of vascular resistances of the afferent and efferent arterioles always showed a decrease in the resistance of the afferent arteriole and an increase or a discrete decrease (sodium depletion) of resistance of the efferent arteriole in the condition of low renal perfusion pressure. In all the cited experiments of Hall, the lack of RAS activity did not lead to a significant change of the decrease of resistance of the vas afferens but to a significant decrease of the resistance of the vas efferens. These characteristics of vascular resistance were independent of the assumption of a filtration pressure equilibrium or disequilibrium (HALL 1986; HALL et al. 1977a, b, 1980). Additional experiments with the AII antagonist des-Asp^1 Ile^8-AII demonstrated that the intrarenal hemodynamic effects were essentially due to AII but not to AIII (HALL et al. 1979).

Data and calculations by Hall et al. support the hypothesis that AII preferentially constricts the efferent arteriole in low renal perfusion pressure states. This assumption is congruent with the data of MYERS et al. (OMAE and MASSON 1960). When AII was infused and the resultant systemic blood pressure increase eliminated by aortic constriction. AII preferentially constricted the vas efferens. In vivo observations of the glomerular microcirculation in the model of the hydronephrotic rat kidney showed that an AII infusion in a low-dose range (0.2–0.4 µg/min/kg body wt. i.v.) decreased the diameter of the efferent arteriole by about 22% but did not cause a consistent reaction in the vas afferens (STEINHAUSEN et al. 1986).

A further indication of the preferential interaction between the efferent arteriole and AII was obtained by studies on isolated pre- and postglomerular arterioles of the rat kidney. Edwards et al. (1983) measured a high reactivity of the efferent arteriole, but not of the isolated afferent arteriole, to AII. The

◄────────────────────────────────────

Fig. 12a–f. Co-expression of the intermediate filaments keratin and vimentin in tubular epithelia of atrophic and cystic kidneys as shown by double immunofluorescence. **a, b** Expression of keratin in tubular epithelia (**a**) and of vimentin in the interstitium but not in the tubular epithelia in control rats. **c–f** Co-expression of keratin (**c, e**) and vimentin (**d, f**) in cystic tubules of a solitary kidney in daunomycin nephrosis (37 days after daunomycin injection, diet C; **c, d**) and in tubular epithelia of an atrophic clipped kidney after 14 days of angiotensin concerting enzyme inhibition (MK 421 therapy). **a–d** – 100 µm, **e, f** – 50 µm

preferential effect of AII on the efferent arteriole in comparison to the effect of AII on the afferent arteriole may be explained, at least to some degree, by the fact that prostacyclin synthesis of the afferent arteriole may antagonize the constrictive action of AII (EDWARDS 1985).

Other investigations in vitro and in vivo indicated that the preferential effect of AII on the vas efferens could be explained at least partially by a stimulated synthesis of the vasconstrictor thromboxane A_2 (TXA_2) in the glomerulus or the vas efferens (GOTO et al. 1987; SHIBOUTA et al. 1979).

Our investigations can best be explained when one assumes a significant constrictive effect of AII on the efferent arteriole in states of low intrarenal perfusion pressure (GRÖNE and HELMCHEN 1986; HELLER and HORACEK 1986; ICHIKAWA and BRENNER 1980, 1987). The inhibition of ACE led to a decrease in AII synthesis and a systemic decrease of arterial pressure in rats with two-kidney, one-clip, RAS-dependent hypertension. During systemic normotension and simultaneous low renal perfusion pressure, RPF decreased by about 30%, GFR by about 95%, and FF by more than 95%. Antihypertensive therapy with dihydralazine without blockade of AII effects resulted in a fall of RBF by only about 40%, of GFR by about 70%, and of FF by about 50% in comparison to the clipped kidney of hypertensive control animals.

Navar et al. have repeatedly stressed that the resistances of pre- and postglomerular vessels show mostly unidirectional alterations (CARMINES et al. 1987; NAVAR and ROSIVALL 1984). With the help of a computer model based on representative experimental micropuncture data of glomerular hemodynamics, it was shown that changes of FF do not necessarily prove a selective change in the resistance of a specific vascular segment. Combined changes of resistances of afferent and efferent vessels, as well as sole changes in the resistance of one arteriole, can alter the FF. In addition, it has to be considered that the glomerular filtration coefficient can also influence FF. Despite these objections, it must be kept in mind that the resistance of the vas efferens can influence FF to a significantly greater degree than the resistance of the vas afferens. A fall of FF to such a drastic extent as in our own experiments in the clipped kidney of rats with RAS inhibition can probably be explained only by a preferential decrease of resistance in the vas efferens, even in consideration of the normogram to the effects of vascular resistances of vas afferens and efferens to CARMINES et al. (1987).

The contribution of direct glomerular changes to the decrease in filtration did not seem to be of importance in our experiments. The ultrafiltration coefficient, the product of glomerular capillary filtration, surface area, and hydraulic conductivity, can be decreased by AII (DEEN et al. 1974). Independent of the mechanism by which AII influences the ultrafiltration coefficient, inhibition of RAS should have increased the coefficient and filtration.

Our data on the hemodynamics of the clipped kidney during chronic RAS blockade are supported by investigations into the acute effect of RAS inhibition in rats with two-kidney, one-clip hypertension. Huang et al. described a significant fall of GFR in clipped kidneys of two-kidney, one-clip rats after intravenous administration of the ACE inhibitor SQ 20881 and the AII antagonist saralasin, and after oral administration of the ACE inhibitor captopril; in the contralateral kidney GFR increased during RAS blockade (HUANG 1986; HUANG and NAVAR 1983; HUANG et al. 1981, 1982a). The systemic mean arterial pressure fell to values between 125 and 135 mmHg and was significantly higher than in our experiments. The reduction of GFR was therefore probably less than in our experiments. Huang et al. stated that the reduction of the GFR was due essentially to the decrease in intrarenal perfusion pressure and was not caused by an inhibition of intrarenal AII effects (HUANG et al. 1991).

This interpretation is in contrast to our own experiments, to the experiments of SCHWIETZER et al. (1988) on patients with acute ACE inhibition, and to those of TEXTOR et al. (1984) on dogs with unilateral renal artery stenosis. During acute reduction of systemic arterial pressure to values below 100 mmHg by the vasodilator sodium nitroprusside, GFR of the clipped kidney was reduced only minimally in the experiments of Textor et al.; with the AII antagonist Sar^1-Ala^8-AII, GFR fell markedly, while RBF increased slightly and blood pressure reduction was comparable to that in the vasodilator experiments.

Frei et al. reported a decrease in filtration fraction and a higher reduction of resistance of the efferent than of the afferent arteriole during acute MK 421 administration, while systemic arterial pressures were even significantly higher than in our experiments; the ultrafiltration coefficient increased significantly (FREI et al. 1987).

Our investigations broaden these data from acute experiments. The functional and morphological results after chronic inhibition of AII synthesis support the pathogenetic concept that a constriction of the efferent arteriole is essential for the maintenance of glomerular filtration in states of low renal perfusion pressure; AII is the main vasoconstrictor for this process.

Effective antihypertensive therapy with dihydralazine and MK 421 was given under simultaneous sodium depletion (sodium-deficient diet). A sufficient and continuous normalization of arterial pressure was not achieved without sodium depletion. Sodium depletion causes significant alterations of vascular reactivity and renal hemodynamics (TUCKER and BLANTZ 1983).

In the experiments of SCHIFFRIN et al. (1983) receptor density of vascular smooth muscle for angiotensin II was diminished by sodium deficiency; these results were obtained in sodium-depleted normotensive and in sodium-depleted rats with two-kidney, one-clip hypertension. Although these results apply to mesenteric arteries, they are probably also valid for intrarenal preglomerular vessels. Also, the AII receptor number in glomeruli decreased during sodium depletion.

Captopril, an ACE inhibitor, inhibited the decrease of glomerular AII receptors in animals with sodium chloride depletion. These experiments were performed by DOUGLAS (1987). The characteristics of angiotensin receptors in preglomerular vessels and glomeruli during chronic ACE inhibition and simultaneous sodium depletion were also investigated in our experiments. It is apparent that sodium depletion and ACE inhibition increased glomerular AII receptor number and did not alter the affinity of AII receptors (SIMON et al. 1993).

Clinical case reports confirm the assumption that sodium chloride depletion contributes to the loss of excretory function of the clipped kidney during ACE inhibition. The glomerular filtration of a transplanted kidney with a 90% stenosis of the renal artery decreased by about 50% during ACE inhibition, sodium depeletion, and blood pressure normalization. GFR increased, however, to 70% of control values after correction of sodium depletion but continued ACE inhibition and blood pressure reduction (HRICIK 1985).

Ploth et al. observed that during low perfusion pressure GFR can easily be disturbed by intravascular volume depletion (PLOTH and WOOLVERTON 1987). The hematocrit values of kidneys treated by MK 421 did not differ significantly from those of dihydralazine-treated animals or those of hypertensive control rats. Volume depletion therefore did not seem to be essential for the drastic reduction of GFR in MK 421 animals in our own experiments.

The inhibition of bradykinin degradation by ACE inhibition can be assessed in its significance for our results; bradykinin, however, does not seem to be important for the systemic hemodynamic effects of ACE inhibition (GRÖNE and DUNN 1985).

4.1.2 Differential Diagnosis, Cellular Mechanisms and Relevance of Inactivity Atrophy

The drastic reduction of glomerular filtration during chronic ACE inhibition was accompanied by an atrophy of proximal tubular epithelia. As the arrangement of the clear atrophic cells in a trabescular and rosette-like pattern imitates the appearance of the adrenal cortex, Selye and Stone described such kidneys as endocrine kidneys. SELYE and STONE (1946) first reported this form of tubular atrophy in rats with kidneys with high-grade stenosis and chronic severe, two-kidney, one-clip hypertension.

BOHLE (1954) described small tubules and clear epithelia in rat kidneys distal to a renal artery stenosis and coined the term "collapsed kidney". In agreement with SELYE and STONE (1946) and our results, Bohle did not find necrosis of tubular epithelia. ZOLLINGER (1966) interpreted the appearance of the endocrine kidney in human kidneys distal to a severe renal artery stenosis as a subinfarct, and therefore as an ischemic epithelial alteration. This pathogenetic explanation of the "collapsed kidney" does not apply to our experiments. The tubular atrophy was not caused by a critically reduced renal blood flow.

In our experiments, the majority of atrophic kidneys of animals with RAS blockade were characterized by this special form of tubular atrophy as described by SELYE and STONE (1946). The interstitium was not widened, and an inflammatory interstitial infiltrate was not found. These morphological results parallel those of Michel et al. after 9 weeks of ACE inhibition therapy. In this study, clear atrophy of tubular epithelia and no or only a focally slight fibrosis was observed in the clipped kidneys of animals that were not salt depleted. Functional data on the extent of renal insufficiency were not supplied (MICHEL et al. 1986, 1987).

This type of tubular atrophy should be clearly separated from tubular atrophy that is often observed in chronic renal disease. Tubules in chronic renal disease are usually dilated or collapsed; the epithelia are without tubular segment differentiation and are surrounded by a broad, convoluted basement membrane. The interstitium is expanded and fibrosed. In contrast to this tubular atrophy, the tubules of the clipped kidney in rats with chronic RAS blockade were surrounded by a normal tubular basement membrane and a normal interstitium; the epithelia had only partly lost their characteristics. Clear-cut separation of these two forms of atrophy seems to be necessary with regard to pathogenetic and prognostic aspects. As will be discussed in detail, clear atrophy of tubular epithelia in clipped kidneys is potentially reversible. In contrast to the usual atrophy of tubular epithelia in chronic renal disease, the clear atrophy of proximal tubules during RAS blockade can be pathogenetically explained with the help of functional data.

During a state of low or nonexistent glomerular filtration, the resorptive and energetic capacities of the proximal tubules were drastically lowered. Sodium potassium ATPase activity and the number of mitochondria and lysosomes, as well as the activity of catabolic lysosomal enzymes (cathepsin B and L) decreased. Tubular atrophy in the clipped kidneys of hypertensive rats after chronic RAS inhibition can therefore be described as *inactivity atrophy*. Former experiments of EVAN et al. and SCHLEIFER and ZOLLINGER did not clearly differentiate between ischemic tubular lesions and atrophy that was due to a lack of ultrafiltrate (EVAN and TANNER 1986; SCHLEIFER 1962; ZOLLINGER et al. 1973).

The atrophy of tubules was concentrated in proximal parts in our models; this was probably due to the fact that the proximal tubules have quantitatively the largest resorptive workload of all tubular epithelia of the nephron. More than 70% of the primary filtrate is reabsorbed in the proximal tubule (WACHSMUTH 1985).

The atrophy of tubular epithelia could have occurred only by an imbalance between anabolic and catabolic intracellular processes. Principally, three cellular mechanisms can lead to atrophy:

1. An increased cellular autophagy
2. A loss of cellular parts by extralysosomal mechanisms
3. A decrease in synthesis of cytoplasmic structures (PFEIFER 1982)

Ultrastructurally, there were no indications for degradation of cell organelles by an increased cellular autophagy; also, the functional data of the decreased cathepsin activity in proximal tubular segments do not support an increased cellular autophagy. An extracellular loss of cytoplasm and intracytoplasmic structures was not observed after 14 days of RAS blockade. Only after prolonged RAS blockade for several weeks and severe tubular atrophy in the clipped kidneys was cellular debris noted within the tiny lumina of numerous tubules. A decreased synthesis of intracytoplasmic substances and physiologic autophagy were probably the main factors for the inactivity atrophy of the tubular epithelia. Experiments are currently being conducted to test whether apoptotic events change. Also, the cellular biology of this form of atrophy will be analyzed in future studies.

Risdon et al. and Bohle et al. pointed to the tight correlation between excretory renal function and tubular interstitial changes (BOHLE et al. 1986; MACKENSEN-HAEN et al. 1981; RIEMENSCHNEIDER et al. 1980; RISDEN et al. 1968). Lesions of the tubulointerstitial compartment were correlated with a decrease in GFR or an increase in plasma creatinine concentration, while there was only a loose correlation between glomerular lesions and excretory renal function. In numerous detailed morphometric investigations, especially by MACKENSEN-HAEN et al. (1981), the correlations between interstitial fibrosis, lesions of the tubular epithelium, and excretory renal function were documented. The main focus of these studies was the analysis of the interstitium and its relation to an effect on excretory renal function. The pathogenetic interpretation of these data was that interstitial edema and interstitial fibrosis are important modulators of excretory renal function. Tubular atrophy was seen as a consequence of the interstitial changes.

It is conceivable that interstitial lesions can significantly influence excretory renal function in states of advanced chronic inflammatory and metabolic glomerular diseases. BOHLE et al. (1986) were able to show a good correlation between interstitial fibrosis and decreased GFR in many different renal diseases; nevertheless, this correlation does not hold true for the inactivity atrophy described here. On the basis of the data obtained, other factors are the primary determinants for excretory renal function in our tubular atrophy model. Primarily, intrarenal and glomerular hemodynamics were the determining parameter for a decrease in excretory renal function. The interstitium was not altered. The intrarenal and postglomerular blood flow seemed to be sufficient during the hypotensive period of antihypertensive therapy; ischemic lesions did not occur. Cell necrosis was seen very seldom. The alterations of the tubular epithelia were caused by factors from the luminal side of the tubule, that is, by a lack of primary urine, and were not a consequence of interstitial alterations like edema or interstitial fibrosis. The atrophic epithelia were a major factor in the decrease of excretory function 2 days after the end of ACE inhibition and unclipping of the renal artery stenosis (Table 2).

The question remains whether the inhibition of AII had a direct effect on the tubular epithelia. The tubular epithelia of the nephron possess luminal- and basolateral-specific AII receptors (BROWN and DOUGLAS 1987; MUJAIS et al. 1986). The proximal tubules have the highest receptor density of all tubular segments.

During chronic RAS blockade the stimulating effect of AII on the proximal epithelia was lacking. Even the reabsorption of a very low primary urinary filtrate could thus be hindered, and inactivity atrophy of the tubular epithelium could have been fostered. Angiotensin II probably has hypertrophic effects on tubular epithelia (WINTERBOURNE and MORA 1978; WOLF and NEILSON 1990a, b; WOLF and NEILSON, this volume). In in vitro experiments on proximal tubular cells a hypertrophic effect of AII was noted (WINTERBOURNE and MORA 1978).

The atrophy of the proximal tubular epithelia could thus have been increased by a lack of trophic influence of AII on tubules.

4.1.3 Reversibility of Inactivity Atrophy

Reversibility of inactivity atrophy was tested after antihypertensive therapy under three different conditions:

1. Unclipping of the renal artery stenosis and contralateral nephrectomy
2. Unclipping of the renal artery stenosis
3. Stopping of antihypertensive therapy without surgical manipulation

The atrophy of the tubular epithelia disappeared within a week after unclipping of the renal artery stenosis and contralateral nephrectomy.

Omae and Masson reported that during the course of renal vascular hypertension with a high-grade stenosis of the renal artery, poststenotic tubular atrophy was reversible only after contralateral nephrectomy (OMAE and MASSON 1960). Uninephrectomy increases renal blood flow and raises the effective transcapillary pressure gradient within the glomerulus and the filtration rate— conditions which apparently promote the reversibility of tubular atrophy (FINE 1987; FINE et al. 1985a). Wright's view that increased "stress" exerts positive effects on the kidney ("the kidney thrives on work") seems to be valid for this experimental condition (WRIGHT 1982). The experimental situation discussed, of simultaneous nephrectomy and unclipping of the renal artery, does not imitate practical clinical situations, because under normal conditions the contralateral, untouched kidney is not removed in the case of unilateral renal artery stenosis. When only the renal artery stenosis was unclipped, GFR increased to a third of that of the contralateral kidney after 15 days. The tubular epithelia regenerated in only about 60% of all animals within 3 weeks. In the remaining animals, relatively large foci of atrophic or incompletely regenerated tubules with surrounding slight interstitial fibrosis were observed. Apparently, contralateral nephrectomy is an additional important stimulus to cell hypertrophy. When after ACE inhibition no surgical manipulation was performed, renal atrophy did not fully reverse. Renal weights did not increase. The relatively small tubular epithelia, however, were regularly differentiated 10 days after ACE inhibition with regard to brush borders and the existence of segmentally differentiated enzyme patterns. Only small foci of fully atrophic tubules remained. An interstitial fibrosis was seen only focally.

During the course of the observation period atrophic foci increased in the group in whom only the renal artery clip was removed after discontinuation of antihypertensive therapy. Atrophy and fibrosis developed a "dynamic" that could not be pathogenetically explained; this may have an important influence on renal function in the long term also in human beings.

These data on only partially reversible atrophy of clipped kidneys after unclipping support Hinman's concept of renal counterbalance and renal "atrophy of disuse." In Hinman's investigations on the atrophy of hydronephrosis, tubular atrophy reversed only if a working stimulus to tubular regeneration was set via contralateral nephrectomy (HINMAN 1943).

4.1.4 Clinical Relevance of the Model of Tubular Inactivity Atrophy

ACE inhibitors were developed because the blockade of the RAS—shown to be of major pathogenetic importance in several experimental and clinical forms of hypertension—seems to be a causal and effective antihypertensive therapy strategy (CUSHMAN et al. 1980). Synthesis of orally effective ACE inhibitors enabled the routine use of ACE inhibitors in clinical practice.

Renovascular hypertension was assumed to be the most appropriate form of hypertension for ACE inhibition treatment. The fact was, however, largely neglected that the RAS may have intrarenal effects that are essential for the maintenance of renal function under certain conditions. These conditions have been discussed in detail in the foregoing sections. In several case reports, acute decline in renal function was reported during ACE inhibition in patients with bilateral renal artery stenosis or in patients with stenosed single functional kidneys (renal transplant patients) (CHRYSANT et al. 1983; COLISTE et al. 1979; COULIE et al. 1983; CURTIS et al. 1983; FARROW and WILKINSON 1979; GRÖNE et al. 1982; GROSSMAN et al. 1980; HOLLENBERG 1983; HRICIK et al. 1983; JACKSON et al. 1984; KAWAMURA et al. 1982; KINDLER et al. 1981; KREMER-HOVINGA et al. 1984; LUDERER et al. 1981; PLANZ and BUNDSCHU 1980; SILAS et al. 1983; VETTER et al. 1984; WAEBER et al. 1984).

Although Textor et al. pointed out the significant and critical influence of renal perfusion pressure on RBF and GFR in stenosed kidneys in patients with bilateral renal artery stenosis, other studies indicated that RAS inhibition in itself has an important role in causing the decrease of excretory function in these patients (HOLLIFIELD et al. 1982; HRICIK et al. 1983; TEXTOR et al. 1985; VAN DER WOUDE et al. 1985). Equivalent reductions of systemic arterial pressure by nitroprusside, minoxidil, or diuretics and vasodilators did not cause a similarly significant reduction of GFR as occurred during RAS blockade.

Our data show convincingly that in unilateral renal artery stenosis the clipped kidney can suffer severely during ACE inhibition. Our own clinical case observations and functional investigations of other clinical groups confirm the clinical relevance of our experimental data (BENDER et al. 1984; GRÖNE et al. 1982; MIYAMORI et al. 1986; SCHELER and GRÖNE 1982; WENTING et al. 1984). In contrast to the systemic effect of ACE therapy in bilateral renal artery stenosis, there is no increase in plasma creatinine concentration. The lesions of the clipped kidney in unilateral renal artery stenosis cannot be recognized by routine clinical functional parameters (LEVENSON and DZAU 1987). The untouched contralateral kidney compensates for the loss of function of the clipped kidney. Plasma creatinine and urea concentrations remain in the normal range. Hollenberg (1984) observed an increase in plasma creatinine concentration of more than

0.3 mg% in only about 25% of patients with unilateral renal artery stenosis during ACE inhibition. Similarly moderate decreases in GFR were reported by other clinical groups (LEVENSON and DZAU 1987). Only Textor observed a more significant decrease of total GFR, from 78 to 58 ml/min (25%) (TEXTOR et al. 1983, 1984). Wenting et al. performed split renal functional measurements in patients with unilateral renal artery stenosis and prolonged ACE inhibition. During ACE inhibition with captopril, GFR in the clipped kidney fell in seven of 14 patients to nonmeasurable values. In other patients, no alteration in GFR of the clipped kidney occurred during RAS blockade. The arterial pressure or the GFR of the clipped kidney before treatment did not differ significantly between these two patient groups (WENTING et al. 1984).

Five determinants seem to be of importance for occurrence of lesions of the clipped kidney during RAS blockade:

1. Extent of reduction of systemic arterial pressure
2. Extent of renal artery stenosis
3. Phase of arterial hypertension and functional reserve of the contralateral kidney that may be damaged by nephrosclerosis
4. Activity of the RAS before therapy
5. Extent of volume and sodium depletion

In patients with unilateral renal artery stenosis, a prolonged RAS blockade may damage the clipped kidney permanently, as is shown in our experiments on the reversibility of tubular atrophy of the clipped kidney. Even in patients in whom the renal artery stenosis has been eliminated after RAS inhibition therapy, partially irreversible functional loss of the clipped kidney could occur. In patients with heart failure, ACE inhibitor therapy may have a beneficial effect, causing vasodilatation and reduction of cardiac postload (CLELAND and DARGIE 1987). According to clinical case reports, some of these patients with a stimulated RAS and sodium depletion induced by diuretics are predisposed to develop a decrease in excretory renal functional during RAS blockade (CLELAND and DARGIE 1987; PACKER et al. 1987). Pathogenetic aspects to those similar discussed for the clipped kidney can be assumed to play a part if a nephrosclerofic kidney has peripheral stenoses. In summary, a chronic blockade of the RAS in states of pre- or intrarenal fixed artery stenosis must be regarded as an antihypertensive therapy that can potentially lead to irreversible renal lesions.

4.2 Models of Cystic Tubular Cell Hyperplasia

4.2.1 General Association Between Proteinuria and Cystogenesis

The hyperplasia of tubular epithelia is a constant and readily apparent characteristic of polycystic diseases, especially if micropapillary epithelial hyperplasia is present (BERNSTEIN 1985; BERNSTEIN et al. 1987; EVAN et al. 1979). Detailed scanning electron-microscopic investigations of human polycystic kidneys have confirmed that tubular cysts are always associated with epithelial proliferation, that is, an increased number of epithelial cells per original tubule length (GRANTHAM et al. 1987). As shown in Fig. 1, numerous influences on the tubular epithelia can stimulate epithelial proliferation. A disturbed permselectivity of the glomerular filter with consecutive glomerular proteinuria can be observed in multiple renal diseases and in those that are accompanied by dilatations and cysts of tubular segments. Our observations in animals with renovascular hypertension, glomerular proteinuria, and tubular dilatation indicated that proteinuria may play a role in the dilatation of nephron segments. In addition, it is known that in congenital nephrotic syndrome of the Finnish type, tubular dilation and cysts can be decumented only after glomerular lesions and glomerular proteinuria have occurred (RISDEN and TURNER 1980). Pinocytotic and metabolic activity of proximal tubular epithelia increase with glomerular proteinuria. Experiments on cells in culture point to the possibility that a higher pinocytotic activity may be accompanied by cell proliferation (BAR-SAGI and FERAMISCO 1986). Glomerular proteinuria could perhaps be a stimulus for proliferation of tubular epithelia and tubular cystogenesis.

4.2.2 Heterologous Proteinuria

4.2.2.1 Proteinuria and Cystogenesis

In the rat, proteinuria can be observed after parenteral administration of large amounts of proteins (KARL et al. 1964; KURTZ and FELDMAN 1962; MARKS and DRUMMOND 1970). In numerous studies on the rat, BSA was injected intraperitoneally to elucidate the mechanisms and morphology of so-called protein overload proteinuria (ANDERSON and RECANT 1961; BLISS and BREWER 1985a, b; DAVIES and BREWER 1977; DAVIES et al. 1978; LAWRENCE and BREWER 1981, 1982, 1984). Considering these reports, increased glomerular transcapillary flow of proteins led to an augmented protein absorption in glomerular visceral epithelia; lysosomal activity of these cells rose. The epithelial cells became edematous; vacuoles were generated, the typical foot processes were lost, and some epithelial cells were detached from the glomerular basement membrane. With prolonged administration of BSA, a focal and segmental sclerosis of glomeruli occurred.

These well-known glomerular alterations after high-dose BSA administration were confirmed and supplemented in our own experiments. After 4–8 weeks of BSA administration, the extent of glomerular sclerosis exceeded significantly the extent of sclerosis indices that were described after short-term BSA administration (Fig. 9). In agreement with other groups, our data showed that proteinuria was a mixture of heterologous BSA and homologous proteins with nominal molecular weights, larger and smaller than albumin.

The tubular effects of protein overload proteinuria were not analyzed in detail in the aforementioned investigations of BSA effects on glomerular structure. In rats, Baxter et al. described an increase in kidney size after prolonged intraperitoneal administration of human albumin (BAXTER and CORTZIAS 1949). After parenteral heterologous protein administration, kidney weights increased significantly in our studies (Fig. 7). Tubular dilatations and casts were formed preferentially in proximal tubular segments (Fig. 8). Significantly increased ^{3}H-thymidine incorporation into the nuclei of tubular epithelia was observed already on the fourth day of high daily BSA administration (Fig. 8). Although an increased ^{3}H-thymidine DNA content cannot automatically be equated with cell proliferation, we regarded a rise in nuclear ^{3}H-thymidine incorporation or an increase in numbers of mitoses that paralleled ^{3}H-thymidine incorporation (HUTCHISON and MUNRO 1961) as indicators of epithelial proliferation. Parallel to tubular epithelial hyperplasia, dilated and cystic tubular segments were demonstrated. The inner medulla was free of dilated tubules. The almost simultaneous occurrence of tubular epithelial proliferation and dilatation hindered an exact analysis of whether one phenomenon was due to the other, or vice versa; nevertheless, it is probable that the hyperplasia of tubular cells caused the dilatation of tubular segments.

4.2.2.2 Proteinuria and Tubular Cell Hyperplasia

The glomerular proteinuria led to a significantly increased pinocytotic activity of epithelia in proximal tubules. In the edematous epithelia, numerous protein reabsorption droplets were observed by light microscopy. OLBRICHT et al. (1986) reported that with heterologous proteinuria, lysosomal enzyme activity of proximal tubular epithelia increased significantly. It is conceivable that an increased protein reabsorption not only stimulates cell metabolism, but may also be a stimulus for a proliferation of tubular epithelia. This idea is supported by the previously cited study on cells in culture that found increased cell proliferation accompanying elevated pinocytotic cell activity (BAR-SAGI and FERAMISCO 1986). Several plasma peptides that are known as potential mitogens, like insulin, are normally filtered in the glomerulus and degraded after reabsorption in the proximal tubular epithelium (KAYSEN et al. 1986; SUMPIO and MAACK 1982). In states of glomerular proteinuria, these peptides cannot be assumed to be responsible for tubular epithelial hyperplasia. Potent insulin-like growth factors such as IGF I and IGF II, which are supposed to play a role in renal growth after uninephrectomy, are filtered in the glomerulus only if glomerular permselectivity is disturbed (FAGIN and MELMED 1987; HAMMERNAN 1989; STILES et al. 1985). Growth factors IGF I and IGF II are bound to specific carrier proteins in plasma. The IGF carrier protein complexes have molecular weights between 150 000 and 45 000 and can therefore be detected only in traces in the glomerular ultrafiltrate under normal conditions. The brush border of proximal tubular epithelia possesses specific IGF II and, to a smaller degree, IGF I receptors (HAMMERMAN and ROGERS 1987). In glomerular proteinuria, the quantity of IGF I and IGF II molecules would be augmented in the primary urine; these molecules could then specifically bind to the proximal tubular epithelia and could function as so-called progression factors on growth-competent epithelia (D'ERCOLE et al. 1984; HIRSCHBERG 1993). Further experiments must confirm this assumption.

The possible relevance of growth factors for tubular cell hyperplasia was also indicated by a model of homologous protein-overload proteinuria which was described by MORI et al. (1986). In rats with prolactin, growth hormone, and ACTH-secreting tumors of the hypophysis, liver hyperplasia was induced with consecutive excessive albumin production. Pronounced homologous proteinuria occurred with an increase in kidney size and the genesis of tubular cysts. The authors did not perform quantitative morphometric or hormonal analysis, which would have allowed assessment of the role of the secreted growth factors and hormones, and of the role of the homologous proteinuria on the tubular alterations.

It also must be considered that glomerular cells and macrophages located in partially sclerosed mesangial areas can synthesize eicosanoids and leukotrienes, substances which can exert hypertrophic and hyperplastic effects (BAND et al. 1985).

The glomerular sclerosis started to increase in the late phase of our experiments. Therefore, it does not seem to be the primary stimulus for cell hyperplasia and tubular dilatation. Our considerations on the induction of tubular epithelial proliferation by proteins of the glomerular ultrafiltrate are confirmed by investigations of BRODKIN and NOBLE (1986). These studies were performed to test a possible mitogenic effect of immunoglobulins on tubular epithelia. The immunoglobulins bound onto specific receptors of proximal tubular epithelia and led to an increased proliferation of tubular epithelia in vivo. In this study, a so-called nonspecific albuminuria also stimulated the proliferation of tubular epithelium, although to a lesser extent than immunoglobulins.

4.2.2.3 Tubular Cell Hyperplasia and Cystogenesis

Postulated causal relationships between tubular cell proliferation and tubular cystogenesis are supported by studies on transgenic mice. MACKAY et al. (1987) investigated lines of transgenic mice with the so-called early region of the SV 40 virus. It was known that gene products of the early region of SV 40 could induce a malignant transformation of cells in culture. The transforming gene coded the large T-antigen. In vivo, proliferation of epithelia was observed when the large T-antigen was produced in tubular epithelia of the mouse kidney. The tubular cell hyperplasia was associated with tubular dilatation and cysts.

KOLLIAS et al. (1987) described the ectopic renal expression of Thy-1 genes in transgenic mice. The proximal tubular epithelium exhibited an increased mitotic activity. Dilated tubules and tubular cysts were observed. Also in transgenic mice c-myc overexpression or bcl-2 deficiency resulted in tubular cell proliferation and polycystic kidneys (TRUDEL et al. 1991; VEIS et al. 1993).

The association of the two phenomena, tubular cell proliferation and cysts, does not indicate a direct causal correlation. The expression of the large T-antigen and other oncogenes could alter the production of proteoglycans and collagen, as well as stimulate DNA synthesis (BANKOWSKI et al. 1978; IOZZO 1985; SUNDARRAJ and CHURCH 1978; WINTER BOURNE and MORA 1978). The compliance of tubular basement membranes thus could have been increased in the cited experiments and dilatation of tubules could have occurred. It can therefore only be assumed that a causal relation between epithelial hyperplasia and cystogenesis does exist. The expression of proto-oncogenes has not yet been studied in the model described here, in contrast to other models with oncogene overexpression (COWLEY et al. 1987, 1991; HARDING et al. 1992; HERRERA 1991).

4.2.2.4 Excretory Renal Function and Cystogenesis

Increased GFR, with a consequent increase in electrolyte and water transport, activated Na^+/H^+ antiport, and Na-K-ATPase of tubular epithelia, can be regarded as a stimulus for the hypertrophy and hyperplasia of tubular epithelia (FINE et al. 1985a, b; GRANTHAM et al. 1989; MOOLENAAR et al. 1983; NORD et al. 1984). According to our functional measurements, in agreement with those of WEENING et al. (1987), no significant differences in GFR were obtained between BSA and control groups; thus, an increased electrolyte transport does not seem probable as a cause of cell hyperplasia.

An obstruction of the ureter, which may cause tubular cell hyperplasia and segmental dilatation, was excluded in our experiments (BENITZ and SHAKA 1964; FETTERMAN et al. 1974; SHEEHAN and DAVIS 1959). There were no macroscopic or microscopic indications for postrenal obstruction. On the other hand, homogenous eosinophil precipitates were observed in proximal and distal tubules in the course of massive proteinuria. A temporary partial or total obstruction of urine flow in the region of entry of the tubules into the medulla could thus not be definitely excluded and might have fostered a tubular dilatation.

4.2.3 Homologous Proteinuria, Models of Acquired Cystic Kidney Disease

4.2.3.1 Proteinuria and Cystogenesis

Daunomycin (D) and puromycinaminonucleoside (PAN) directly damage the visceral epithelial cells of the glomeruli (ANDREWS 1977; BAKKER et al. 1987; ERICSSON and ANDRES 1961; FISHMAN and KARNOVSKY 1985; GLASSER et al. 1977; PINTO and BREWER 1975; SCHWARTZ et al. 1984; SPINELLI and BRÜCHER 1975). MESSINA et al. (1987) and CAULFIELD et al. (1976) have investigated the glomerular alterations after PAN sequentially and in detail. Before proteinuria occurred, the podocytes showed a general loss of foot processes. The start of the proteinuria happened at the time at which the visceral epithelial cells partly detached from the glomerular basement membrane. In the course of proteinuria, the number of glomerular basement membrane segments that were denuded from visceral epithelial cells increased. The cytoplasm of the podocytes showed varyingly large, partly ruptured vacuoles. These light-microscopic and ultra-structural features of the glomeruli after D and PAN were confirmed by our studies (FISHER and HELLSTROM 1962; FRENK et al. 1955; GRÖNE et al. 1980b; GROND et al. 1984, 1985).

Daunomycin induced a severe nephrotic syndrome with a continuously high homologous proteinuria (Table 4a, c). In a relatively short time of 7 weeks, pronounced polycystic kidneys were generated, dependent on the diet fed to the rats. Uninephrectomy exacerbated the cystic tubular alterations.

Cystogenesis was not due to a substance-specific effect of D. Cystic renal alterations also occurred after PAN injection. The extent of tubular cysts, however, was smaller than in animals with D-nephrosis. This phenomenon is probably due to a less pronounced nephrosis after PAN injection. PAN-treated animals showed pronounced proteinuria only at the end of the experiment; proteinuria was always less than in D-treated rats. Metabolic alterations such as hypercholesterolemia and hypertriglyceridemia were also less severe in PAN-treated than in D-treated rats.

The proliferative activity of the tubular epithelia increased with glomerular proteinuria. The significant rise in cell hyperplasia and the tubular dilatations and tubular cysts occurred at different points of time. Therefore, it can be assumed that the increased proliferation of tubular epithelia was not secondary to the dilation of tubules. The scanning electron microscopy of the tubular dilatations demonstrated the probable association between tubular dilatation and tubular hyperplasia. The proliferative epithelia seemed to distend the tubules with the formation of colon-like structures. Polypoid proliferations and tubular ridges formed partial obstructions to urine flow. Thus, the intratubular pressure could have increased with continued glomerular filtration and, in addition, could have dilated the tubules.

4.2.3.2 Cell Toxicity of Daunomycin and Puromycinaminounucleoside and Cystogenesis

According to the literature, D and PAN seem to have a direct tubular toxic effect (FAJARDO et al. 1980). NAGLE et al. (1972) described at 8 days after the start of daily intramuscular PAN injections (50 mg/kg body wt.) that proximal tubular epithelia appeared swollen and numerous lysosomes and damaged mitochondria could be seen. The tubular epithelia demonstrated an increased protein permeability to peroxidase. Cell necrosis, and increased number of epithelial mitoses per area, and cell debris in the lumina of tubules were observed.

In contrast to our data, the PAN dose applied in the experiments of Nagle et al. was high.

Cell apoptosis nevertheless may be an important factor in the development of tubular lesions (GOBE and AXELSEN 1987). Cell necrosis and cell apoptosis, along with glomerular proteinuria, could well have exerted a proliferative stimulus in our experiments. Similar phenomena have been observed after chronic application of hydrocarbons (ADEN et al. 1985; SHORT et al. 1987).

4.2.3.3 Excretory Renal Function and Cystogenesis

The excretory renal function decreased during tubular cystogenesis, independent of the specific diet. GFR fell continuously to about 10% of control values during the experimental period. This decrease in excretory renal function was not caused solely by the cystic nephron parts; only about one third of all tubules were cystically dilated. Numerous tubules with very small lumina that were covered by atrophic and hyperplastic epithelia were observed. Tubular cysts apparently decreased total renal function by a compression of surrounding nephron segments that finally became atrophic (CARONE et al. 1988). A morphological study in human cystic kidneys confirmed these experimental observations (BIRENBOIM et al. 1987). The number and the size of tubular cysts were directly correlated with the serum creatinine concentrations in two studies on patients with genetically determined cystic kidneys (GABOW et al. 1984; REUBI 1985).

According to our sequential hemodynamic data, it does not seem probable that a primarily increased electrolyte and water transport of tubular epithelia with a simultaneous increase of GFR constituted a cause of the tubular epithelial hyperplasia. On the other hand, it is possible that in the course of cystogenesis, tubular epithelia changed not only their morphological phenotype but also their functional characteristics. An abnormal tubular transport with accumulation of osmotically active substances and a consequent accumulation of fluid within the tubules could be conceived. Avner et al. induced proximal tubular cysts by cortisone administration and triiodothyronine in metanephric tissue cultures (AVNER 1988; AVNER et al. 1984). The induction of cysts was directly dependent on the activity of the epithelial sodium potassium ATPase. A blockade of sodium potassium ATPase by ouabain suppressed cystogenesis completely (AVNER et al. 1985, 1987).

4.2.3.4 Tubular Basement Membranes and Cystogenesis

The basement membranes of dilated tubules were thickened even in areas with large tubular cysts. An abnormally increased compliance of tubular basement membrane has been assumed as the dominant pathogenetic factor during cystogenesis (CARONE et al. 1974; HAY 1983; WALDHERR et al. 1982; WINSTON and SAFIRSTEIN 1985). If an increased deformability of the tubular basement membrane were the only stimulus to cystogenesis, an increase of the tubular segment by a factor of 1000 should lead to an extremely thin basement membrane; this has been stated in detail by WELLING and GRANTHAM (1986). Thin tubular basement membranes have not been observed, either in cysts of human polycystic kidneys or in experimentally induced cystic kidneys of animals (AVNER 1988; BERNSTEIN et al. 1987; GRANTHAM et al. 1989). GRANTHAM et al. (1987) measured the viscoelastic properties of microdissected tubular segments in tubular cysts in two experimental cystic kidney disease models (cystic kidneys induced by diphenylthiazol and nordihydroguaretic acid) and in experimental hereditary cystic kidney disease models. The mechanical features of tubular basement membranes were similar in cystically altered tubules and in normal tubules. Also in our studies, there were no direct indications for a large deformability of tubular basement membranes as judged by light microscopy and ultrastructure. The tubular basement membranes were always thicker than normal. This increase in the tubular basement membrane could have been due to an elevated synthesis or to a decreased degradation of basement membrane components (MADRI et al. 1980; ROHDE et al. 1979). Studies of KANWAR and CARONE (1984) and EBIHARA et al. (1988) in the diphenylthiazole cystic kidney disease model of the rat pointed to an increased synthesis of proteoglycans by tubular epithelial cells. The pronounced increase in rough endoplasmic reticulum in the hyperplastic tubular epithelia favor an elevated production of basement membrane components in our cystic kidney disease model; also, the synthesis of a new intermediate filament (vimentin) speaks in favor of an increased synthesis of structural proteins. It cannot be excluded that a synthesis of altered basement membrane components (BEAVAN et al. 1991) thus fostered a dilatation of the tubules, as a changed tubular basement membrane could have had altered viscoelastic properties. In addition, an altered extracellular matrix can lead to an increase in tubular epithelial proliferation (TAUB et al. 1990; WILSON et al. 1992).

4.2.3.5 Interstitial Cells and Cystogenesis

The formation of cysts in D- and PAN-nephrosis was accompanied by focal tubular atrophy, interstitial fibrosis, and interstitial mononuclear infiltration. BERTANI et al. KELLY et al. proposed that the interstitial inflammatory infiltrate had an important role in cystogenesis (BERTANI et al. 1982, 1986; KELLY and NEILSON 1987). Kelly et al. hypothesized that the tubular microcysts in Kd-Kd mice with interstitial nephritis were initiated by an interstitial inflammation. Macrophages can synthesize proteases such as collagenase and elastase and secrete these enzymes, which could potentially damage the extracellular matrix and tubular basement membrane (NATHAN 1987). Tubular dilatations thus could occur more easily (WERB et al. 1980). T lymphocytes synthesize β-transforming growth factor (TFG), a peptide that may influence cell proliferation, cell differentiation, (WANG and HSU 1986) and matrix synthesis. The development of renal cysts in a transgenic mouse with immunodeficiency argues against a significant role of lymphacytes.

Gardner et al. reported that a positive correlation could be established between an infiltration of the interstitium and tubules by granulocytes and cystogenesis in the mouse (GARDNER et al. 1986, 1987; WERDER et al. 1984). The interstitium was not infiltrated by granulocytes in our experimental model. Thus, granulocytes did not seem to be a part of the pathogenesis of tubular cysts. An interstitial nephritis was not seen in the early stages of our studies. A cystogenic influence of interstitial cells in later phases of our studies, however, cannot be definitely excluded, although it does not seem to be the dominant cystogenic factor.

4.2.4 Influence of Diet on Cystogenesis

It is known that one can modulate glomerular function and glomerular structure by diet. This has been extensively investigated and is uniformly accepted (FINE 1987). A high-protein diet increases renal blood flow in many mammals, including man, and increases the effective transcapillary glomerular filtration pressure and glomerular filtration. These hemodynamic effects contribute significantly to glomerular sclerosis, especially in states of reduced kidney mass (BRENNER et al. 1982). In experiments on the growth characteristics of rats it was noted that a high-casein and -fat diet could modulate kidney growth (BLATHERWICK and MEDLAR 1937; FERNANDES et al. 1978; FINE 1987; HALLIBURTON 1969; NEW BURGH and CURTIS 1928; RUMSFELD 1956; SAXTON and KIMBALL 1941). As we assumed a central role of tubular epithelial hyperplasia in cystogenesis, it seemed reasonable to also assess the effect of casein and dietary fats in cystogenesis. A casein- and fat-rich diet led to a significant increase of tubular cysts in comparison to a regular diet that was a mixture of vegetable and animal proteins and had a low amount of fat. This tubular cyst enhancement was especially notable in states of homologous proteinuria (daunomycin nephrosis). A diet containing only casein was accompanied by an enhancement of tubular cysts only in D- and PAN-nephrosis; cyst size was not stimulated by casein in states of heterologous proteinuria. The tubuloproliferative effects of the synthetic casein and fat diet were seen, although to a slight degree, in control animals. Control animals with a casein- and fat-enriched diet (CF) had significantly higher proteinuria than control animals with diets P and C. The proteinuria of the control group CF was caused by an increased glomerular membrane permeability after a lipid-rich diet; the pathogenesis of this increased protein permeability has been described in detail in another report (GRÖNE et al. 1989). The proteinuria and tubular cell hyperplasia were nevertheless small in comparison to those in animals with nephrosis and heterologous and homologous proteinuria. Thus, tubular cysts were not observed in the course of the experiment in control animals.

Rats treated with BSA had significantly higher proteinuria with the casein- and fat-rich diet than with regular rat chow. At least part of the tubular effect of the CF diet could thus be explained by an increased proteinuria. On the other hand, an analysis of the data in D-nephrosis showed that the C and CF diets had a proliferative and cystogenic effect independent of the extent of proteinuria. We can only speculate on the molecular mechanisms of the proliferative action of a diet rich in casein or casein and fat. The alimentary status of an animal can have a significant effect on growth factors such as insulin-like growth factors (IGF) that probably exert a central influence on kidney growth (HALL et al. 1981; JOBIN and BONJOUR 1986; STILES et al. 1979, 1985). It remains unclear if the high proline and low glycine content of the casein diet in important (JACQUES et al. 1986). Also, our data on plasma lipids and plasma lipoproteins did not contribute to an explanation of the dietary effects. Fasting plasma cholesterol and triglyceride concentrations were always elevated above normal values, independent of the diet in nephrotic animals (DE MENDOZA et al. 1976). Nevertheless, a detailed analysis of lipoprotein profiles has to be done to recognize possible differences between diet groups. Recent studies on cells in culture, including human glomerular mesangial cells, point to a proliferative action of lipoproteins via stimulation of autocrine growth factors (FROSTEGARD et al. 1990; GRÖNE et al. 1992); also, lipids may modulate the transport characteristics of proximal tubular epithelia for electrolytes and thereby influence epithelial growth (LEVI et al. 1990). Lipids may enhance the effect oxidative processes seem to have on the genesis of tubular cysts (HOCKENBERG et al. 1993; HJELLE et al. 1990).

Our results on the dietary effects were confirmed by LAOUARI et al. (1983), who conducted experiments on rats to test the influence of a protein-enriched diet on glomerular function. A diet with a high protein and a high casein content led to impressive cystic tubular degeneration in addition to pronounced glomerular sclerosis.

4.2.5 Coexpression of the Intermediate Filaments Vimentin and Keratin in Epithelia of Atrophic and Cystic Tubules

An increased incidence of renal cell carcinoma has been noted in acquired cystic kidney disease of human beings in retrospective studies (HUGHSON et al. 1986). The acquired cystic kidneys in daunomycin nephrosis could perhaps contribute to an understanding of the pathogenesis of renal carcinomas (STERUBERG et al. 1972).

The immunohistologic documentation of tissue-specific different inter-mediate filament proteins can aid considerably in the histopathologic classifica-tion of malignant tumors. Carcinomas synthesize keratins; sarcomas are almost always kertain-negative but positive for vimentin or desmin (MOLL et al. 1982). The coexpression of vimentin and keratin can be found in relatively few organs and tumors (CASELITZ et al. 1981; CZERNOBILINSKY et al. 1985; GATTER et al. 1986; HENZEN-LOGMANS et al. 1987; LANE 1982; LANE et al. 1983; LA ROCCA and RHEINWALD 1984; MCMUTT et al. 1985; MIETTINEN et al. 1984). Renal cell carcinomas can coexpress keratin and vimentin. A simultaneous synthesis of vimentin and keratin in renal cell carcinomas has been found in 57–100% of studied cases (HERMANN et al. 1983; HOLTHÖFER et al. 1983). We found that 80% of renal cell carcinomas showed a coexpression of vimentin and keratin (GRÖNE et al. 1986a). The coexpression of vimentin and keratin in renal cell carcinomas is difficult to explain because tubular epithelia of the adult human and rat kidney exclusively synthesize keratin-intermediate filaments (BACHMANN et al. 1983; HOLTHÖFER et al. 1983). Renal cell carcinomas originate from tubular epithelia; the majority of carcinomas have their origin from proximal tubular epithelia (GRÖNE et al. 1986a).

A simultaneous synthesis of keratin and vimentin was shown in altered epithelia by double-immunofluorescence (Fig. 12a–d). This coexpression was observed only in damaged epithelia with partial or complete loss of the brush border or the basolateral labyrinth or with pronounced flattening, but not in regularly differentiated tubular epithelia. The reasons for this synthesis of vimentin in epithelial cells could correspond to those that have been postulated for vimentin production in many lines of cultured epithelial cells (VIRTANEN et al. 1981). The three-dimensional organization of a cell and the mode of cell-to-cell interaction apparently influenced the differential expression of intermediate filaments in these cell culture experiments. When certain epithelia were cultured in suspension, only keratin was synthesized. Epithelia in culture increased their vimentin RNA and vimentin protein synthesis with decreasing cell number, but increased their keratin synthesis with increasing cell number (BEN-ZE'EV 1983, 1984). When desmosomal cell contacts were destroyed, the vimentin synthesis of epithelial cells rose (BEN-ZE'EV 1986).

The vimentin synthesis of cultured cells also seemed to be growth regulated (CONNELL and RHEINWALD 1983; FARBER and WILKINSON 1987; FERRARI et al. 1986). Vimentin expression was especially noticeable in kidneys with high proliferative activity. This close association between epithelial proliferation and vimentin expression also became apparent in parallel experiments conducted on rats with acute renal failure induced by mercury chloride. Only regenerating and proliferating epithelia expressed vimentin and keratin (GRÖNE et al. 1987). The experiments also showed the dynamics of filament expression, since vimentin synthesis decreased and vanished after regeneration of tubular epithelia was complete. The coexpression of keratin and vimentin was also found in damaged tubules of human kidneys.

The question arises whether tubular epithelia with a simultaneous synthesis of keratin and vimentin constitute the precursor cells of renal cell carcinomas. The fact that rats with daunomyocin nephrosis develop renal cell adenomas and carcinomas in a significantly higher proportion than normal rats of the same age could point to a relationship between damaged tubular epithelia with vimentin and keratin coexpression and these renal tumors. The coexpression of keratin and vimentin in damaged tubular epithelia in human renal diseases that do not have an increased incidence of renal cell carcinoma speaks against this assumption.

4.2.6 Clinical Relevance of the Studies on Tubular Cell Hyperplasia and Cystogenesis

Polycystic kidney diseases are partly genetically determined, partly acquired. In animal experiments, cystic kidneys were generated by drugs, toxins and bacterial infections. Morphological and functional investigations on human cystic kidneys and experimental cystic kidney disease models have analyzed different aspects of the pathogenesis of tubular cysts. Numerous theories on cystogenesis resulted which were quite often discussed in a manner claiming absolute validity (AVNER 1988; BERNSTEIN et al. 1987; GARDNER and EVANS 1984; GRANTHAM et al. 1989; GRANTHAM 1985). It is probable that differences in environmental factors, extracellular factors and intracellular alterations of the tubular epithelia interact to generate tubular cysts.

Our studies therefore do not attempt to point to two factors of tubular cystogenesis as the only important modulators of tubular cystogenesis. In contrast, we tried to analyze two conditions, glomerular proteinuria and dietetic influences, which may have modulatory effects on the genesis and enlargement of renal cysts, also under clinical conditions.

The cystic kidneys in D- and PAN-nephrosis could also serve as a cystic kidney disease model for further studies on cystogenesis. One advantage of the model is that it is consistently reproducible in a short time period.

We found morphological and functional similarities between acquired cystic kidney disease in chronic renal disease and also similarities to genetically determined cystic kidneys (FARAGGIANA et al. 1985). Immunohistologic results in human acquired cystic kidney disease point to the fact that the majority of cysts originate from proximal tubular segments, as in our model (FINLEY and DABBS 1988). The drastic reduction of GFR at the end of our experiments corresponds to the significantly reduced excretory function in human acquired cystic kidney disease (GRANTHAM 1985).

Patients with genetically determined autosomal recessive or dominant polycystic kidney disease differ extensively in the phenotypic expression of their disease; some patients develop only a few cysts and do not suffer from a decline in excretory renal function, while other patients develop numerous and large renal cysts in proximal and distal tubular segments and, finally, severe renal insufficiency (FINLEY and DABB 1988; GARDNER and EVANS 1984; GRANTHAM et al. 1989). Because of this variable clinical expression of genetically determined cysts, one can reasonably argue that endogenous and exogenous influences modulate the severity of cystic kidneys. Infections of the urinary tract and arterial hypertension have already been noted as important factors in the progression of cystic disease (CHURCHILL et al. 1989; KIME et al. 1962).

Proteinuria and dietary influences could perhaps be additional modulators of cystogenesis. Although the direct mitogenic stimuli of the diets on tubular epithelia are unknown, the cystogenic characteristics of diets in our animal experiments could be a stimulus for further studies. It should especially be investigated whether the cystogenesis of human kidneys depends on dietary influences; this could have relevance for the prophylaxis of cystic kidneys in either genetically determined or acquired cystic kidney disease.

Acknowledgements. This work was supported by a grant of the German Research Foundation (Deutsche Forschungsgemeinschaft, SFB 330, C7) to Dr. H.-J. Gröne. The studies are part of the *Habilitation* of H.-J. Gröne. The author is indebted to Professor Dr. U. Helmchen, Director of the Institute of Pathology, University of Hamburg, for his helpful advice; to Professor Dr. Mary Osborn and Professor Dr. K. Weber, Max Planck Institute of Biophysical Chemistry, Göttingen, for providing the antibodies to intermediate filaments and for their constructive criticism; to Professor Dr. P.J. Olbricht, Department of Internal Medicine, University of Hannover, for his help in the measurement of enzyme activities, and to Dr. P. Schwartz, Department of Anatomy, University of Göttingen, for his help with the scanning electron microscopy studies. The technical assistance of E. Gutjahr, N. Rasch, and B. Reinelt is appreciated.

References

Aden CL, Ridder G, Stone L, Kanerva RL (1985) Pathology of petrochemical fuels in male rats. Acute toxicity. In: Bach PH, Lock EA (eds) Renal heterogeneity and target cell toxicity. Wiley, Chichester, p 461

Anderson MS, Recant L (1961) Fine structural alterations in the rat kindey following intraperitoneal bovine albumin. Am J Pathol 40: 555

Anderson WP, Korner PI, Johnston CI (1979) Acute angiotensin II-mediated restoration of distal renal artery pressure in renal artery stenosis and its relationship to the development of sustained one-kidney hypertension in conscious dogs. Hypertension 1: 292

Anderson WP, Korner PI, Angus JA, Johnston CI (1981) Contribution of stenosis resistance to the rise in total peripheral resistance during experimental renal hypertension in conscious dogs. Clin Sci 61: 663

Andrews PM (1977) A scanning and transmission electron microscopic comparison of puromycin aminonucleoside-induced nephrosis to hyperalbuminemia-induced proteinuria with emphasis on kindney podocyte pedicle loss. Lab Invest 36: 183

Atkinson AB, Robertson JIS (1979) Captopril in the trestment of clinical hypertension and cardiac failure. Lancet 2: 836

Autio-Harmainen H, Väänänen R, Rapola J (1981) Scanning electron microscopic study of normal human glomerulogenesis and of fetal glomeruli in congenital nephrotic syndrome of the Finnish type. Kidney Int 20: 747

Avner ED, Piesco NP, Sweeney WE, Studnicki FM, Fetterman GH, Ellis D (1984) Hydrocortisone-induced cystic metanephric maldevelopment in serum-free organ culture. Lab Invest 50: 208

Avner ED (1988) Renal cystic disease. Insights from recent experimental investigations. Nephron 48: 89

Avner ED, Sweeney WE, Finegold DN, Piesco NP, Ellis D (1985) Sodium potassium ATPase activity mediates cyst formation in metanephric organ culture. Kidney Int 28: 447

Avner ED, Sweeney WE, Ellis D (1987) Increased organic anion uptake mediates proximal tubular cyst formation in metanephric organ culture. Kidney Int 31: 159(A)

Avner ED, Studnicki FE, Young MC, Sweeney WE jr, Piesco NP, Ellis D, Fetterman GH (1988) Congenital murine polycystic kidney disease. II. Pathogenesis of tubular cyst formation. Pediatr Nephrol 2: 210

Bachmann S, Kriz W, Kuhn C, Franke WW (1983) Differentiation of cell types in the mammalian kidney by immunofluorescence microscopy using antibodies to intermediate filament proteins and desmoplakins. Histrochemistry 77: 365

Bakker WW, Kalicharan D, Donga J, Hulstaert CE, Hardonk MK (1987) Decreased ATPase activity in adriamycin nephrosis is independent of proteinuria. Kidney Int 31: 704

Bankowski E, Rzecyzycki W, Nowak HKF, Jodczyk KJ (1978) Decrease of collagen biosynthesis ability of rat kidney fibroblasts transformed with SV40 virus. Mol Cell Biochem 20: 77

Bar-Sagi D, Feramisco JR (1986) Induction of membrane ruffling and fluid-phase pinocytosis in quiescent fibroblasts by rats proteins. Science 233: 1061

Band L, Sraer J, Perez J, Nivez M-P, Ardaillou R (1985) Leukotriene C4 binds to human glomerular epithelial cells and promotes their proliferation in vitro. J Clin Invest 76: 374

Bauer JH, Reams GP (1985) Hemodynamic and renal function in essential hypertension during treatment with enalapril. Am J Med 79 [Suppl 3C]: 10

Baxter TJ (1960) Cortisone-induced renal changes in the rabbit: a microdissection study. Br J Exp Pathol 41: 140

Baxter JH, Cotzias GC (1949) Effects of proteinuria on the kidney. J Exp Med 89: 643

Beavan LA, Carone FA, Nakamura S, Jones JK, Reindel JF, Price RG (1991) Comparison of proteoglycans synthesized by porcine normal and polycystic renal tubular epithelial cells in vitro. Arch Biochem Biophys 284: 392

Bender W, LaFrance N, Walker WG (1984) Mechanism of deterioration in renal function in patients with renovascular hypertension treated with enalapril. Hypertension 6 [Suppl I]: I-93–I-97

Benitez L, Shaka JA (1964) Cell proliferation in experimental hydronephrosis and compensatory renal hyperplasia. Am J Pathol 44: 961

Bennett WM (1985) Evaluation and management of renal infection. In: Grantham JJ, Gardner KD (eds) Problems in diagnosis and management of polycystic kidney disease. Intercollegiate Press, Kansas City, p 98

Ben-Ze'ev A (1983) Cell configuration-related control of vimentin biosynthesis and phosphorylation in cultured mammalian cells. J Cell Biol 97: 858

Ben-Ze'ev A (1984) Differential control of cytokeratins and vimentin synthesis by cell-cell contact and cell spreading in cultured epithelial cells. J Cell Biol 99: 1424

Ben-Ze'ev A (1986) Tumor promoter-induced disruption of junctional complexes in cultured epithelial cells is followed by the inhibition of cytokeratin and desmoplakin synthesis. Exp Cell Res 164: 335

Bernstein J (1985) Morphology of human renal cystic disease. In: Cumming ND, Klahr S (eds) Chronic renal disease: causes, complications and treatment. Plenum Medical Book, New York, p 47

Bernstein J, Evan AP, Gardner KD (1987) Epithelial hyperplasia in human polycystic kidney diseases. Am J Pathol 129: 92

Bertani T, Poggi A, Pozzoni R, Delaini F, Sacchi G, Thoua Y, Mecca G, Remuzzi G, Donati MB (1982) Adriamycin-induced nephrotic syndrome in rats. Lab Invest 46: 16

Bertani T, Cutillo F, Zoja C, Broggini M, Remuzzi G (1986) Tubulo-interstitial lesions mediate renal damage in adriamycin glomerulopathy. Kidney Int 30: 488

Birenboim N, Donoso VS, Huseman RA, Grantham JJ (1987) The renal excretion and cyst accumulation of β_2-micro-globulin in autosomal dominant polycystic kidney disease. Kidney Int 31: 85

Blatherwick NR, Medlar EM (1937) Chronic nephritis in rats fed high protein diets. Arch Int Med 59: 572

Bliss DJ, Brewer DB (1985a) Increased albumin and normal dextran clearances in protein-overload proteinuria in the rat. Clin Sci 69: 321

Bliss DJ, Brewer DB (1985b) Glomerular lysozyme binding in protein-overload proteinuria. Virchows Arch [B] 48: 351

Bohle A (1954) Kritischer Beitrag zur Morphologie einer endokrinen Nierenfunktion und deren Bedeutung für den Hochdruck. Arch Kreislaufforsch 20: 193

Bohle A, Mackensen-Haen S, von Giese H (1986) Über die Bedeutung tubulo-interstitieller Veränderungen für die Ausscheidefunktion und die Konzentrationsleistung der Niere. Zentralbl Allg Pathol Pathol Anat 132: 351

Boylan JW, Deetjen P, Kramer K (1970) Niere und Wasserhaushalt. In: Gauer OH, Kramer K, Jung R (eds) Physiologie des Menschen. Urban and Schwarzenberg, Munich

Brenner BM, Meyer TW, Hostetter TH (1982) Dietary protein intake and the progressive nature of kidney disease: the role of hemodynamically mediated glomerular injury in the pathogenesis of progressive glomerular sclerosis in aging renal ablation and intrinsic renal disease. N Engl J Med 307: 652

Bricker NS, Patton JF (1955) Cystic disease of the kidneys. A study of dynamics and chemical composition of cyst fluid. Am J Med 18: 207

Brodkin M, Noble B (1986) Increased cell proliferation as a proximal tubule response to immunological injury. Kidney Int 29: 267(A)

Brown CP, Douglas JG (1987) Influence of transmembrane potential differences of renal tubular epithelial cells on ANG II binding. Am J Physiol 252: F209

Brunette DM (1984) Mechanical stretching increases the number of epithelial cells synthetizing DNA in culture. J Cell Sci 69: 35

Carmines PK, Perry MD, Hazelrig JB, Navar LG (1987) Effects of preglomerular and postglomerular vascular resistance alterations on filtration fraction. Kidney Int 31 [Suppl 20]: S229

Carone FA, Rowland RG, Perlman SG, Ganote CE (1974) The pathogenesis of drug-induced renal cystic disease. Kidney Int 5: 411

Carone FA, Ozon S, Samma S, Kanwar YS, Oyasu R (1988) Renal functional changes in experimental cystic disease are tubular in origin. Kidney Int 33: 8

Carone FA, Hollenberg PF, Nakamura S, Punyarit P, Glogowski W, Flouret G (1989) Tubular basement membrane change occurs pari passu with the development of cyst formation. Kidney Int 35: 1034

Caselitz J, Osborn M, Seifert G, Weber K (1981) Intermediate-sized filament proteins (prekeratin, vimentin, desmin) in the normal parotid gland and parotid gland tumors: immunofluorescence study. Virchows Arch [A] 393: 273

Caulfield JP, Reid JJ, Farquhar MG (1976) Alterations of the glomerular epithelium in acute aminonucleoside nephrosis. Lab Invest 34: 43

Christensen EI, Maunsbach AB (1980) Digestion of protein in lysosomes of proximal tubule cells. In: Maunsbach AB, Olsen TS, Christensen EI (eds) Functional ultrastructure of the kidney. Academic, London, p 341

Chrysant SG, Dunn M, Marples D, Demasters K (1983) Severe reversible azotemia from captopril therapy. Arch Intern Med 143: 437

Chung-Park M, Ricanati E, Lankerani M et al (1983) Acquired renal cysts and multiple renal cell and urothelial tumors. Am J Clin Pathol 79: 238

Churchill DN, Bear JC, Morgan J, Payne RH, McManamon PJ, Gault MH (1989) Prognosis of adult onset polycystic kidney disease reevaluated. Kidney Int 26: 190

Cleland JGF, Dargie HJ (1987) Heart failure, renal function and angiotensin-converting-enzyme inhibitors. Kidney Int 31 [Suppl 20]: S220

Cohen AH, Hoyer JR (1986) Nephronophthisis. A primary tubular basement membrane defect. Lab Invest 55: 564

Collste P, Haglund L, Lundgren G, Mangusson G, Östman J (1979) Reversible renal failure during treatment with captopril. Br Med J 2: 612

Cowley BD jr, Smardo FL Jr, Grantham JJ, Calvet JP (1987) Elevated c-myc proto-oncogene expression in autosomal recessive polycystic kidney disease. Proc Natl Acad Sci USA 84: 8394

Cowley BD jr, Chadwick LJ, Grantham JJ, Calvet JP (1991) Elevated proto-oncogene expression in polycystic kidney of the C57BL/6J(c pk) mouse. J Am Soc Nephrol 1: 1048

Cowley BD jr, Gudapaty S. Kraybill AL, Barash BD, Harding MA, Calvet JP, Gattone VH II (1993) Autosomal-dominant polycystic kidney disease in the rat. Kidney Int 43: 522

Cushman DW, Cheung HS, Sabo EF, Ondette MA (1980) Angiotensin-converting-enzyme inhibitors: evolution of a new class of antihypertensive drugs. In: Horowitz ZP (ed) Angiotensin-converting-enzyme inhibitors. Urban and Schwarzenberg, Baltimore, p 3

Connell ND, Rheinwald JG (1983) Regulation of the cytoskeleton in mesothelial cells: reversible loss of keratin and increase in vimentin during rapid growth in culture. Cell 34: 245

Coulie P, Deplaen JF, Van Ypersele de Strihou C (1983) Captopril-induced acute reversible renal failure. Naphron 35: 108

Crocker JFS, Brown DM, Borch RF, Vernier RL (1972) Renal cystic disease induced in newborn rats by diphenylamine derivates. Am J Pathol 66: 343

Crocker FS, Blecher SR, Givner ML, McCarthy SC (1987) Polycystic kidney and liver disease and corticosterone changes in the cpK mouse. Kidney Int 31: 1088

Cuppage FE, Huseman RA, Chapman A, Grantham JJ (1980) Ultrastructure and function of cysts from human adult polycystic kidneys. Kidney Int 17: 372

Curtis JJ, Luke RG, Whelchel JD, Diethelm AG, Jones P, Dustain HP (1983) Inhibition of angiotensin-converting enzyme in renal transplant recipients with hypertension. N Engl J Med 308: 377

Czernobilinsky B, Moll R, Levy R, Franke WW (1985) Coexpression of cytokeratin and vimentin filaments in mesothelial, granulosa and rete ovarii cells of the human ovary. Eur J Cell Biol 37: 175

Dalgaard OZ (1957) Bilateral polycystic disease of the kidneys: a follow-up of two hundred and eighty-four patients and their families. Acta Med Scand [Suppl] 328: 1

Davies DJ, Brewer DB (1977) Irreversible glomerular damage following heterologous serum albumin overload. J Pathol 123: 45

Davies DJ, Brewer DB, Hardwicke J (1978) Urinary proteins and glomerular morphometry in protein overload proteinuria. Lab Invest 38: 232

Deen WM, Robertson CR, Brenner BM (1972) A model of glomerular ultrafiltration in the rat. Am J Physiol 232: F477

Deen WM, Robertson CR, Brenner BM (1974) Glomerular ultrafiltration. Fed Proc 33: 14

D'Ercole JA, Stiles AD, Underwood LE (1984) Tissue concentrations of somatomedian C: further evidence for multiple sites of synthesis and paracrine or autocrine mechanisms of action. Proc Natl Acad Sci USA 81: 935

De Mendoza SG, Kashyap ML, Chen CY, Lutmer RF (1976) High-density lipoproteinuria in nephrotic syndrome. Metabolism 25: 1143

Dobyan DC, Hill D, Lewis T, Bulger RE (1981) Cyst formation in rat kidney induced by cis-platinum administration. Lab Invest 45: 260

Douglas JG (1987) Angiotensin receptor subtypes of the kidney cortex. Am J Physiol 253: F1

Dunnill MS (1985) Acquired Cystic Disease. In: Grantham JJ, Gardner KD (eds) Problems in diagnosis and management of polycystic kidney disease. Intercollegiate Press, Kansas City, p 211

Dunnill MS, Millard PR, Oliver D (1977) Acquired cystic disease of the kidneys: a hazard of long-term intermittent maintenance haemodialysis. J Clin Pathol 30: 868

Ebihara J, Killen PD, Laurie GW, Huang T, Yamada Y, Martin GR, Brown KS (1988) Altered m-RNA expression of basement membrane components in a murine model of polycystic kidney disease. Lab Invest 58: 262

Edwards RM (1983) Segmental effects of norepinephrine and angiotensin II on isolated renal microvessels. Am J Physiol 244: F526

Edwards RM (1985) Effects of prostaglandins on vasoconstrictor action in isolated renal arterioles. Am J Physiol 248: F779

Elliott HL, Macdougall AI, Buchanan WM (1977) Acquired cystic disease of kidney. Lancet 2: 1359

Ericsson JLE, Andres GA (1961) Electron microscopic studies on the development of the glomerular lesions in aminonucleoside nephrosis. Am J Pathol 39: 643

Evan AP, Gardner KD Jr (1976) Comparison of human polycystic and medullary cystic kidney disease with diphenylamine-induced cystic disease. Lab Invest 35: 93

Evan AP, Gardner KD Jr (1979) Nephron obstruction in norhydroguaiaretic acid-induced renal cystic disease. Kidney Int 15: 7

Evan AP, Tanner GA (1986) Proximal tubule morphology after single nephron obstruction in the rat. Kidney Int 30: 818

Evan AP, Hong SK, Gardner K Jr, Park YS, Itgaki R (1978) Evolution of the collecting tubular lesion in diphenylamine-induced renal disease. Lab Invest 38: 244

Evan AP, Gardner KD, Bernstein J (1979) Polypoid and papillary epithelial hyperplasia: a potential cause of ductal obstruction in adult polycystic kidney disease. Kidney Int 16: 743

Fagin JA, Melmed S (1987) Relative increase in insulin-like growth factor I messenger ribonucleic acid levels in compensatory renal hypertrophy. Endocrinology 120: 718

Fajardo LF, Eltringham JR, Stewart JR, Klauber MR (1980) Adriamycin nephrotoxicity. Lab Invest 43: 242

Faraggiana T, Bernstein J, Strauss L, Churg J (1985) Use of lectins in the study of histogenesis of renal cysts. Lab Invest 53: 575

Farber E, Wilkinson R (1987) Hepatocarcinogenesis: a dynamic cellular perspective. Lab Invest 56: 4

Farrow PR, Wilkinson R (1979) Reversible renal failure during treatment with captopril, Br Med J 1: 1680

Fayemi AL, Ali M (1980) Acquired renal cysts and tumors superimposed on chronic primary kidney diseases. Pathol Res Pract 168: 73

Feiner HD, Katz LA, Gallo GR (1981) Acquired cystic disease of kidney in chronic dialysis patients. Urology 12: 260

Fernandes G, Yunis EJ, Miranda M, Smith J, Good RA (1978) Nutritional inhibition of genetically determined renal disease and autoimmunity with prolongation of life in kdkd mice. Proc Natl Acad Sci USA 75: 2888

Ferrari S, Battinin R, Leszek K, Rittling S, Calabretta B, De Riel JK, Philiponis V, Wei J-F, Baserga R (1986) Coding sequence and growth regulation of the human vimentin gene. Mol Cell Biol 6: 3614

Fetterman GH, Ravitch MM, Sherman FE (1974) Cystic changes in fetal kidneys following ureteral ligation: studies by microdissection. Kidney Int 5: 11

Fine LG, Badie-Dezfooly B, Lowe AG, Hamzeh A, Wells J, Salehmoghaddam S (1985a) Stimulation of Na$^+$/H$^+$ antiport is an early event in hypertrophy of renal proximal tubular cells. Proc Natl Acad Sci USA 82: 1736

Fine LG, Holley RW, Nasri H, Badie-Dezfooly B (1985b) BSC-1 growth inhibitor transforms a mitogenic stimulus into a hypertrophic stimulus for renal proximal tubular cells. Relationship to Na$^+$/H$^+$ antiport activity. Proc Natl Acad Sci USA 82: 6163

Fine LG (1987) The role of nutrition in hypertrophy of renal tissue. Kidney Int 32 [Suppl 22]: S2

Finley JL, Dabbs DJ (1988) The histogenesis of acquireed cystic disease of the end-stage kidney. An immunoperoxidase and lectin-binding study. Lab Ivest 58: abstract 29

Fisher ER, Hellstrom HR (1962) Mechanism of proteinuria. Lab Invest 11: 617

Fishman JA, Karnovsky MJ (1985) Effects of the aminonucleoside of puromycin on glomerular epithelial cells in vitro. Am J Pathol 118: 398

Frei U, Schindler R, Graf S, Koch KM (1987) Glomerular hemodynamics of the elipped kidney: Effects of calcium-antagonist (CA) and coverting enzyme inhibition (CEI). Xth international congress of nephrology, London, abstract 277

Frenk S, Antonowicz I, Craig JM, Metcoff J (1955) Experimental nephrotic syndrome induced in rats by aminonucleoside. Renal lesions and body electrolyte composition. Proc Soc Exp Biol Med 89: 424

Frostegard J, Hamsten A, Gidlund M, Nilsson J (1990) Low-denisity lipoprotein-induced growth of U937 cells: a novel method to determined the receptor binding of low-density lipoprotein. J Lipid Res 31: 37

Gabow PA, Ikle DW, Holmes JH (1984) Polycystic kidney disease: prospective analysis of nonazotemic patients and family members. Ann Intern Med 101: 238

Gardner KD Jr (1969) Composition of fluid in twelve cysts of a polycystic kidney. N Engl J Med 282: 985

Gardner KD Jr (1976) An overview of the cystic renal diseases. In: Gardner KD (ed) Cystic diseases of the kidney, Wiley, New York, p 1

Gardner KD (1984) Acquired renal cystic disease and renal adenocarcinoma in patients on long-term hemodialysis. N Engl J Med 310: 390

Gardner KD Jr, Evan AP (1983) Renal cystic disease induced by diphenylthiazone. Kidney Int 24: 43

Gardner KD, Evan AP (1984) Cystic kidneys: an enigma evolves. Am J Kidney Dis 3: 403

Gardner KD Jr, Solomon S, Fitzgerrel WW, Evan AP (1976) Function and structure in the diphenylamine-exposed kidney. J Clin Invest 57: 796

Gardner KD Jr, Evan AP, Reed WP (1986) Accelerated renal cyst development in deconditioned germ-free rats. Kidney Int 29: 1116

Gardner KD Jr, Reed WP, Evan AP, Zedalis J, Hylarides MD, Leon AA (1987) Endotoxin provocation of experimental renal cystic disease. Kidney Int 32: 329

Garg LC, Knepper MA, Burg MB (1981) Mineralocorticoid effects on NA-K-ATPase in individual-nephron segments. Am J Physiol 240: F536

Gatter KC, Dunill MS, Van Muijen GNP, Mason DY (1986) Human lung tumours may coexpress different classes of intermediate filaments. J Clin Pathol 39: 950

Giroux L, Smeeesters C, Boury F, Faure MP, Jean G (1984) Adriamycin and adriamycin-DNA nephrotoxicity in rats. Lab Invest 50: 190

Glasser RJ, Velosa JA, Michael AF (1977) Experimental model of focal sclerosis. Lab Invest 36: 519

Gobe GC, Axelsen RA (1987) Genesis of renal tubular atrophy in experimental hydronephrosis in the rat. Role of apoptosis. Lab Invest 56: 273

Goodman T, Grice HC, Becking GC, Salem FA (1970) A cystic nephropathy induced by nordihy-droguaiaretic acid in the rat. Lab Invest 23: 93

Goto F, Jackson EK, Ohnishi A, Herzer W, Branch RA (1987) Effect of cyclooxygenase and thromboxane synthase inhibition on the response to angiotensin II in the hypoperfused canine kidney. J Pharmacol Exp Ther 243: 799

Grantham JJ (1983) Polycystic kidney disease: a predominance of giant nephrons. Am J Physiol 244: F3

Grantham JJ, Uchic M, Cragoe EJ, Kornhaus J, Grantham JA, Donoso V, Mangoo-Kaarim R, Evan A, McAteer J (1989) Chemical modification of cell proliferation and fluid secretion in renal cysts. Kidney Int 35: 1379

Grantham J (1985) Acquired cystic disease: replacing one kidney disease with another. Kidney Int 28: 99

Grantham JJ, Geiser JL, Evan AP (1987) Scanning electron microscope study of cyst formation and growth in autosomal dominant polycystic kidney disease. Kidney Int 31: 1145

Grantham JJ, Donoso VS, Evan AP, Carone FA, Cardner KD Jr (1987) Viscoelastic properties of tubule basement membranes in experimental renal cystic disease. Kidney Int 32: 187

Gröne H-J, Dunn MJ (1985) The role of prostaglandins in arterial hypertension: a critical review. In: Grünfeld JP, Maxwell MH (eds) Advances in nephrology, vol 14, Year Book Medical Publishers, Chicago, p 241

Groñe H-J, Helmchen U (1982) Renal insufficiency in two-kidney, two-clip hypertensive rats treated with captopril and sarcosine[1]-isoleucine[8]-angiotensin II. In: Seybold D, Gessle U (eds) Acute renal failure. Karger, Basel, p 178

Gröne H-J, Helmchen U (1986) Impairment and recovery of the clipped kidney in two-kidney, one-clip hypertensive rats during and after antihypertensive therapy. Lab Invest 54: 645

Gröne H-J, Helmchen U, Kirchertz EJ, Rieger J, Scheler F (1982) Captopril bei Nierenarterienstenosen. Verh Dtsch Ges Inner Medizin 88: 769

Gröne HJ, Weber K, Helmchen U, Osborn M (1986a) Villin—a marker of brush border differentiation and cellular origin in human renal cell carcinoma. Am J Pathol 124: 294

Gröne H-J, Gröne E, Schwartz P, Weber MH, Helmchen U (1986b) Experimentelles Modell fur erworbene multiple Nierenzysten. Verch Dtsch Ges Pathol 70: 640

Gröne H-J, Weber K, Gröne E, Helmchen U, Osborn M (1987) Coexpression of keratin and vimentin in damaged and regenerating tubular epithelia of the kidney. Am J Pathol 129: 1

Gröne H-H, Walli AK, Gröne E, Niedmann P, Thiery J, Seidel D, Helmchen U (1989) Induction of glomerulosclerosis, A functional and morphological study in the rat. Lab Invest 60: 433

Gröne H-J, Simon M, Fuchs E (1992) Autoradiographic characterization of angiotensin receptor subtypes in fetal and adult human kidney. Am J Physiol 263: F326

Gröne EF, Abboud HE, Höhne M, Walli AK, Gröne H-J, Stüker D, Robenek H, Wieland E, Seidel D (1992) Actions of lipoproteins in cultured human mesangial cells; modulation by mitogenic vasoconstrictiors. Am J Physiol 263: F 686

Grond J, Weening JJ, Elema JD (1984) Glomerular sclerosis in nephrotic rats. Lab Invest 51: 277

Grond J, Kondstaal J, Elema JD (1985) Mesangial function and glomerular sclerosis in rats with aminonucleoside nephrosis. Kidney Int 27: 405

Gross DM, Sweet CS, Ulm EH, Bcklund EP, Morris AA, Weitz D, Bohn DL, Wenger HC, Vassil TC, Stone CA (1981) Effect of N-(S)-1-carboxy-3-phenylpropyl-L-Ala-L-Pro and its ethyl ester (MK-421) on angiotensin-converting enzyme in vitro and angiotensin I pressor responses in vivo. J Pharmacol Exp Ther 216: 552

Grossman A, Echland D, Price P, Edwards CRW (1980) Captopril; reversible renal failure with severe hyperkalemia. Lancet 1: 712

Haase H, Rother KO, Uebel H (1965) Erzeugung von Krankheitszuständen durch das Experiment, part 4: Niere, nierenbecken, Blase. In: Eichler O, Farch A, Herven H, Welch AD (eds) Handbuch der experimentellen Pharmakologie. Springer, Berlin Heidelberg New York, p 5

Hall JE (1986) Control of sodium excretion by angiotensin II: intrarenal mechanisms and blood pressure regulation. Am J Physiol 250; R960

Hall JE, Guyton AC, Cowley AW jr (1977) Dissociation of renal blood flow and filtration rate autoregulation by renin depletion. Am J Physiol 232: F215

Hall JE, Guyton AC, Jackson TE, Coleman TG, Lohmeier TE, Trippodo NC (1977b) Control of glomerular filtration rate by renin-angiotensin system. Am J Physiol 233: F366

Hall JE, Coleman TG, Guyton AC, Balfe JW, Salgado HC (1979) Intrarenal role of angiotensin II and des-Asp[1] angiotensin II. Am J Physiol 236: F252

Hall JE, Guyton AC, Smith MJ, Coleman TG (1980) Blood pressure and renal function during chronic changes in sodium intake: role of angiotensin. Am J Physiol 239: F271

Hall K, Sara VR, Enberg G, Ritzen EM (1981) Somatomedins and postnatal growth. In: Ritzen M, Aperia A (eds) The biology of normal human growth. Raven, New York, p 275

Halliburton IW (1969) The effect of unilateral nephrectomy and of diet on the composition of the kidney. In: Nowinski WW, Goss RJ (eds) Compensatory renal hypertrophy, Academic, New York, p 101

Hammernan MR (1989) The growth factor hormone–insulin-like growth factor axis in the kidney. Am J Physiol 257: F503

Hammerman MR, Rogers S (1987) Distribution of IGF receptors in the plasma membrane of proximal tubular cells. Am J Physiol 253: F841

Harding MA, Gattone VH II, Grantham JJ, Calvet JP (1992) Localization of overexpressed c-myc mRNA in polycystic kidneys of the cpK mouse. Kidney lnt 41: 317

Harris PJ, Navar LG (1985) Tubular transport responses to angiotensin. Am J Physiol 248: F621

Hay EH (1983) Cell and extracellular matrix: Their organization and mutual dependence. In: Satir BH (ed) Modern cell biology, vol 2, Liss, New York, p 509

Heller J, Horacek V (1986) Angiotensin II: preferential efferent constriction. Renal Physiol 9: 357

Helmchen U, Kneissler U (1976) Role of the renin-angiotensin system in renal hypertension. An experimental approach. Curr Top Pathol 61: 203

Helmchen U, Gröne H-J, Kirchertz EJ, Bader H, Bohle RM, Kneissler U, Khosla MC (1982) Contrasting renal effects of different antihypertensive agents in hypertensive rats with bilaterally constricted renal arteries. Kidney Int 22 [Suppl 12]: S198

Henzen-Logmans SC, Mullink H, Ramaekers FCS, Tadema T, Meijer CJLM (1987) Expression of cytokeratins and vimentin in epithelial cells of normal and pathologic thyroid tissue. Virchows Arch [A] 410: 347

Herman CJ, Mosecker O, Kant A, Huysmans A, Vooijs GP, Ramaekers FCS (1983) Is renal (Grawitz) tumor a carcinosarcoma? Evidence from analysis of intermediate filament types. Virchows Arch [B] 44: 73

Herrera GA (1991) C-erb B-2 anuplification in cystic renal disease. Kidney Int 40: 509

Hirschberg R (1993) IGF-1 is ultrafiltered into the urinary space and may exert biological effects in proximal tubues in the nephrotic syndrome. J Am Soc Nephrol 4: 771 (abstract)

Hjelle JT, Guenthner TM, Bell K, Whalen R, Fouret G, Carone FA (1990) Inhibition of catalese and epoxide hydrolase by the renal cystogen 2-amino-4.5 diphenyl thiazole and its metabolites. Toxicology 60: 211

Hoch-Ligeti C (1960) Sequence of tissue, serum and urine changes in rats treated with aminonucleo-side. Br J Exp Pathol 41: 119

Hockenberg DM, Oltvai ZN, Yin X-M, Milliman CL, Korsmeyer SJ (1993) Bcl-2 functions in an antioxidant pathway to prevent apoptosis. Cell 75: 241

Hollenberg NK (1983) Medical therapy of renovascular hypertension: efficacy and safety of captopril in 269 patients. Cardiovase Rev Rep 4: 854

Hollenberg NK (1984) Renal hemodynamics in essential and renovascular hypertension. Influence of captopril. Am J Med 76 (B): 22

Hollified JW, Moore LC, Winn SD (1982) Angiotensin-converting enzyme inhibition in renovascular hypertension. Cardiovase Rev Rep 3: 673

Holthofer H, Miettinen A, Passivuo, R, Lehto VP, Linder E, Altthan O, Virtanen I (1983) Cellular origin and differentiation of renal carcinomas. a fluoresecence microscopic study with kidney-specific antibodies, anti-intermediate filament antibodies and lectins. Lab Invest 49: 317

Hricik DE (1985) Captopril-induced renal insufficiency and the role of sodium balance. Ann Intern Med 103: 222

Hricik DE, Browning PJ, Kopelman R, Goorno WE, Madias NE, Dzau VJ (1983) Captopril-induced functional renal insufficiency in patients with bilateral renal artery stenosis or renal artery stenosis in a solitary kidney. N Engl J Med 308: 373

Huang W-C (1986) Effects of verapamil alone and with captopril on blood pressure and bilateral renal function in Goldblatt hypertensive rats. Clin Sci 70: 453

Huang W-C, Navar LG (1983) Effects of unclipping and converting-enzyme inhibition on bilateral renal function in Goldblatt hypertensive rats. Kidney Int 23: 816

Haung W-C, Ploth DW, Bell PD, Work J, Navar LG (1981) Bilateral renal function responses to converting enzyme inhibitor (SQ 20, 881) in two-kidney, one-clip Goldblatt hypertensive rats. Hyertension 3: 285

Huang W-C, Ploth DW, Navar LG (1982) Effects of saralasin infusion on bilateral renal function in two-kidney, one-clip Goldblatt hypertensive rats. Clin Sci 62: 573

Hughson MD (1985) Cancer in acquired cystic disease. In: Grantham JJ, Gardner KD (eds) Problems in diagnosis and management of polycystic kidney disease. Intercollegiate Press, Kansas City, p 211

Hughson MD, Hennigar GR, McManus JFA (1980) Atypical cysts, acquired renal cystic disease, and renal cell tumors in end-stage dialysis kidneys. Lab Invest 42: 475

Hughson MD, Buchwald D, Fox M (1986) Renal neoplasia and acquired cystic kidney disease in patients receiving long-term dialysis. Arch Pathol Lab Med 110: 592

Hutchison WC, Munro HN (1961) The determination of nucleic acids in biological materials. Methods Enzymol 86: 768

Huttunen NP (1976) Congenital nephrotic syndrome of Finnish type: study of 75 patients. Arch Dis Child 51: 344

Ichikawa I, Brenner BM (1984) Glomerular actions of angiotensin II. Am J Med 76 (B) 43

Ichikawa J, Brenner BM (1980) Importance of efferent arteriolar vascular tone in regulation of proximal tubule fluid reabsorption and glomerulotubular balance in the rat. J Clin Invest 65: 1192

Iglesias CG, Torres VE, Offord KP (1983) Epidemiology of adult polycystic kidney disease, Olmsted County, Minnesota: 1935–1980. Am J Kidney Dis 2: 630

Iozzo RV (1985) Biology of disease. Proteoglycans: structure, function, and role in neoplasia. Lab Invest 53: 373

Ishikawa I, Saito Y, Onouchi Z, Kitada H, Suzuki S, Kurihara S, Yuri T, Shinoda A (1980) Development of acquired cystic disease and adenocarcinoma of the kidney of glomerulonephritic chronic hemodialysis patients. Clin Nephrol 14: 1

Jacques H, Deshaies Y, Savoie L (1986) Relationship between dietary proteins, their in vitro digestion products, and serum cholesterol in rats. Atherosclerosis 61: 89

Jobin JR, Bonjour JP (1986) Compensatory renal growth: modulation by calcium PTH and 1,25-$(OH)_2D_3$. Kidney Int 29: 1124

Kanwar YS, Carone FA (1984) Reversible changes of tubular cell and basement membrane in drug-induced renal cystic disease. Kidney Int 26: 35

Karl IE, Garcia P, White WL, Recant L, Kissane JM (1964) Proteinuria induced by albumin injection. Lab Invest 13: 1600

Kawamura J, Okada Y, Nishibuchi S, Yoshida O (1982) Transient anuria following administration of angiotension II-converting enzyme inhibitor (SQ 14225) in a patient with renal artery stenosis of the solitary kidney successfully treated with renal autotransplantation. J Urol 127: 111

Kaysen GA, Myers BD, Courser WG, Rabkin R, Felts JM (1986) Biology of disease: mechanisms and consequences of proteinuria. Lab Invest 54: 479

Kelly CJ, Neilson EG (1987) Medullary cystic disease: an inherited form of autoimmune interstitial nephritis? Am J Kidney Dis 10: 389

Kime SQ, McNamara JJ, Lose S, Farmer S, Silbert C, Bricker NS (1962) Experimental polycystic renal disease in rats: electron microscopy, function and susceptibility to pyelonephritis. J Lab Clin Med 60: 64

Kindler J, Konrads A, Meurer KA, Sieberth HG (1981) Progrediente reversible Nierenisuffizienz nach Blutdrucksenkung mit Captopril. Internist 22: 360

Koch-Weser J (1976) Drug therapy: hydralazine. N Engl J Med 295: 320

Kollias G, Evans DJ, Ritter M, Beech J, Morris R, Grosveld F (1987) Ectopic expression of Thy-1 in the kidney of transgenic mice induces functional and proliferative abnormalities. Cell 51: 21

Kramer P, Broyer M, Brunner FP (1982) Combined report on regular dialysis and transplantation in Europe, XII, 1981. Proc EDTA 19: 4

Kremer-Hovinga TK, Donker AJN, Piers DA (1984) Converting enzyme-induced reversible deterioration of renal function in a patient with unilateral renal artery stenoses. Clin Nephrol 22: 106

Krempien B, Ritz E (1980) Acquired cystic transformation of the kidneys of hemodialysed patients. Virchows Arch [A] 386: 189

Kurtz SM, Feldman JD (1962) Morphologic studies of the normal and injured rat kidney following protein overload. Lab Invest 11: 167

Lane EB (1982) Monoclonal antibodies provide specific intramolecular markers for the study of epithelial tonofilament organization. J Cell Biol 92: 665

Lane EB, Hogan BL, Kurkinen M, Garrels JI (1983) Co-expression of vimentin and cytokeratins in parietal endoderm cells of early mouse embryo. Nature 303: 701

Laouari D, Kleinknecht C, Gubler M-C, Broyer M (1983) Adverse effect of proteins on remnant kidney: dissociation from that of other nutrients. Kidney Int 24 [Suppl 16]: S248

La Rocca RJ, Pheinwald JG (1984) Coexpression of simple epithelial keratins and vimentin by human mesothelium and mesotheliomas in vivo and in culture. Cancer Res 44: 2991

Lawrence GM, Brewer DB (1981) Effect of strain and sex on the induction of hyperalbuminaemic proteinuria in the rat. Clin Sci 61: 751

Lawrence GM, Brewer DB (1982) A biochemical and immunological investigation into the physiological basis of the increased albumin filtration induced in hyperalbuminaemic female Wistar rats. Clin Sci 62: 495

Lawrence GM, Brewer DB (1984) Glomerular ultrafiltration and tubular reabsorption of bovine serum albumin and derivatives with increased negative charge in the normal female Wister rat. Clin Sci 66: 47

Levenson DJ, Dzau VJ (1987) Effects of angiotensin-converting enzyme inhibition on renal hemodynamics in renal artery stenosis. Kidney Int 31 [Suppl 20]: S173

Levi M, Baird BM, Wilson PV (1990) Cholesterol modulates rat renal brush border membrane phosphate transport. J Clin Invest 85: 231

Luderer JR, Schoolwerth SC, Sinicrope RA, Ballard JO, Lookingbill DP, Hayes AH (1981) Acute renal failure, hemolytic anemia and skin rash associated with captopril therapy. Am J Med 71: 493

Maack T, Park CH, Camargo MJ (1985) Renal filtration, transport and metabolism of proteins. In: Seldin DW, Giebisch G (eds) The kidney: physiology and pathophysiology. Raven, New York, p 1773

MacKay K, Striker LJ, Pinkert CA, Brinster RL, Striker GE (1987) Glomerulosclerosis and renal cysts in mice transgenic for the early region of SV40. Kidney Int 32: 827

Mackensen-Haen S, Bader R, Grund KE, Bohle A (1981) Correlations between renal cortical interstitial fibrosis, atrophy of the proximal tubules and impairment of the glomerular filtration rate. Clin Nephrol 15: 167

Madri JA, Roll JR, Furthmayr H, Foidart J (1980) Ultrastructural localization of fibronectin and laminin in the basement membranes of the murine kidney. J Cell Biol 86: 682

Marks MI, Drummond KN (1970) Nephropathy and persistent proteinuria after albumin administration in the rat. Lab Invest 23: 416

Martinez-Maldonado M (1985) General features of autosomal dominant polycystic kidney disease. Functional aspects: Electrolyte and uric acid excretion with a comment on stone formation. In: Grantham JJ, Gardner KD (eds) Problems in diagnosis and management of polycystic kidney disease. Intercollegiate Press, Kansas City, p 70

Matas AJ, Kjellstrand CM, Simmons RL (1975) Increased incidence of malignancy during chronic renal failure. Lancet 1: 883

Maunsbach AB (1966) Observations on the segmentation of the proximal tubule in the rat kidney. Comparison of results from phase contrast, fluorescence and electron microscopy. J Ultrastruct Res 16: 239

McGeoch JEM, Darmady EM (1973) Enzyme changes in experimental renal microcystic disease. Br J Exp Pathol 54: 555

McKinley CA (1920) Epithelial hyperplasia in congenital cystic kidneys. J Urol 4: 195

McNutt MA, Bolen JW, Gown AM, Hammar SP, Vogel AM (1985) Coexpression of intermediate filaments in human epithelial neoplasms. Ultrastruct Pathol 9: 31

Messina A, Davies DJ, Dillane PC, Ryan GB (1987) Glomerular epithelial abnormalities associated with the onset of proteinuria in aminonucleoside nephrosis. Am J Pathol 126: 220

Michel J-B, Dussaule J-C, Choudat L, Auzan C, Nochy D, Corvol P, Menard J (1986) Effects of antihypertensive treatment in one-clip, two-kidney hypertension in rats. Kidney Int 29: 1011

Michel J-B, Dussaule J-C, Choudat L, Nochy D, Corvol P, Menard J (1987) Renal damage induced in the clipped kidney of one-clip, two-kidney hypertensive rats during normalization of blood pressure by converting enzyme inhibition. Kidney Int 31 [Suppl 20]: S 168

Miettinen M, Franssila K, Lehto V-P, Passivuo R, Virtanen I (1984) Expression of intermediate filament protein in thyroid gland and thyroid tumors. Lab Invest 50: 262

Milutinovic J, Agodoa LCY, Cutler RE, Striker GE (1980) Autosomal dominant polycystic kidney disease. Early diagnosis and consideration of pathogenesis. Am J Clin Pathol 73: 740

Mimran A (1983) Renal aspects of treatment by converting-enzyme inhibitors in hypertension. Clin Exp Hypertens [A] 5: 1381

Miyamori I, Yasuhara S, Takeda Y, Koshida H, Ikeda M, Nagai K, Okamoto H, Morise T, Takeda R, Aburano T (1986) Effects of converting enzyme inhibition on split renal function in renovascular hypertension. Hypertension 8: 415

Moolenaar WH, Tsien RY, van Der Saag PT, De Laat SW (1983) Na^+/H^+ exchange and cytoplasmic pH in the action of growth factors in human fibroblasts. Nature 304: 645

Mori H, Yamashita H, Nakanishi C, Koizumi K, Makino S, Kishimoto Y, Hayashi Y (1986) Proteinuria induced by transplantable rat pituitary tumor MtT SA5. Lab Invest 54: 636

Mujais SK, Kauffman S, Katz AI (1986) Angiotensin II binding sites in individual segments of the rat nephron. J Clin Invest 77: 315

Nagle RB, Bulger RE, Striker GE, Benditt EP (1972) Renal tubular effects of the aminonucleoside of puromycin. Lab Invest 26: 558

Narasimhan N, Golper TA, Wolfson M, Rahatzad M, Bennett WM (1986) Clinical characteristics and diagnostic considerations in acquired renal cystic disease. Kidney Int 30: 748

Nathan CF (1987) Secretory products of macrophages. J Clin Invest 79: 319

Navar LG, Rosivall L (1984) Contribution of the renin-angiotensin system to the control of intrarenal hemodynamics. Kidney Int 25: 857

Newburgh LH, Curtis AC (1928) Production of renal injury in the white rat by the protein of the diet. Arch Intern Med 42: 801

Nord EP, Hafezi A, Wright EM, Fine LG (1984) Mechanism of Na$^+$ uptake into renal brush border membrane vesicles. Am J Physiol 247: F548

Norman J, Badie-Dezfooly B, Nord EP, Kurtz I, Schlosser J, Chaudhari A, Fine LG (1987) EGF-induced mitogenesis in proximal tubular cells: potentiation by angiotensin II. Am J Physiol 253: F299

Olbricht CJ, Cannon JK, Gard LC, Tisher CC (1986) Activities of cathepsin B and L in isolated nephron segments from proteinuric and nonproteinuric rats. Am J Physiol 250: F1055

Omae T, Masson GMC (1960) Reversibility of renal atrophy caused by unilateral reduction of renal blood supply. J Clin Invest 39: 21

Osswald H, Haas JA, Marchand GR, Knox FG (1979) Glomerular dynamics in dogs at reduced renal artery pressure. Am J Physiol 236: F25

Packer M, Lee WH, Medina N, Yushak M, Kessler PD (1987) Functional renal insufficiency during long-term therapy with captopril and enalapril in severe chronic heart failure. Ann Intern Med 106: 346

Pederson J Chr, Persson AEG, Maunsbach AB (1980) Ultrastructure and quantitative characterization of the cortical interstitium in the rat kidney. In: Maunsbach AB, Olsen TS, Christensen EJ (eds) Functional ultrastructure of the kidney. Academic, London, p 443

Pfeffer JM, Pfeffer MA, Frohlich ED (1971) Validity of an tail-cuff method for determining systolic arterial pressure in unanesthetized normotensive and spontaneously hypertensive rats. J Lab Clin Med 78: 957

Pfeifer U (1982) Kinetic and subcellular aspects of hypertrophy and atrophy. Exp Pathol 23: 1

Pinto JA, Brewer DB (1975) Combined light- and electron-microscope morphometric studies of acute puromycin aminonucleoside nephropathy in rats. J Pathol 116: 149

Planz G, Bundschu HD (1980) Zunehmende Niereninsuffizienz nach Blutdrucksenkung mit Captopril bei maligner Hypertonie. Klin Wochenschr 58: 897

Ploth DW, Woolverton V (1987) Acute renal dysfunction in 1-kidney, 1-clip hypertension (1-K, 1C HT) during Na-nitroprusside-reduced blood pressure (BP). Kidney Int 31: 306 (abstract)

Popper H, Mandel E, Mayer H (1937) Zur Kreatininbestimmung im Blute. Biochem 291: 354

Preuss H, Geoly K, Johnson M, Chester A, Kliger A, Schreinger G (1979) Tubular function in adult polycystic kidney disease. Naphron 24: 198

Rahilly MA, Samuel K, Ansell JD, Micklem HG, Fleming S (1992) Polycystic kidney disease in CBA/N immunodeficient mouse. J Pathol 168: 335

Resnick JS, Brown DM, Vernier RL (1976) Normal development and experimental models of cystic renal disease. In: Gardner KD (ed) Cystic disease of the kidney. Wiley, New York, p 221

Reubi FC (1985) Pathophysiology of renal failure. In: Grantham JJ, Gardner KD (eds) Problems in diagnosis and management of polycystic kidney disease. Intercollegiate Press, Kansas City p 81

Riemenschneider T, Mackensen-Haen S, Christ H, Bohle A (1980) Correlation between endogenous creatinine clearance and relative interstitial volume of the renal cortex in patients with diffuse membranous glomerulonephritis having a normal serum creatinine concentration. Lab Invest 43: 145

Risdon RA, Sloper JC, De Wardener HE (1968) Relationship between renal function and histological changes found in renal-biopsy specimens from patients with persistent glomerular nephritis. Lancet 2: 363

Risdon RA, Turner DR (1980) Atlas of renal pathology. Lippincott, Philadelphia, p 83

Rohde H, Wick G, Timpl R (1979) Immunochemical characterization of the basement membrane glycoprotein laminin. Eur J Biochem 102: 195

Rossier BC, Geering K, Kraehenbuhl JP (1987) Regulation of the sodium pump: how and why? TIBS 12: 483

Rumsfeld HWJr (1956) Role of dietary protein in normal rat proteinuria. Am J Physiol 184: 473

Safouh M, Crocker JF, Vernier RL (1970) Experimental cystic diesease of the kidney. Lab Invest 23: 392

Saxton JA, Kimball GC (1941) Relation of nephrosis and other diseases of albino rats to age and to modification of diet. Arch Pathol 32: 951

Scheler F, Gröne H-J (1982) Typische Risiken bei der Behandlung der arteriellen Hypertonie. Internist 23: 127

Schiffrin EL, Thome FS, Genest J (1983) Vascular angiotensin II receptors in renal and Docasalt hypertensive rats. Hypertension 5 [Suppl V]: 16

Schimke RN (1985) Hereditary features of autosomal dominant polycystic kidney disease. A genetic approach. In: Grantham JJ, Gardner KD (eds) Problems in diagnosis and management of polycystic kidney disease. Intercollegiate Press, Kansas City, p 187

Schwietzer G (1980) Angiotensin II dependency of vascular resistance in the untouched kidney of renal hypertensive rats. Nephron 26: 195

Schwietzer G, Lessmann J, Oelkers W, Bähr V, Distler A (1988) Influence of captopril on the control of glomerular filtration rate (GFR) during acute hypotension in normal man. Kidney Int 33 (abstract): 305

Schleifer D (1962) Histologische Untersuchungen über die Sekretions-leistung einzelner Nierentubuli nach mechanischer Abtrennung von ihren Glomerula. Z Zellforsch 57: 597

Schwartz MM, Sharon Z, Pauli BU, Lewis EJ (1984) Inhibition of glomerular visceral epithelial cell endocytosis during nephrosis induced by puromycin aminonucleoside. Lab Invest 51: 690

Selye H, Stone H (1946) Pathogenesis of the cardiovascular and renal changes which usually accompany malignant hypertension. J Urol 56: 399

Sheehan HL, Davis JC (1959) Experimental hydronephrosis. Arch Pathol 68: 185

Shibouta Y, Inada Y, Terashita Z, Nishikawa K, Shintaro K, Shimamoto K (1979) Angiotensin-II-stimulated release of thromboxane A_2 and prostacyclin (PGI_2) in isolated, perfused kidneys of spontaneously hypertensive rats. Biochem Pharmacol 28: 3601

Shiraiwa K, Tsutsumi M, Konishi Y (1986) Daunomycin-induced nephropathy, rat. In: Jones TC, Mohr U, Hunt RD (eds) Urinary system. Springer, Berlin Heidelberg New York, p 239

Short BG, Burnett VL, Cox MG, Bus JS, Swenberg JA (1987) Site-specific renal cytotoxicity and cell proliferation in male rats exposed to petroleum hydrocarbons. Lab Invest 57: 564

Siles JN, Klenka Z, Soloman SA, Bone JM (1983) Captopril-induced reversible renal failure: a marker of renal artery stenosis affecting a solitary kidney. Br Med J 286: 1702

Simon M, Fuchs E, Gröne H-J (1993) In situ characterization of renal angiotensin II (Ang II) receptors in renovascular hypertension and chronic angiotensin-converting enzyme blockade. Kidney Int 44: 245 (abstract)

Spertini F, Brunner HR, Waeber B, Gavras H (1981) The opposing effects of chronic angiotensin-converting enzyme blockade by captopril on the responses to exogenous angiotensin II and vasopressin vs. norepinephrine in rats. Circ Res 48: 612

Spinelli F, Brucher C (1975) Structural changes of the podocytes in different states of experimentally induced proteinura in the rat. Contr Nephrol 1: 86

Steinhausen M (1987) Physiologie und Pathophysiologie der Nierendurchblutung. Z Kardiol 76 [Suppl 4]: 71

Steinhausen M, Snoei H, Parekh N, Baker R, Johnson PC (1983) Hydronephrosis: a new method to visualize vas afferens, efferens, and glomerular network. Kidney Int 23: 794

Steinhausen M, Kucherer H, Parekh N, Weis S. Wiegman DL, Wilhelm K-R (1986) Angiotensin II control of the renal microcirculation: effect of blockade by saralasin. Kidney Int 30: 56

Sternberg SS (1970) Cross-striated fibrils and other ultrastructural alterations in glomeruli of rats with daunomycin nephrosis. Lab Invest 23: 39

Sternberg SS, Philips FS, Cronin AP (1972) Renal tumors and other lesions in rats following a single intravenous injection of daunomycin. Cancer Res 32: 1029

Stiles CD, Capone GT, Scher CD, Antoniades HN, Van WYK JJ, Pledger WJ (1979) Dual control of cell growth by somatomedins and platelet-derived growth factors. Cell Biol 76: 1279

Stiles AD, Sosenko IRS, D'Ercole AJ, Smith BT (1985) Relation of kidney tissue somatomedin-C/insulin-like growth factor I to postenphrectomy renal growth in the rat. Endocrinology 117: 2397

Strum P (1875) Über das Adenom der Niere und über die Beziehung desselben zu einigen anderen Neubildungen der Niere. Arch Heilk 16: 193

Sumpio BE, Maack T (1982) Kinetics, competition, and selectivity of tubular absorption of proteins. Am J Physiol 243: F379

Sundarraj N, Church RL (1978) Alterations of post-translational modifications of procollagen by SV40-transformed human fibroblasts. FEBS Lett 85: 47

Sweet CS, Gross DM, Arbegast PT, Gaul SL, Britt PM, Ludden CT, Weitz D, Stone CA (1981) Antihypertensive activity of N-(S)-1-(ethoxycarboxyl)-3-phenylpropyl-L-Ala-Pro (MK-421), an orally active converting-enzyme inhibitor. J Pharmacol Exp Ther 216: 558

Sweet R, Keane WF (1979) Perinephric abscess in patients with polycystic kidney disease undergoing chronic hemodialysis. Naphron 23: 237

Takahashi H, Calvet JP, Dittemore-Hoover D, Yoshida K, Grantham JJ, Gattone VH (1991) A hereditary model of slowly progressive polycystic kidney disease in the mouse. J Am Soc Nephrol 1: 980

Taub M, Laurie GW, Martin GR, Kleiman HK (1990) Altered basement membrane protein biosynthesis by primary cultures of cpk/cpk mouse kidney. Kidney Int 37: 1090

Textor SC, Novick A, Mujais SK Ross R, Bravo EL, Fouad FM, Tarazi RC (1983) Response of the stenosed and contralateral kidneys to Sar-1-Thr-8-All in human renovascular hypertension. Hypertension 5: 796

Textor SC, Tarazi RC, Novick AC, Bravo EL, Fouad FM (1984) Regulation of renal hemodynamics and glomerular filtration in patients with renovascular hypertension during converting enzyme inhibition with captoprial. Am J Med 76 (B): 29

Textor SC, Novick AC, Tarazi RC, Klimas V, Vidt DG, Pohl M (1985) Critical perfusion pressure for renal function in patients with bilateral atherosclerotic renal vascular disease. Ann Intern Med 102: 308

Thomson BJ, Jenkins DAS, Allan PL, Elton RA, Winney RJ (1986) Acqured cystic disease of the kidney in patients with end-stage chronic renal failure: a study of prevalence and aetiology. Naphrol Dial Transplant 1: 38

Torres VE, Holley KE, Offord KP (1985) General features of autosomal dominant polycystic kidney disease. Epidemiology. In: Grantham JJ, Gardner KD (eds) Problems in diagnosis and management of polycystic kidney disease. Intercollegiate Press, Kansas City p 49

Trudel M, D'Agati V, Costantini F (1991) C-myc as an inducer of polycystic kidney disease in transgenic mice. Kidney Int 39: 665

Trump BF, Berezesky IK, Lipsky MM, Jones TW (1985) Heterogeneity of the nephron: significance of nephrotoxicity. In: Bach PH, Lock EA (eds) Renal heterogeneity and target cell toxicity. Wiley, Chichester, p 31

Tucker BJ, Blantz RC (1983) Mechanism of altered glomerular hemodynamics during chronic sodium depletion. Am J Physiol 244: F11

Van der Woude FJ, Van Son WJ, Tegzess AM, Donker AJM, Scoff MJH, Van Der Slikke LB, Hoorntje SJ (1985) Effect of captopril on blood pressure and renal function in patients with transplant renal artery stenosis. Nephron 39: 184

Veis DJ, Sorenson CM, Shutter JR, Korsmeyer SJ (1993) Bcl-2-deficient mice demonstrate fulminant lymphoid apoptosis, polycystic kidneys and hypopigmented hair. Cell 75: 229

Vetter W, Wehling M, Foerster E-C, Kuhlmann U, Boentin H-J, Greninger P, Vetter H (1984) Long-term effect of captopril on kidney function in various forms of hypertension. Klin Wochenschr 62: 731

Virtanen I, Lehto V-P, Lethonen E, Vartio T, Stenman S, Kurki P, Wager O, Small JV, Dahl D, Badley RA (1981) Expression of intermediate filaments in cultured cells. J Cell Sci 50: 45

Von Möllendorf W (1930) Der Exkretions-apparat. In: Von Mollendrof W, Bargmann W (eds) Handbuch der mikroskipischen Anatomic des Menschen, part 1. Springer, Berlin, p 1

Wachsmuth ED (1985) Renal cell heterogeneity at a light microscopic level. In: Bach PH, Lock EA (eds) Renal heterogeneity and target cell toxicity, Wiley, Chichester, p 13

Waeber B, Schaller M-D, Wauters, J-P, Brunner HR (1984) Deterioration of renal function in hypertensive patients with scleroderma despite blood presure normalization with captopril. Kiln Wochenschr 62: 728

Waldherr R, Lennert T, Weber H-P, Födisch HJ, Schärer K (1982) The nephronophthisis complex. A clinicopathologic study in children. Virchows Arch [A] 394: 235

Wang, JL, Hsu Y-M (1986) Negative regulators of cell growth. TIBS 11: 24

Weber, MH, Cheong K-S, Schott KJ, Neuhoff V (1986) Microelectrophoresis in the differential diagnosis of proteinuric diseases. Electorphoresis 7: 134

Weening JJ, Van Guldener C, Daha MR, Klar N, Van Der Wal A, Prins FA (1987) The pathophysiology of protein-overload proteinuria. Am J Pathol 129: 64

Welling LW, Grantham JJ (1986) Cystic and developmental diseases of the kidney. In: Brenner BM, Rector FC (eds) The kidney. Saunders, Philadelphia, p 1341

Wenting GJ, Tan-Tjiong HL, Derkx FHM, DeBruyn JHB, man in't Veld AJ, Schalekamp MADH (1984) Split renal function after captopril in unilateral renal artery stenosis. Br Med J 288: 886

Werb Z, Band MJ, Jones PA (1980) Degradation of connective tissue matrices by macrophages. I. Proteolysis of elastin, glycoproteins and collagen by proteinases isolated from macrophages. J Exp Med 152: 1340

Werder AA, Amos MA, Nielsen AH, Wolfe GH (1984) Comparative effects of germ-free and ambient environments on the development of cystic kidney disease in CFW mice. J Lab Clin Med 103: 399

Wilson PD, Sherwood AC (1991) Tubulocystic epithelium. Kidney Int 39: 450

Wilson PD, Schrier RW, Breckon RD, Gabow PA (1986) A new method for studying human polycystic kidney disease epithelia in culture. Kidney Int 30: 371

Wilson PD, Hreniuk D, Gabow PA (1992) Abnormal extracellular matrix and excessive growth of human adult polycystic kidney disease epithelia. J Cell Physiol 150: 360

Winston JA, Safirstein R (1985) Reduced renal blood flow in early cisplatin-induced acute renal failure in the rat. Am J Physiol 249: F490

Winterbourne DJ, Mora PT (1978) Altered metabolism of heparan sulfate in simian virus 40 transformed clones mouse cells. J Biol Chem 253: 5109

Wolf G, Neilson EG (1990a) Angiotensin II induces cellular hypertrophy in cultured murine proximal tubular cells. Am J Physiol 259: F768

Wolf G, Neilson EG (1990b) Angiotensin II induces cellular hypertrophy and hyperplasia. Kidney Int 39: 401

Wright RS (1982) Effects of urinary tract obstruction on glomerular filtration rate and renal blood flow. Semin Nephrol 2: 5

Zeier M, Waldherr R, Geberth S, Ritz E (1987) Extrarenal pathology and renal cell carcinoma in adult polycystic kidney disease (PCKD). 17th annual meeting of the National Kidney Foundation, Washington, abstract 25

Zollinger HU (1966) Niere und ableitende Harnwege. In: Doerr W, Uchlinger E (eds) Spezielle pathologische Anatomie, vol 3. Springer, Berlin, Heidelberg New York, p 144

Zollinger HU, Tohorst J, Riede UN, von Toenges V, Geering B, Rohr HP (1973) Der inkomplette order Sub-Infarkt der Niere (einseitige zentral-arterielle Schrumpfniere). Pathologisch anatomische, morphometrische und elektronenmikroskopische Untersuchungen). Beitr Pathol 148: 15

Mechanisms of Renal Damage
in Chronic Pyelonephritis (Reflux Nephropathy)*

J.A. ROBERTS

1 Introduction

The relation between vesicoureteral reflux and pyelonephritis was first pointed out in a study of patients with neurogenic bladder (HUTCH 1952). Almost 10 years later, studies done by HODSON and EDWARDS (1960) indicated the importance of intrarenal reflux in the pathogenesis of chronic pyelonephritis. Further studies by HODSON et al. (1975), using the pig as an experimental animal, showed that sterile reflux could produce renal scars in the areas of intrarenal reflux. His model, however, required bladder neck obstruction and a high voiding pressure in order to produce the high-grade reflux. While Hodson felt that sterile reflux damages the kidney, RANSLEY and RISDON's study (1978) in the same model did not confirm Hodson's work, and they showed that scarring from sterile reflux would occur only if the bladder neck obstruction was severe enough to cause high-pressure reflux. This has been confirmed in another pig model of obstructive reflux (JORGENSON 1986). We also confirmed these latter studies in the monkey, showing that after bladder neck obstruction, increased voiding and resting bladder pressure as well as peristaltic failure of the ureter led to transmission of these high pressures to the kidney with renal damage and interstitial nephritis (MENDOZA and ROBERTS 1983). Neurogenic sphincteric dysfunction such as that which occurs in myelodysplasia may also cause high-pressure voiding, which will cause renal damage whether reflux is present or not, as shown in studies of myelodysplastic patients (McGUIRE et al. 1981). The studies of ALLEN (1977), HINMAN (1973), KOFF and MURTAGH (1984), and VAN GOOL (1979) all showed

*Supported by USPHS grant RR00164 and DK14681.

that the dysfunctional voiding which can occur in neurologically normal children, may cause not only reflux, but also renal damage from voiding pressures as high as 150 cm of water.

In the absence of these abnormalities low-pressure sterile reflux should not lead to renal damage. However, it may allow any bacteria colonizing the bladder to reach the kidney and cause intrarenal reflux and pyelonephritis. Thus, usually nonvirulent *Escherichia coli* or other Enterobacteriaceae may cause pyelonephritis in the presence of reflux (LOMBERG et al. 1983). Indeed, these bacteria may lead to severe renal damage, probably because the host reaction to them is not as marked and the diagnosis is not made as rapidly as with nephropathogenic P-fimbriated *E. coli*, which cause a marked inflammatory response with fever and symptoms (LOMBERG et al. 1989).

The study of reflux, led to the recommendation that the term "chronic atrophic pyelonephritis", used to describe renal scarring from infection and vesicoureteral reflux, should be replaced by the term "reflux nephropathy" (BAILEY 1973). This term has been widely accepted, showing that many commonly assume that vesicoureteral reflux is the primary cause for the acquired renal scarring of chronic pyelonephritis. Many studies of patients with vesicoureteral reflux have demonstrated that renal scars are almost always associated with previous urinary tract infections (FILLY et al. 1974; SMELLIE et al. 1975, 1985; WINBERG et al. 1982; WINTER et al. 1983). Moreover, it has been demonstrated by several authors that new renal scarring can be prevented by keeping the patients free of urinary tract infections (EDWARDS et al. 1977; SKOOG et al. 1987; SMELLIE and NORMAND 1975). It has now been shown that new renal scars after urinary tract infection also occur in the absence of demonstrable reflux (BISSETT et al. 1987; WINBERG et al. 1982; WINTER et al. 1983).

In most cases the renal damage and scars from vesicoureteral reflux, whether alone or in combination with infection, are thought to be acquired. However, in an early study by MACKIE and STEPHENS (1975) renal dysplasia and vesicoureteral reflux were thought to be related or separate expressions of a malformation of the urinary tract during intrauterine fetal development. Attention has been focused once more on the contribution of renal dysplasia to the pathology of reflux nephropathy. Recently, due to the common use of fetal ultrasound for other purposes, hydronephrosis has been diagnosed prior to birth. Cystograms done in the immediate postoperative period have identified vesicoureteral reflux as responsible for the hydronephrosis in some cases. In this situation, the reflux is often high grade and is usually found in males. In these patients the kidneys tend to be small with smooth outlines, rather than exhibiting segmental scarring. (GORDON et al. 1990; ROSENBERG 1991; STEELE et al. 1989). In the recent study of RISDON et al. (1993) of small kidneys removed for nonfunction, renal dysplasia was the usual pathologic picture in 62% of male infants with hydronephrosis, often diagnosed in utro. Some, however, did show segmental renal scarring, thought to be associated with infection. The kidneys removed from female infants showed changes that appeared to be completely acquired, with segmental scarring overlying dilated calyces and with evidence of infection. Renal dysplasia, therefore, may be a cause for the pathological diagnosis of reflux nephropathy in a large number of infants presenting with intrauterine hydronephrosis as opposed to the acquired pathology following low grades of reflux and infection.

With the advent of computed tomodensitometry (CT) (ROSENFIELD et al. 1979), it has been found that adults whose acute pyelonephritis can be well characterized by CT frequently develop renal scarring in the same areas as those identified during acute disease (MEYRIER et al. 1989). Similarly, studies using DTPA (^{99m}technetium-dimercaptosuccinic acid) renal scans in children with acute pyelonephritis showed that the areas of the kidney involved with acute pyelonephritis on initial scan during the acute disease are the same areas that end with renal scars (RUSHTON et al. 1992). In this latter study, the incidence of vesicoureteral reflux was actually lower in those who developed renal scars than in the children with reflux who later developed renal scars. Taken together, these facts would suggest that the term "reflux nephropathy", used to replace the diagnosis "chronic atrophic pyelonephritis", may not be the preferable term since renal scarring following acute pyelonephritis may occur in the absence as well as in the presence of reflux.

Nonobstructive pyelonephritis refers to those bacterial renal infections which occur in the absence of bladder neck or ureteral obstruction or other abnormalities such as stone. It does not preclude the presence of vesicoureteral reflux unless the vesicoureteral reflux causes an obstructive abnormality (high-grade reflux with ureterectasis, pyelectasias, and calyectasis). It also includes the terms "acute bacterial pyelonephritis" and "chronic pyelonephritis." Since there appears to be no difference in the end result of treatment of high-grade vesicoureteral reflux by medical therapy alone or by ureteral reimplantation plus medical therapy (ALLEN et al. 1992; BIRMINGHAM REFLUX STUDY GROUP 1983; WALKER 1994; OLBING 1992, personal communication), it would seem likely that urinary tract infection is the more important part of this combination of vesicoureteral reflux and urinary tract infection. The studies to be reported here reinforce the hypothesis that "chronic pyelonephritis = reflux nephropathy" is due to bacterial infection of the kidney, either with or without vesicoureteral reflux. The unit nephron theory of Bricker has been shown to be operative in experimental chronic pyelonephritis in the dog (BRICKER et al. 1958) and more recently in our studies in the monkey (JANSON and ROBERTS 1978), wherein renal damage led to the loss of entire nephrons. End-stage renal disease from chronic pyelonephritis is associated with both tubulointerstitial disease and focal glomerulosclerosis and albuminuria (KINCAID-SMITH 1973), as is end-stage renal disease from glomerulonephritis (SCHRIER et al. 1988).

Chronic pyelonephritis is reported as the cause of end-stage renal disease in 15–25% of children and young adults coming to end-stage renal disease either with or without reflux (SCHARER 1971). It is thought that end-stage renal disease from bacterial infection is probably the result of renal damage from acute infection occurring during early childhood; however, recent studies (MEYRIER et al. 1989) show that adults also develop cortical scars from acute pyelonephritis. When renal damage is severe enough in children, the remnant kidney may well be insufficient to maintain the increased load for renal function occurring during adolescence, leading to end-stage renal disease. It has been suggested that either glomerular hyperfiltration or hypertension of the remaining nephrons is the cause of end-stage renal disease (BRENNER 1983). This leads to progressive destruction of the remaining nephrons with focal glomerulosclerosis and further tubulointerstitial disease.

2 Bacterial Adherence

Most experimental studies of urinary tract infection are of *E. coli*, since this is the etiologic agent for urinary tract infection in over 90% of cases and in over 80% of cases of acute pyelonephritis. *E. coli* which cause disease begin with bacteria normally resident in the fecal stream, and then colonize either the perineum of females or prepuce of uncircumcised males, prior to causing an ascending urinary tract infection (FOWLER and STAMEY 1977; WISWELL et al. 1985). Adhesion may occur because of a nonspecific characteristic such as hydrophobicity but more frequently is due to a specific receptor-lectin interaction. The mechanism by which adhesion occurs follows multiple physicochemical events (JONES and ISAACSON 1983). While the negative charges of both bacteria and epithelial cells at first attract, they then repel as the cells approach each other. Forces of attraction are greatest when they are more than 10 nm apart. Closer than this, adhesion is repelled. The magnitude of the repulsive force increases with the radius of the cell. Therefore, bacterial fimbriae, hair-like appendages on the surface of bacteria having a radius of 2–10 nm, are not repelled as much as the bacteria, whose radius approaches 250 nm (ROBERTS 1987). These appendages have been termed either fimbriae (DUGUID et al. 1966) or pili (BRINTON 1965). Fimbriae are not the only means of attachment, as carbohydrate polymers can also overcome the repulsive forces (JONES and ISAACSON 1983).

It was not until 1976 that studies by SVANBORG-EDÉN et al. (1976) showed that adherence to urinary tract epithelial cells by *E. coli* was a possible initiating step in the onset of urinary tract infection. FOWLER and STAMEY (1977) showed that introital colonization by bacterial adherence preceded urinary tract infections in women; at about the same time, BOLLGREN and WINBERG (1976) reported on the periurethral and preputial bacterial flora in children susceptible to urinary tract infections. This work was continued by Källenius, who correlated bacterial adhesion to mannose-resistant agglutination of human erythrocytes (KÄLLENIUS et al. 1980) in patients with nonobstructive pyelonephritis.

Nonobstructive acute pyelonephritis is caused most often by P-fimbriated *E. coli*, being reported in over 95% of children (ELO et al. 1985; KÄLLENIUS et al. 1981; VÄISÄNEN et al. 1981) and in 50–90% of adults (DOWLING et al. 1987; LATHAM and STAMM 1984). P-fimbriae were thus named because they act as lectins for urothelial receptors which are the P blood-group antigens (KÄLLENIUS et al. 1980; LEFFLER and SVANBORG-EDÉN 1980) (Fig. 1a).

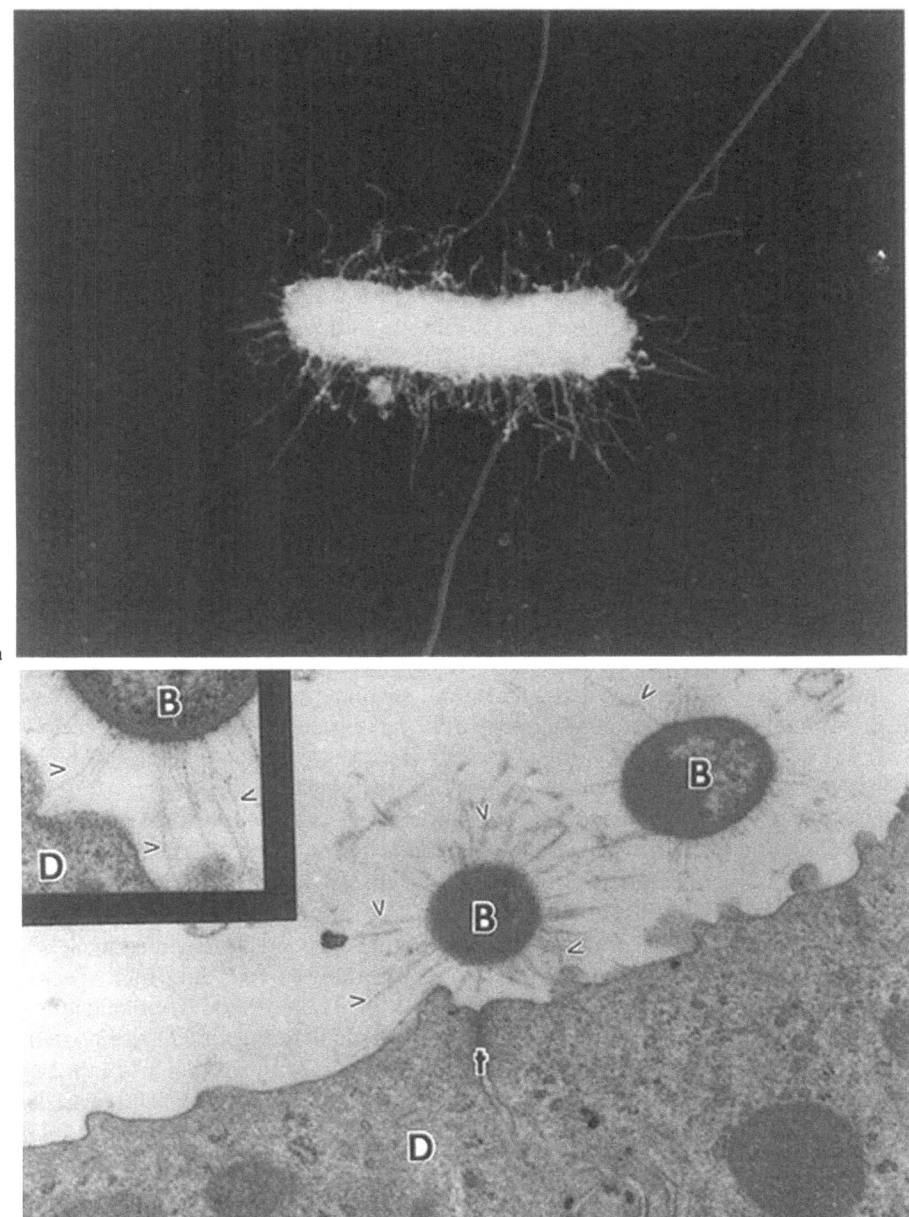

Fig. 1. a Shadow cast of P-fimbriated *E. coli* with platinum carbon. ×30 000. b P-fimbriated (*arrows*) *E. coli* (*B*) adhering to a distal tubular cell (*D*) by means of fimbriae. The tight junction between tubular cells is evident (*t*). × 18 000. Inset: TEM, × 95 000

P-fibriae are heteropolymeric structures composed of a rigid stalk. It contains the major protein linked end to end with a flexible-tip fibrillum consisting of four proteins, of which PapG, the receptor binding adhesin, is located at the distal end of the fimbriae (KUEHN et al. 1992; LINDBERG et al. 1987; LUND et al. 1987).

The tip adhesin may recognize one of three different α-Galp-(1-4)-β-Galp-containing receptors. Class-I adhesins adhere to globotriaosylceramide, class-II adhesins adhere to globotetraosylceramide (globoside), and class-III adhesins adhere to globopentaosylceramide (Globo A or the Forssman antigen). P-fimbriae with either class-II or -III adhesins are found in both fecal and urine isolates, but pyelonephritogenic strains carry the class-II adhesin and those associated with cystitis, the class-III adhesin. This suggest a greater density of Globo A receptors on urothelium of the bladder and a greater density of globoside receptors on urothelium from the upper urinary tract and kidney. A *pap*G mutant with deletion of the tip adhesin is still able to express morphologically normal fimbriae that, however, cannot mediate α-Galp-1-4-β-Galp-specific attachment in vitro (HULTGREN et al. 1993).

My interest in bacterial adhesion began when an ultrastructural study of chronic pyelonephritis by T.W. Smith, Jr., in our laboratory showed fimbriated *E. coli* reaching renal tubular epithelium during experimental pyelonephritis (SMITH and ROBERTS 1978) (Fig. 1b). We later found that these were P-fimbriae (ROBERTS et al. 1984).

P-fimbriated *E. coli* often also have other proposed virulence factors such as bacterial hemolysin, type-1 fimbriae, and aerobactin and are resistant to serum bactericidal activity. A clonal theory has been advanced to explain the concomitant presence of these factors (ACHTMAN et al. 1983; PLOS et al. 1989). Thus, the presence of P-fimbriae is probably not the only virulence factor important in the etiology of acute pyelonephritis. P-fimbriae have been found to be important in experimental studies with monkeys and the Balb/c mouse. These animals are known to have the same urothelial cell receptor for *E. coli* with P-fimbriae. In both the Balb/c mouse and the nonhuman primate, immunization with both homologous and heterologous purified P-fimbriae protected against pyelonephritis, following either a bladder infection in the mouse or a kidney infection in the monkey (O'HANLEY et al. 1985; ROBERTS et al. 1984; 1989). After reaching the bladder, colonization of the ureter can occur from P-fimbriated *E. coli* even in the absence of vesicoureteral reflux, as has been shown by studies in the monkey (ROBERTS et al. 1985). Studies of patients also suggest that this would be so, since early (WINBERG et al. 1974), as well as more recent ones (WINTER et al. 1983) showing that only one third of children with nonobstructive pyelonephritis had vesicoureteral reflux. Once within the ureter, colonization of transitional cells affects ureteral peristalis (ROBERTS 1975). When such *E. coli* colonize the ureter and its function ceases, this produces ureteral dilatation in a physiologic obstruction as first suggested by MICHIE (1959). Such obstruction would be expected to lead to a change in the shape of the renal papilla, by which intrarenal reflux of the bacteria within the ureter into the kidney could occur at a very low pressure (ANGEL et al. 1979).

In a recent paper by MOBLEY et al. (1993), a double-deletion pap mutant without the tip protein of a human pyelonephritic *E. coli* isolate remained able to provoke development of acute pyelitis or pyelonephritis in the CBA mouse model. These data suggest either that P-fimbriae are not required for human pyelonephritis, or that the mouse model is not relevant for human disease, as the mouse normally has vesicoureteral reflux by which a bladder inoculate may reach the kidney. In the primate, the P-fimbriated *E. coli* strain JR1 will reach the kidney and cause pyelonephritis even in the absence of vesicoureteral reflux, whereas non-P-fimbriated *E. coli* will not (ROBERTS et al. 1985).

The pattern of receptor glycolipids in the monkey and the human kidney is similar and in both cases dominated by globoside, arguing that the monkey model used is more relevant as an animal model for urinary tract infection than the mouse. A mutant strain, DS17-8, expressing P-fimbriae lacking the PapG adhesin, was constructed by allelic replacement, introducing a 1-bp deletion early in the *pap*G gene. In cynomolgus monkeys the wild-type strain DS17 and DS17-8 were equally able to cause bladder infection, whereas only the wild-type strain DS17 was able to cause pyelonephritis, as monitored by bacteriologic, functional, and histopathologic criteria. Since DS17, but not DS17-8, adheres to renal tissue in vitro these data underscore the critical role of microbial adherence to host tissues in infectious disease and strongly suggest that the PapG tip adhesin of P-fimbriae is essential in the pathogenesis of human kidney infection (unpublished data).

3 Cytokines and Vascular Events

It has been shown in human beings that *E. coli* bacteria stimulate urothelial cells to secrete interleukin-6 into the urine concomitantly with elevation of serum levels (DE MAN et al. 1989). After infection, complement activation of C5a is a chemotactic event (WARD et al. 1965), and formation of C3b both opsonizes *E. coli* (MEYLAN and GLAUSER 1989) and activates receptors for *E. coli* on polymorphonuclear cells (GLAUSER et al. 1991) (Fig. 2).

Previous studies in animals with kidney infection have also shown suppression of splenic lymphocytes' response to mitogens (MILLER and NORTH 1979), and the human T-lymphocyte response to phytohemagglutinin was suppressed by bacterial lipopolysaccharide (ELLNER and SPAGNUOLO 1979). Our recent studies suggest that suppressor T cells may be responsible for this suppression early in the course of experimental pyelonephritis (unpublished data). The CD4 + Leu8-subpopulation has been demonstrated to contain helper-inducer activity (GATENBY et al. 1982), and in our study there was a significant drop in these helper-induced cells which coincided with the increase in suppressor cells. The CD4 + CD29 + subpopulation has been shown to more clearly delineate helper-inducer cells, separating helper-inducer and suppressor- inducer activities (MORIMOTO et al. 1985). CD4 + CD29 + cells have been demon-

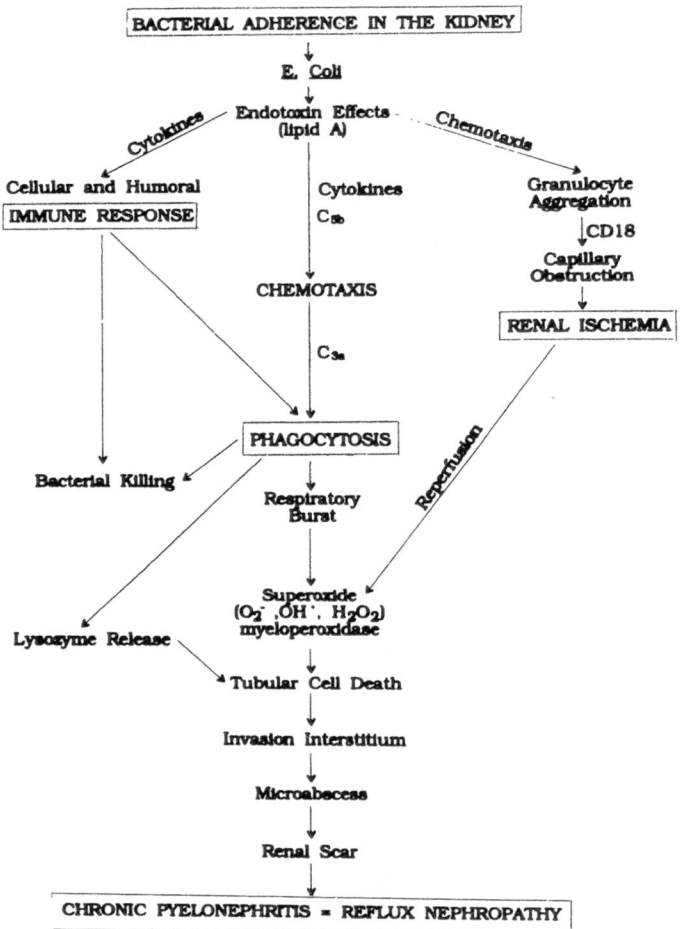

Fig. 2. Events leading to chronic pyelonephritis (reflux nephropathy)

strated to be previously activated cells containing memory activity and having a propensity to localize at sites of tissue inflammation (DAIMLE and DOYLE 1990; SANDERS et al. 1988). The Leu8 monoclonal antibody identifies cells that have the surface receptor (LAM-1, L-selectin) for high endothelial cells of the postcapillary venules of lymph nodes (CAMERINI et al. 1989). The CD8 + Leu8 + population may therefore have unique recirculatory properties.

Interleukin-6 levels in the blood increase markedly within hours after bacteria reach the kidney (ROBERTS et al. 1993), being responsible for the initiation of the acute-phase response in the liver (RICHARDS et al. 1991). Bacterial lipopolysaccharide predominantly induces interleukin-1 and tumor

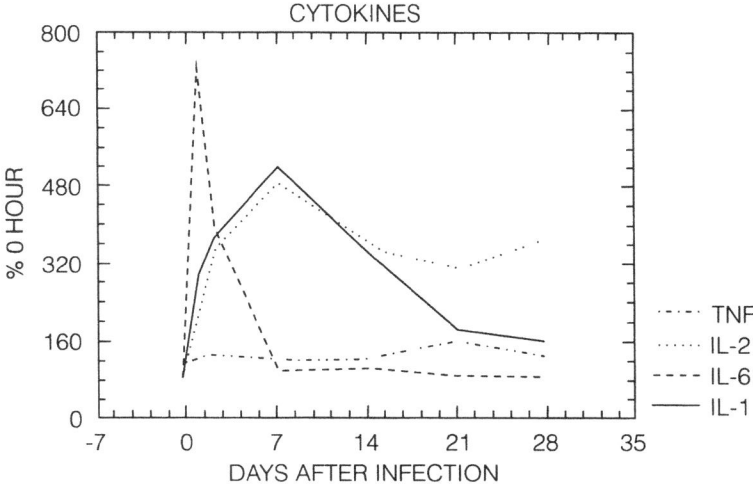

Fig. 3. Cytokine cascade occurring in monkeys following an ascending renal infection with P-fimbriated *E. coli*

necrosis factor production in monocytes. The monocyte has a receptor for the bacterial endotoxin (CD14) which initiates the cytokine cascade to involve endothelial cells, neutrophils, lymphocytes, and fibroblasts (BILLIAU and VANDEKERCKHOVE 1991) (Fig. 3). The effect on endothelial cells is important, in that it increases adhesion of granulocytes to endothelial surfaces, and this can lead to renal ischemia (KAACK et al. 1986). While ischemia itself may be damaging, it is during reperfusion that maximum damage appears to occur. Reperfusion injury is due to a great extent to neutrophil-mediated damage from oxygen free radicals (GRISHAM et al. 1986). In the kidney, however, injury from warm ischemia is not mediated by neutrophils alone (PALLER 1989). The neutrophilic response following renal ischemia may be only a secondary response, or one secondary to activation of interleukin-1 (DINARELLO 1992). The adhesion of the granulocytes to the endothelium is mediated by leukocyte adhesion molecules such as CD11a and CD18 (PATARROYO and MAKGOBA 1989).

T lymphocytes, as well as polymorphonuclear cells, secrete enzymes that degrade components of extracellular matrix (DAIMLE and DOYLE 1990). The increase in CD4 cells in our acute infection, therefore, may have assisted in capillary transmigration of inflammatory cells to the site of antigen expression by the bacteria. While pro-inflammatory cytokines such as IL-1α and TNFα are unable to modulate endothelial permeability, they may contribute indirectly by increasing endothelial expression of adhesion molecules for polymorphonuclear leukocytes such as ICAMs, causing adhesion and migration of inflammatory cells to the antigenic site where capillary obstruction may occur and where phagocytosis begins, both resulting in release of toxic forms of oxygen which may damage renal tubules, ending in their death (ARNAOUT 1993).

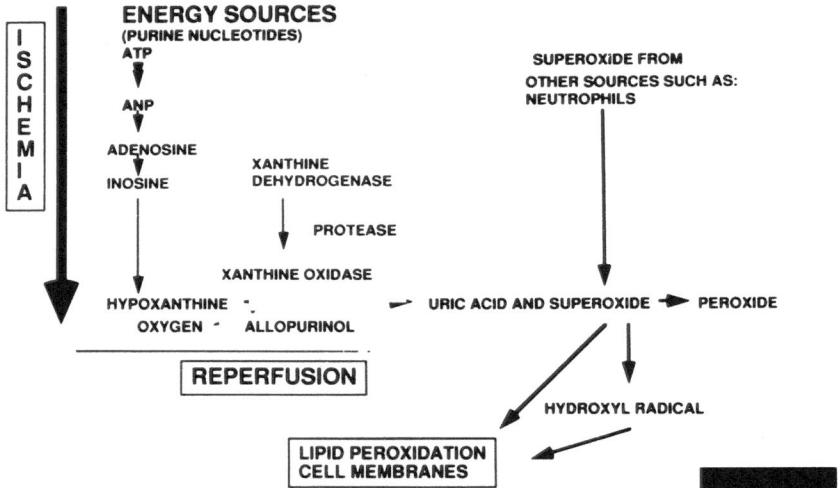

Fig. 4. Events during ischemia and following reperfusion, illustrating the effect of allopurinol in blocking xanthine oxidase and preventing the formation of toxic oxygen radicals

This adhesion, which later leads to penetration of the capillary walls to reach the interstitium and renal tubular spaces, results in granulocytic aggregation, capillary obstruction, and renal ischemia (KAACK et al. 1986). The renal damage which occurs in this instance in the monkey can also be prevented by treatment with allopurinol, which inhibits xanthine oxidase and prevents the reperfusion damage following the ischemic event (ROBERTS et al. 1986). (Fig. 4). Our studies illustrate the unique relationships between cytokines and lymphocytes in the response to bacterial infection, as the inflammatory response is regulated not only by cytokine activity, but by lymphocyte activation as well. Attempts to modulate the inflammatory response and decrease renal damage, while not affecting the ability of the host to eradicate the bacterial parasite, will probably include treatment with monoclonal antibodies to IL-1, TNF, or interferon gamma, or modulation of their effects by treatment with soluble receptors for those cytokines.

4 Sepsis

Some episodes of acute pyelonephritis may progress to septic death. Sepsis is a clinical syndrome which follows an infection; it is a generalized, nonspecific inflammatory response which escapes the anatomical barriers of the host, damaging by its systemic effects. Sepsis mediated by gram-negative bacteria follows release of endotoxin by the bacteria that activates complement, and this leads to generation of the inflammatory mediators, cytokines and arachidonic acid metabolites (BILLIAU and VANDEKERCKHOVE 1991).

Both monocytes and macrophages release a number of cytokines upon stimulation by endotoxin (DINARELLO 1987). The interleukins, together with tumor necrosis factor α, are produced by many different cells but mainly by those of the monocyte/macrophage cell lineage. These cytokines act pleiotropically and exert their effects on many cells. They are particularly important as elicitors of the acute-phase reaction (DINARILLO 1987) and also promote the respiratory burst of phagocytosis (BABIOR et al. 1973; KLEBANOFF et al. 1986; MATSUBARA and ZIFF 1986). During the cytokine-mediated acute-phase reaction and the local respiratory burst that rapidly occurs upon infection, formation of highly reactive free radicals of oxygen such as superoxide, hydroxyl radicals, hydrogen peroxide, myeloperoxide, and singlet oxygen radicals occurs. The generation of toxic nitric oxide through the L-arginine oxidase system and the release into the renal tubules of lysosomal enzymes formed during endocytosis are also associated with this respiratory burst (BEVILACQUA et al. 1985; GOLDSTEIN et al. 1973; IGNARRO 1986). All these substances are not only deleterious to the bacteria but also to the host.

An excessive host response to the bacteria causing acute pyelonephritis results in activation of complement and of certain cytokines, particularly IL-2, IL-2R, and IL-6. The increase in circulatory IL-2R occurs because upon stimulation more of these cellular receptors are expressed, and the cells release IL-2R into the circulation. This might have the untoward effect of binding some of the circulatory IL-2. An excessive increase in IL-2 and IL-6 may be due to the fact that increased IL-1 may in some cases be protective (ROBERTS et al. 1993).

Other proof of the importance of cytokines is the fact that intravenous administration of TNF and IL-1β induces septic shock-like states in both man and animals (NATANSON et al. 1989; OKUSAWA et al. 1988). This activation of the inflammatory response which leads to shock from these cytokines is similar to the activation of neutrophils and cascade systems which occurs after endotoxin challenge (VAN DEVENTER et al. 1990). Further proof is the fact that the lethal cytokine effects may be inhibited in vivo by giving neutralizing antibodies (ALEXANDER et al. 1991) or receptor antagonists (STARNES et al. 1990; OHLSSON et al. 1990). Additional evidence for the initial importance of endotoxin is that both septic shock (VAN DEVENTER et al. 1990) and septic death (WAAGE et al. 1989) have been shown to occur following experimental endotoxin administration. At present, the treatment of septic shock is being evaluated with antibodies to endotoxin (ZIEGLER et al. 1991) and some of the cytokines such as TNF (HINSHAW et al. 1990). The best solution may well involve therapeutic regimens combining the two.

5 Inflammation

Once these polymorphonuclear cells reach the bacteria themselves, phagocytosis begins. It was suggested some time ago that inflammatory events are responsible for renal damage following infection, as opposed to any direct effect of the bacteria themselves (GLAUSER et al. 1978). When the inflammatory response was prevented experimentally by decomplementation with cobra venom factor in the rat (SULLIVAN et al. 1977) and in the monkey (ROBERTS et al. 1983), acute renal damage was prevented. More recent studies also show that renal damage from the respiratory burst of phagocytosis after infection is due to neutrophil-mediated tissue damage, as the extent of renal damage was directly correlated with the numbers of neutrophils and was modulated by treatment with cortico-steroids (ORMROD et al. 1986). In the monkey the leukocytosis is maximal by 24 h, but ultrastructural studies showed no renal damage unitl 48 h after bacterial inoculation (FUSSELL and ROBERTS 1984 (Fig. 5). Without treatment, by 48 h there is a loss of up to 30% of renal function (ROBERTS et al. 1990). Neutrophils that reach the tubular lumen become active phagocytes, opsonizing the bacteria by means of complement activated by the alternative pathway (PAQUET 1984). The receptors for C3 on neutrophils cause this activation and the respiratory burst that occurs within the phagosome but also on the surface of the phagocyte. Recent studies have shown that bacteria associated with acquired renal scarring from acute pyelonephritis cause more active release of superoxide and other toxic oxygen radicals from the surface of the phagocyte than within the phagosome (MUNDI et al. 1991); therefore, adjoining renal tubules would be expected to be damaged. Our recent studies of elastase in polymorphonuclear cells showed that bacterial strains which caused renal scarring from acute pyelonephritis also caused more release of elastase from the surface of the phagocytes during phagocytosis, and this would also be expected to further damage renal tubular cells (Fig. 6). Superoxide production may lead to production of other toxic radicals such as hydrogen peroxide, hydroxyl radicals, singlet oxygen and, in the presence of halides and myeloperoxidase, a secondary toxic effect. These reactions will all eradicate bacteria in the phagosome (KLEBANOFF 1975), but they can damage the renal tubules if they occur in them. While all cells in the body have superoxide dismutase, which ameliorates the effect of these toxic free radicals of oxygen, there is no superoxide dismutase in urine or phagocytes (FRIDOVICH 1978). Thus, the respiratory burst acts unopposed, damaging both neutrophils and tubular cells. This is suggested by the finding that superoxide dismutase prevents the renal damage from renal infection (ROBERTS et al. 1982). These free oxygen radicals have now been shown to activate transcription with the induction of early genes c-fos, c-myc, c-jun, and β-actin, probably by inducing DNA strand breaks. These genes are thought to encode transcription factors to participate in cell growth as well as differentiation and development. The reactive oxygen radicals also have been shown to stimulate the growth of fibroblasts, thus promoting fibrosis and scar formation. Thus, the free radicals of oxygen cause cellular damage by at least two mechanisms: damage of DNA and damage to the cell membrane by lipid peroxidation. The overall effect on the cell membrane is to decrease its fluidity and destabilize membrane receptors, as well as inhibiting protein synthesis, all leading to cell death (WINROW et al. 1993).

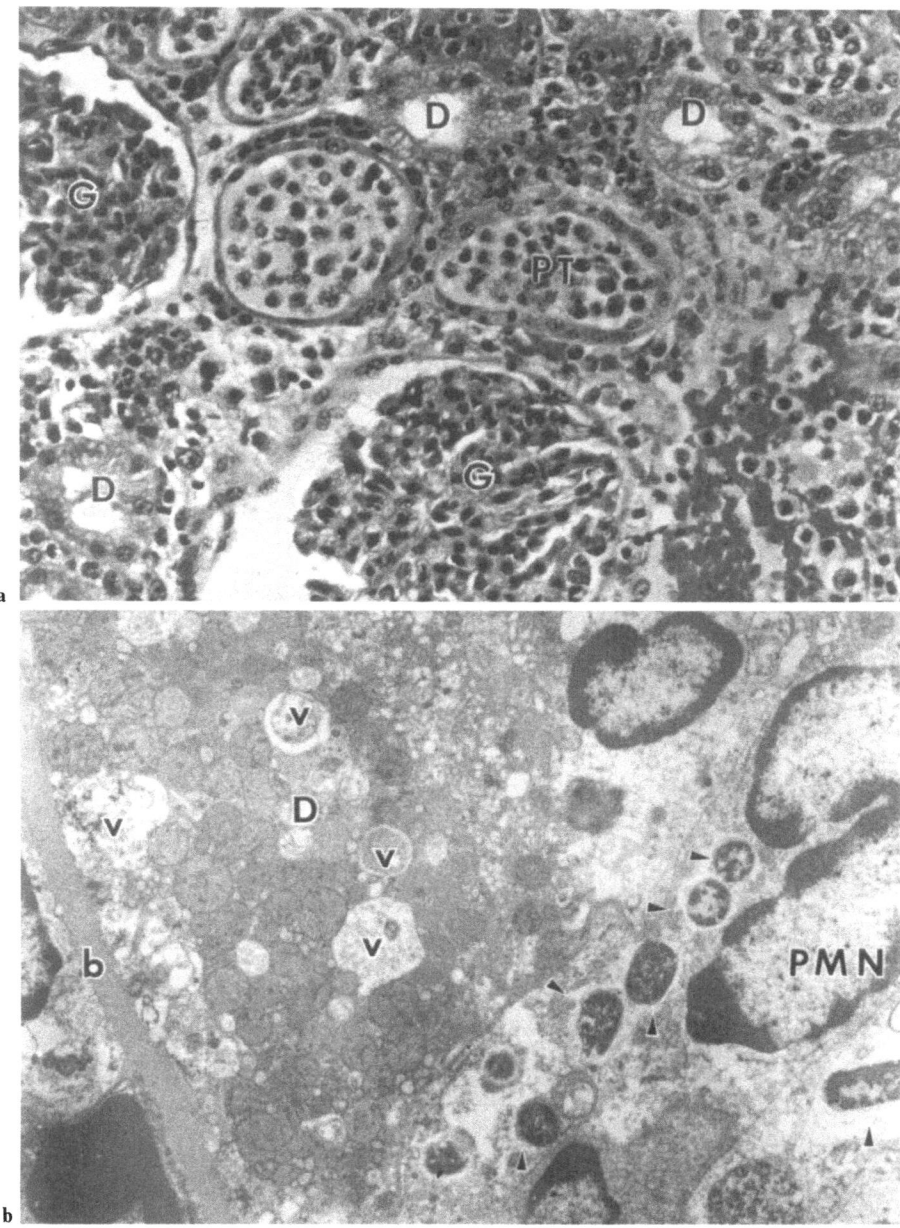

a

b

Fig. 5. a Degenerating renal tubules (*D*) and marked granulocytic aggregation in tubules (*Pt*) in an acute infection (48 h). Note normal glomerulus (*G*). H&E × 750 **b** Granulocyte-phagocytosing bacteria (*arrows*) in tubules with dying adjoining tubular cell (*D*) but intact basement membrane (*B*). Note loss of mitochondrial inner membranes and loss of cristae in others and vacuoles (*V*). TEM × 18 000. **c** Granulocytes within a distal renal tubule, and phagocytosed disintegrated bacteria (*PL*) array and granulocyte in the interstitium with bacteria (*arrows*) (*PI*). Distal tubular cells (*d*). migratory granulocyte between tubular cells (*M*). TEM × 18 000

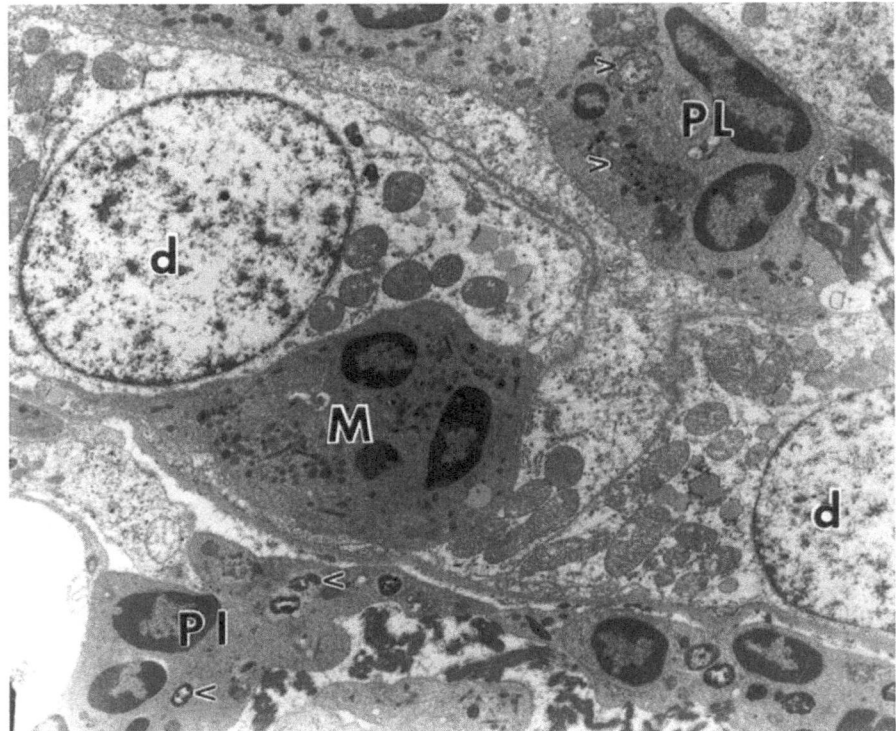

Fig. 5c

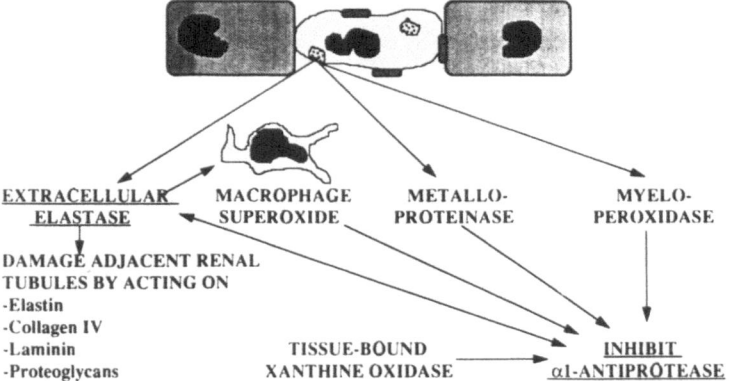

Fig. 6. Mechanism of damage from extracellular release of elastase from granulocytes

6 Effect of Treatment

Studies in a rodent model showed that renal damage can be prevented with antibiotic therapy if begun prior to suppuration (no later than 30 h after the infection) (GLAUSER et al. 1978). This fact was supported by more recent animal studies; however, these showed that therapy must be begun within 24 h to be protective (SLOTKI and ASSCHER 1982), while similar studies showed that treatment could be delayed up to 4 days after the onset of infection and still be effective in preventing renal scarring (MILLER and PHILLIPS 1981). While the studies of RANSLEY and RISDON (1981) in the pig with reflux did not determine when treatment should be started, they did show that antibiotic treatment decreases renal damage from infection even in the presence of reflux. Our recent studies in the monkey showed that renal damage could not be totally prevented when antibiotic therapy was delayed until 72 h after infection. The addition of allopurinol to the antibacterial therapy, however, gave additional protection, probably because of its effect on reperfusion events (ROBERTS et al. 1990). It is of interest that effective antibiotic treatment of pyelonephritis in our model abrogates the immune response, unlike the protective immune response in untreated disease (NEAL et al. 1991). This explains why patients develop recurrent episodes of pyelonephritis. While most patients who develop the renal scars of chronic atrophic pyelonephritis had their first infection within the first 3 years of life, studies by WINBERG et al. (1974) and WINTER et al. (1983) showed that improper or delayed treatment of acute pyelonephritis is responsible for the renal scarring. Studies by SMELLIE et al. (1985) in older children confirmed this fact. Thus, the areas of acute pyelonephritis are those which develop renal scars in chronic disease (Fig. 7).

7 Prevention of Chronic Pyelonephritis

The mode of prevention of the disease by vaccination with P-fimbriae or by oral administration of the receptor or an analogue of the receptor causing competitive inhibition of the receptor-ligand interaction is still under investigation. Following vaccination with P-fimbriae in the monkey, while there was also an antibody reponse to contaminating endotoxin, protection was shown to correlate with antibody titers to P-fimbriae as opposed to the O antigen (ROBERTS et al. 1984). Our studies of immunization with heterologous P-fimbriae in the baboon have shown only partial protection (ROBERTS et al. 1989); thus, a broadly active common vaccine against pyelonephritis may be difficult to obtain. However, SCHMIDT et al. (1984) found that certain fimbrial peptides may be immunogenic epitopes, and O'HANLEY et al. (1985), using the gene probe for the gal-gal binding adhesin and one for the hemolysin gene, showed that the nucleotide sequence for hemolysin and P-fimbriae in many heterologous strains seem to be the same. Thus, a vaccine may well be possible for the prevention of disease from

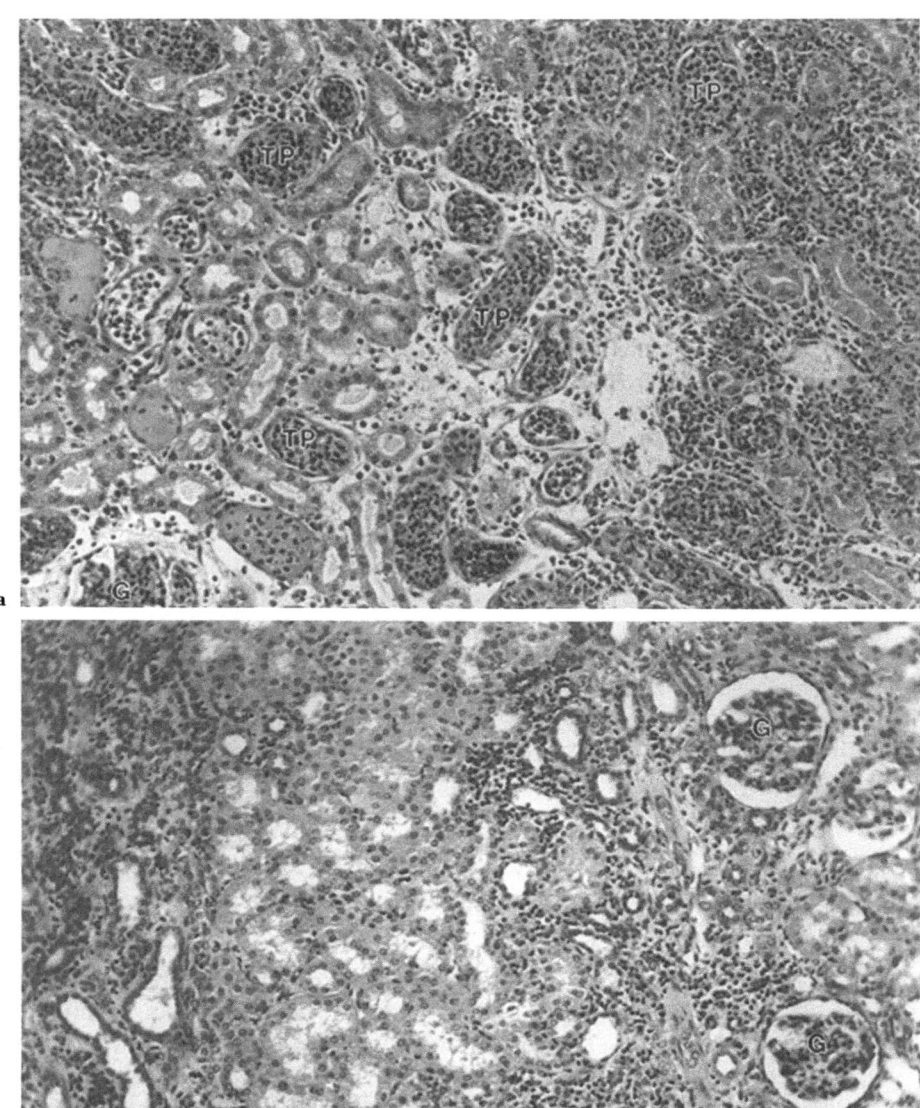

Fig. 7. a Acute pyelonephritis in the monkey at 48 h after infection. Tubules engorged with granulocytes (*TP*), interstitial edema, and leukocyte infiltrate are noted. H&E × 300. **b** Chronic pyelonephritis 4 weeks after infection. Note the patchy nature of scar formation with tubular atrophy and dilation, and interstitial collections of lymphocytes next to normal tubules and glomeruli (*G*). H&E, × 300. **c** Electron micrograph of chronic pyelonephritis, showing infiltrate of granular leukocyte (*GL*) (eosinophil) and lymphocyte (*ly*) into medullary interstitium between irregular basal lamina (*bl*) with floculent densities. Note mitochrondia (*M*) with ruptured inner membranes. × 7500. (From SMITH and ROBERTS (1978), with permission)

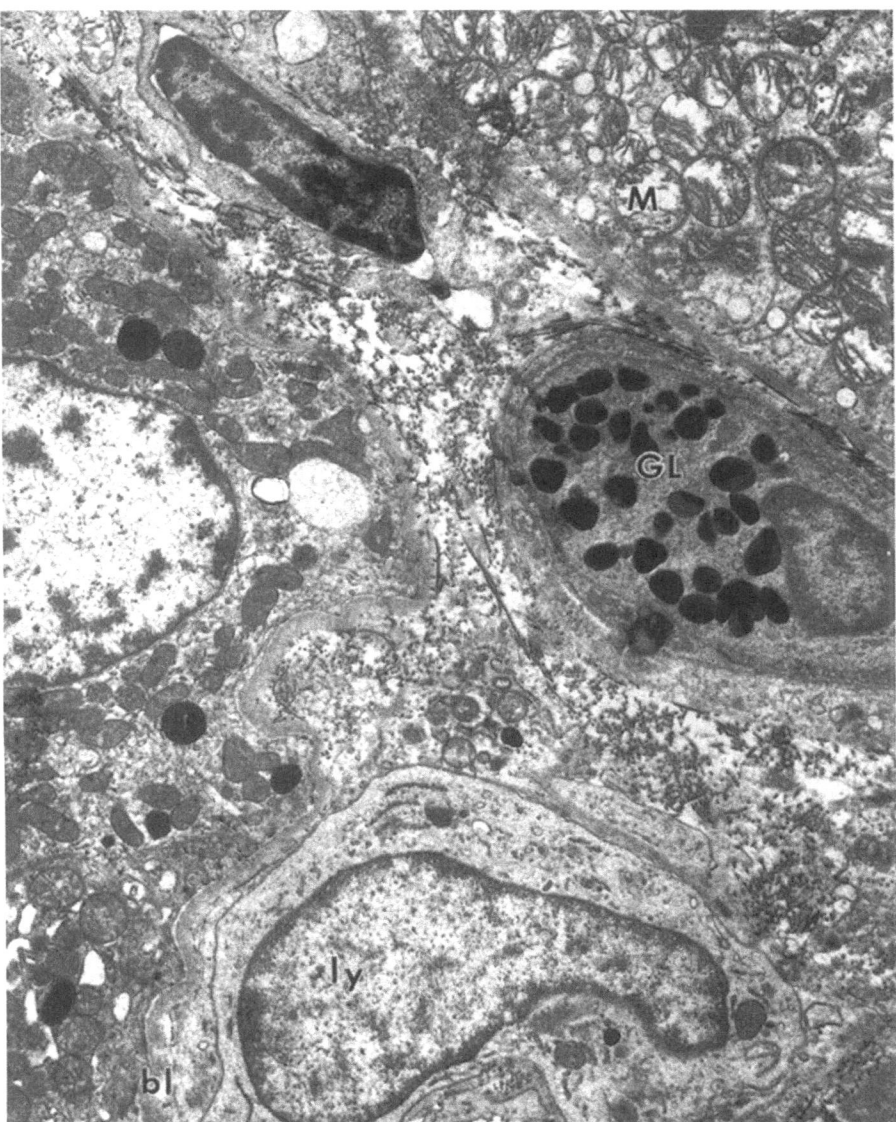

Fig. 7c

many fimbriated strains. Since ascending nonobstructive pyelonephritis occurs
because of adhesion by P-fimbriae, this vaccine will be designed to prevent
bacteria from reaching the kidney. In pyelonephritis associated with obstruction
or vesicoureteral reflux, bacteria would be expected to cause pyelonephritis with
significant renal damage. Thus, in these cases a vaccine to P-fimbriae would not
be helpful. Indeed, in the presence of vesicoureteral reflux it has been shown that

P-fimbriation is not necessary for pyelonephritis to occur (LOMBERG et al. 1984). Both pyelonephritis and renal scars occur more frequently from non-P-fimbriated *E. coli* in children with reflux (LOMBERG et al. 1989). Thus, when vesicoureteral reflux is present, reliance on prophylactic antibiotics until the reflux disappears should be stressed, as originally shown by SMELLIE and NORMAND (1975).

Extensive genetic analyses of *E. coli* for the genes necessary in the production of P-fimbriae have been done in the laboratories of Staffan Normark (NORGREN et al. 1987; HULTGREN et al. 1989). These explain the complex biogenesis of the formation of fimbriae by *E. coli*. It now appears that the tips of P-fimbriae are the specific adhesins. Normark feels that using a combination of the periplasmic transport protein and the tip-associated protein may well be the most effective method of developing a vaccine against heterologous P-fimbriae (LUND et al. 1988), a vaccine that we are at present testing in the monkey.

One difficulty will be in deciding who should be immunized. Individuals who are nonsecretors and thus have more receptors may well be candidates. Berg's studies of children showed that the human kidney appears to be more vulnerable to the damaging effects of infection occurring during the first 3 years of life (BERG and JOHANNSON 1982). This reduction in renal function was not dependent on either the presence or grade of vesicoureteral reflux, but rather was correlated with infection. In a study of adults who had their first infection during infancy, JACOBSON et al. (1989) showed decreased renal function in all, hypertension in one third, and end-stage renal disease in 10%. We have shown in the monkey that maternal immunization leads to passive immunization of their infants, with protective activity against experimental pyelonephritis (KAACK et al. 1988). Thus, if it can be shown that the nonsecretor status is a familial trait, maternal immunization for passive protection of the newborns at risk might even be considered. Until preventive therapy such as vaccination can be developed, early effective bacterial eradication with antibacterials in combination with anti-inflammatory agents or allopurinol remains the best treatment.

Acknowledgement. The electron micrographs were done by Everett Fussell, except for Fig. 7c, which was done by T. Woodie Smith.

References

Achtman M, Mercer A, Kusecek B, Pohl A, Heuzenroeder M, Aaronson W, Sutton A, Silver RP (1983) Six widespread bacterial clones among *Escherichia coli* K1 isolates. Infect Immun 39: 315–335
Alexander HR, Doherty GM, Buresh CM, Venzon DJ, Norton JA (1991) A recombinant human receptor antagonist to interleukin-1 improves survival after lethal endotoxemia in mice. J Exp Med 173: 1029
Allen TD (1977) The non-neurogenic neurogenic bladder. J Urol 117: 232–238
Allen TD, Arant BS Jr, Roberts JA (1992) Commentary: vesicoureteral reflux—1992. J Urol 148: 1758–1760
Angel JR, Smith TW Jr, Roberts JA (1979) The hydrodynamics of pyelorenal reflux. J Urol 122: 20–26

Arnaout MA (1993) Cell adhesion molecules in inflammation and thrombosis: status and prospects. Am J Kidney Dis 21: 72–76

Babior BM, Kipnes RS, Curnette JT (1973) Biological defense mechanisms. The production by leukocytes of superoxide, a potential bactericidal agent. J Clin Invest 52: 741

Bailey RR (1973) The relationship of vesicoureteral reflux to urinary tract infection and chronic pyelonephritis—reflux nephropathy. Clin Nephrol 1: 132–141

Berg UB, Johansson SB (1982) Age as a main determinant of renal functional damage in urinary tract infection. Arch Dis Child 58: 963–969

Bevilacqua MP, Pober JS, Wheeler ME, Cotran RS, Gimbrone MA jr (1985) Interleukin 1 acts on cultured human vascular endothelium to increase the adhesion of polymorphonuclear leukocytes, monocytes, and related leukocyte cell lines. J Clin Invest 76: 2003

Billiau A, Vandekerckhove F (1991) Cytokines and their interactions with other inflammatory mediators in the pathogenesis of sepsis and septic shock. Eur J Clin Invest 21: 559–573

Birmingham Reflux Study Group (1983) Prospective trial of operative versus non-operative treatment of severe vesicoureteral reflux: two years' observation in 96 children. Br Med J 287: 171–174

Bisset GS III, Strife JL, Dunbar JS (1987) Urography and voiding cystourethrography: findings in girls with urinary tract infection. AJR 148: 479

Bollgren I, Winberg J (1976) The periurethral aerobic flora in girls highly susceptible to urinary infections. Acta paediatr Scand 65: 81–87

Brenner BM (1983) Hemodynamically mediated glomerular injury and the progressive nature of kidney disease. Kidney Int 23: 647–655

Bricker NS, Dewey RR, Lubowitz H (1958) Studies in experimental pyelonephritis. Simultaneous and serial investigation of a pyelonephritic and intact kidney in the same animal. Clin Res 6: 292–294

Brinton CC Jr (1965) The structure, function, synthesis and genetic control of bacterial pili and a molecular mechanism for DNA and RNA transport in gram-negative bacteria. Trans NY Acad Sci 27: 1003–1154

Camerini D, James SP, Stamenkovic I, Seed B (1989) Leu8/TQ1 is the human equivalent of the Mel-14 lymph node homing receptor. Nature 342: 78

Daimle NK, Doyle LV (1990) Ability of human T lymphocytes to adhere to vascular endothelial cells and to augment endothelial permeability to macromolecules is linked to their state of post-thymic maturation. J Immunol 144: 1233–1240

de Man P, van Kooten C, Aarden L (1989) Interleukin-6 induced at mucosal surfaces by gram-negative bacterial infection. Infect Immun 57: 3383–3388

Dinarello CA (1987) The biology of interleukin 1 and comparison to tumor necrosis factor. Immunol Lett 16: 227

Dinarello CA (1992) Role of interleukin-1 in infectious diseases. Immunol Rev 127: 119–145

Dowling KJ, Roberts JA, Kaack MB (1987) P-fimbriated E. coli urinary tract infection: a clinical correlation. South Med J 80: 1533–1536

Duguid JP, Anderson ES, Campbell I (1966) Fimbriae and adhesive properties of salmonellae. J Pathol Bacteriol 92: 107–138

Edwards D, Normand ICS, Prescod N, Smellie JM (1977) Disappearance of reflux during long-term prophylaxis of urinary tract infections in children. Br Med J 2: 285–288

Ellner JJ, Spagnuolo PJ (1979) Suppression of antigen- and mitogen-induced human T-lymphocyte DNA synthesis by bacterial lipopolysaccharide: mediation by monocyte activation and production of prostaglandins. J Immunol 123: 2689

Elo J, Tallgren LG, Väisänen V, Korhonen TK, Mäkela PH (1985) Association of P and other fimbriae with clinical pyelonephritis in children. Scand J Urol Nephrol 19: 281–284

Filly RA, Friedland GW, Govan DE, Fair WR (1974) Development and progression of clubbing and scarring in children with recurrent urinary tract infections. Radiology 113: 145

Fowler JE Jr, Stamey TA (1977) Studies of introital colonization in women with recurrent urinary infection. VII. The role of bacterial adherence. J Urol 117: 472–476

Fridovich I (1983) Superoxide radical: an endogenous toxicant: Annu Rev Pharmacol Toxicol 23: 239–257

Fussell EN, Roberts JA (1984) The ultrastructure of acute pyelonephritis in the monkey. J Urol 133: 179–183

Gatenby PA, Kansas GS, Xian CY, Evans RL, Engleman EG (1982) Dissection of immunoregulatory subpopulations of T lymphocytes within the helper and suppressor lineages in man. J Immunol 129: 1997

Glauser M, Lyons JM, Braude AI (1978) Prevention of chronic pyelonephritis by suppression of acute suppuration. J Clin Invest 61: 403–407

Glauser MP, Zanetti G, Baumgartner J-D, Cohen J (1991) Septic shock: pathogenesis. Lancet 338: 732–739

Goldstein IM, Brai M, Osler AG, Weismann G (1973) Lysosomal enzyme release from human leukocytes: mediation by the alternate pathway of complement activation. J Immunol III:35–37

Gordon AC, Thomas DFM, Arthur RJ, Irving HC, Smith SEW (1990) Prenatally diagnosed reflux: a follow-up study. Br J Urol 65: 407–412

Grisham MB, Hernandez LA, Granger DN (1986) Xanthine oxidase and neutrophil infiltration in intestinal ischemia. Am J Physiol 251: G567–G574

Hinman F, Baumann FW (1973) Vesical and ureteral damage from voiding dysfunction in boys without neurologic or obstructive disease. J Urol 109: 727–732

Hinshaw LB, Tekamp-Olsen P, Chang ACK, Lee PA, Taylor FB Jr, Murray CK, Peer GT, Emerson TE jr, Passay RB, Juo GC (1990) Survival of primates in LD100 septic shock following therapy with antibody to tumor necrosis factor (TNFα). Circ Shock 30: 279

Hodson CJ, Edwards D (1960) Chronic pyelonephritis and vesicoureteric reflux. Clin Radiol 11: 219–231

Hodson CJ, Maling TMJ, McManamon PJ, Lewis MG (1975) The pathogenesis of reflux nephropathy (chronic atrophic pyelonephritis). Br J Radiol [Suppl] 13: 1–26

Hultgren SJ, Lindberg F, Magnusson G et al. (1989) The PapG adhesin of uropathogenic *Escherichia coli* contains separate regions for receptor binding and for the incorporation into the pilus. Proc Natl Acad Sci USA 86: 4357–4361

Hultgren SJ, Abraham S, Caparon M, Falk P, St Geme JW III, Normark S (1993) Pilus and nonpilus bacterial adhesins: assembly and function in cell recognition. Cell 73: 887–901

Hutch JA (1952) Vesico-ureteral reflux in the paraplegic: cause and correction. J Urol 68: 457–467

Jacobson SH, Eklof O, Eriksson CG, Lins L-E, Tidgren B, Winberg J (1989) Development of hypertension and uraemia after pyelonephritis in childhood: 27-year follow-up. Br Med J 299: 703–706

Janson KL, Roberts JA (1978) Experimental pyelonephritis. V. Functional characteristics of pyelonephritis. Invest Urol 15: 397–400

Jones GW, Isaacson RW (1983) Proteinaceous bacterial adhesins and their receptor. CRC Crit Rev Microbiol 10: 229–260

Jorgensen TM (1986) Pathogenetic factors in vesicoureteral reflux. Neurourol Urodynam 5: 153–183

Kaack MB, Dowling KJ, Patterson GM, Roberts JA (1986) Immunology of pyelonephritis. VIII. *E. coli* causes granulocytic aggregation and renal ischemia. J Urol 136: 1117–1122

Kaack MB, Roberts JA, Baskin G, Patterson GM (1988) Maternal immunization with P-fimbriae for the prevention of neonatal pyelonephritis. Infect Immun 56: 1–6

Källenius G, Winberg J (1978) Bacterial adherence to periurethral epithelial cells in girls prone to urinary tract infections. Lancet 2: 540–543

Källenius G, Möllby R, Svenson SB, Winberg J, Lundblad A, Svenson S (1980) The pk antigen as receptor of pyelonephritogenic *E. coli*. FEMS Microbiol Lett 7: 297–302

Källenius G, Möllby R, Svenson SB, Helin I, Hultberg H, Cedergren B, Winberg J (1981) Occurrence of P-fimbriated *Escherichia coli* in urinary tract infections. Lancet 2: 1369–1372

Kincaid-Smith P (1975) Glomerular lesions in atrophic pyelonephritis and reflux nephropathy. Kidney Int 8 [Suppl]: 81–83

Klebanoff SJ (1975) Antimicrobial mechanisms in neutrophils of polymorphonuclear leukocytes. Semin Hematol 12: 117–142

Klebanoff SJ, Vadas MA, Harlan JM, Sparks LH, Gamble JR, Agosti JM, Waltersdorph AM (1986) Stimulation of neutrophils by tumor necrosis factor. J Immunol 136: 4220

Koff SA, Murtagh D (1984) The uninhibited bladder in children: effect of treatment on vesicoureteral reflux resolution. Contr Nephrol 39: 211–220

Kuehn M, Heuser J, Normark S, Hultgren S (1992) P pili in uropathogenic *E. coli* are composite fibres with distinct fibrillar adhesive tips. Nature 356: 252–255

Latham R, Stamm W (1984) Role of fimbriated *Escherichia coli* in urinary tract infections in adult women: correlation with localization studies. J Infect Dis 149: 835–840

Leffler H, Svanborg-Edén CS (1980) Chemical identification of a glycosphingolipid receptor for *Escherichia coli* attaching to human urinary tract epithelial cells and agglutinating human erythrocytes. FEMS Microbiol Lett 8: 127–134

Lindberg F, Lund B, Johansson L, Normark S (1987) Localization of the receptor-binding protein adhesin at the tip of the bacterial pilus. Nature 328: 84–87

Lomberg H, Hanson L, Jacobsson B, Jodal N, Leffler H, Eden CS (1983) Correlation of P blood group, vesicoureteral reflux, and bacterial attachment in patients with recurrent pyelonephritis. N Engl J Med 308: 1189–1192

Lomberg H, Hellstrom M, Jodal U, Leffler H, Lincoln K, Eden CS (1984) Virulence-associated traits in Escherichia coli causing first and recurrent episodes of urinary tract infection in children with or without vesicoureteral reflux. J Infect Dis 150: 561–569

Lomberg H, Hellstrom M, Jodal U, Orskov I, Svanborg Edén C (1989) Properties of Escherichia coli in patients with renal scarring. J Infect Dis 159: 579–582

Lund B, Lindberg F, Marklund B-I, Normark S (1987) The PapG protein is the alpha-D-galactopyranosyl (1–4) beta-D-galactopyranose-binding adhesin of uro-pathogenic Escherichia coli Proc Natl Acad Sci USA 84: 5898–5902

Lund B, Linberg F, Marklund B-I, Normark S (1988) Tip proteins of pili associated with pyelonephritis: new candidates for vaccine development. Vaccine 6: 110–112

Mackie GG, Stephens FD (1975) Duplex kidneys: a correlation of renal dysplasia with position of the ureteral orifice. J Urol 114: 274–280

Matsubara T, Ziff M (1986) Increased superoxide anion release from human endothelial cell in response to cytokines. J Immunol 137: 3295

McGuire EJ, Woodside JR, Borden TA, Weiss RM (1981) Prognostic value of urodynamic testing in myelodysplastic patients. J Urol 126: 205–209

Mendoza JM, Roberts JA (1983) Effects of sterile high-pressure vesicoureteral reflux on the monkey. J Urol 130: 602–606

Meylan PR, Glauser MP (1989) Role of complement-derived and bacterial formylpeptide chemotactic factors in the in vivo migration of neutrophils in experimental Escherichia coli pyelonephritis in rats. J Infect Dis 159: 959–965

Meyrier A, Condamin M-C, Fernet M, Labigne-Roussel A, Simon P, Callard P, Rainfray M, Soilleux M, Groc A (1989) Frequency of development of early cortical scarring in acute primary pyelonephritis. Kidney Int 35: 696–703

Michie AJ (1959) Chronic pyelonephritis mimicking ureteral obstructions. Pediatr Surg 6: 1117–1127

Miller T, North D (1979) Immunobiologic factors in the pathogenesis of renal infection. Kidney Int 16: 665

Miller T, Phillips S (1981) Pyelonephritis: the relationship between infection, renal scarring, and antimicrobial therapy. Kidney Int 19: 654–662

Mobley HLT, Jarvis KG, Elwood JP, Whittle DI, Lockatell CV, Russell RG, Johnson DE, Donnenberg MS, Warren JW (1993) Isogenic P-fimbrial deletion mutants of pyelonephritogenic Escherichia coli: the role of αGal(1–4)βGal binding in virulence of a wild-type strain. Mol Microbiol 10: 143–155

Morimoto C, Letvin NL, Boyd AW, Hagan M, Brown HM, Kornacki MM, Schlossman SF (1985) The isolation and characterization of the human helper-inducer T-cell subset. I. Immunol 134: 3762

Mundi H, Bjorksten B, Svanborg C, Ohman L, Dahlgren C (1991) Extracellular release of reactive oxygen species from human neutrophils upon interaction with Escherichia coli strains causing renal scarring. Infect Immun 59: 4168–4172

Murray HW (1990) Gamma interferon, cytokine-induced macrophage activation, and antimicrobial host defense. In vitro in animal models, and in humans. Diagn Microbial Infect Dis 13: 411

Natanson C, Eichenholz PW, Danner RL, Eichacker PQ, Hoffman WD, Kuo GC, Banks SM, macVittie TJ, Parrillo JE (1989) Endotoxin and tumor necrosis factor challenges in dogs simulate the cardiovascular profile of human septic shock. J Exp Med 169: 823

Neal DE Jr, Kaack MB, Baskin G, Roberts JA (1991) Attenuation of antibody response to acute pyelonephritis by treatment with antibiotics. Antimicrob Agents Chemother 35: 2340–2344

Norgren M, Baga M, Tennent JM et al (1987) Nucleotide sequence, regulation and functional analysis of the papC gene required for cell surface localization of Pap pili of uropathogenic Escherichia coli. Mol Microbiol 1: 169–178

Normark S, Lark D, Hull R, Norgren M, Bagga M, O'Hanley P, Schoolnik G, Falkow S (1983) Genetics of digalactoside-binding adhesin from a uropathogenic Escherichia coli strain. Infect Immun 41: 942–949

O'Hanley P, Lark D, Falkow S, Schoolnik G (1985) Molecular basis of Escherichia coli colonization of the upper urinary tract in BALB/c mice: Gal-Gal pili immunization prevents E. coli pyelonephritis in the BALB/c mouse and model of human pyelonephritis. J Clin Invest 75: 347–360

Ohlsson K, Björk P, Bergenfeld M, Hageman R, Thompson RC (1990) Interleukin-1 receptor antagonist reduces mortality from endotoxin shock. Nature 348: 550

Okusawa S, Gelfand JA, Ikejima T, Connolly RJ, Dinarello CA (1988) Interleukin 1 induces a shock-like state in rabbits. J Clin Invest 81: 1162

Ormrod D, Cawley S, Miller T (1986) Neutrophil-mediated tissue destruction in experimental pyelonephritis. In: Kass EH, Svanborg Eden C (eds) Host-parasite interactions in urinary tract infections. University of Chicago, Chicago, pp 365–368

Paller MS (1989) Effect of neutrophil depletion on ischemic renal injury in the rat. J Lab Clin Med 113: 379–386

Paquet N (1984) Detection of complement-coated bacteria in experimental urinary tract infections. Master's thesis, University of Geneva, Geneva

Patarroyo M, Makgoba (1989) Leucocyte adhesion to cells in immune and inflammatory responses. Lancet 2: 1139–1142

Plos K, Hull SI, Hull RA et al (1989) Distribution of the P-associated-pilus (pap) region among E. coli from natural sources. Evidence for horizontal gene transfer. Infect Immun 57: 1604–1611

Ransley PG, Risdon RA (1978) Reflux and renal scarring. Br J Radiol [Suppl] 14: 1–34

Ransley PG, Risdon RA (1981) Reflux nephropathy: effects of antimicrobial therapy on the evolution of the early pyelonephritic scar. Kidney Int 20: 733–742

Richards C, Gauldie J, Baumann H (1991) Cytokine control of acute-phase protein expression. Eur Cytokine Network 2: 89–98

Risdon RA, Yeung CK, Ransley PG (1993) Reflux nephropathy in children submitted to unilateral nephrectomy: a clinicopathological study. Clin Nephrol 40: 308–314

Roberts JA (1975) Experimental pyelonephritis in the monkey. III. Pathophysiology of ureteral malfunction induced by bacteria. Invest Urol 13: 117–120

Roberts JA (1987) Bacterial adherence and urinary tract infection. South Med J 80: 347–351

Roberts JA, Roth JK Jr, Domingue G, Lewis RW, Kaack B, Baskin G (1982) Immunology of pyelonephritis in the primate model. V. Effect of superoxide dismutase. J Urol 128: 1394–1400

Roberts JA, Roth JK Jr, Domingue G, Lewis RW, Kaack B, Baskin GB (1983) Immunology of pyelonephritis in the primate model. VI. Effect of complement depletion. J Urol 129: 193–196

Roberts JA, Kaack B, Källenius G, Möllby R, Winberg J, Svenson SB (1984) Receptors for pyelonephritogenic Escherichia coli in primates. J Urol 131: 163–168

Roberts JA, Suarez GM, Kaack B, Källenius G, Svenson SB (1985) Experimental pyelonephritis in the monkey. VII. Ascending pyelonephritis in the absence of vesicoureteral reflux. J Urol 133: 1068–1075

Roberts JA, Kaack MB, Fussell EF, Baskin G (1986) Immunology of pyelonephritis. VII. Effect of allopurinol. J Urol 136: 960–963

Roberts JA, Kaack MB, Baskin G, Korhonen TK, Svenson SB, Winberg J (1989) P-fimbriae vaccines. II. Cross-reactive protection against pyelonephritis. Pediatr Nephrol 3: 391–396

Roberts JA, Kaack MB, Baskin G (1990) Treatment of experimental pyelonephritis in the monkey. J Urol 143: 150–154

Roberts JA, Kaack MB, Baskin G, Martin LN (1993) Events leading to septic death from experimental acute pyelonephritis in the monkey. J Urol 150: 1030–1033

Rosenberg AR (1991) Vesico-ureteric reflux and antenatal sonography. In: Bailey RR (ed) Proceedings of 2nd CJ Hodson symposium on reflux nephropathy. Design Printing Services, Christchurch pp 1–2

Rosenfield AT, Glickman MG, Taylor KJW, Crade M, Hopson J (1979) Acute focal bacterial nephritis (acute lobar nephronia). Radiology 132: 553–561

Rushton HG, Majd M, Jantausch B, Wiedermann BL, Belman AB (1992) Renal scarring following reflux and nonreflux pyelonephritis in children: evaluation with ^{99m}technetium-dimercaptosuccinic and scintigraphy. J Urol 147: 1327–1332

Sanders ME, Makgoba MW, Sharrow SO, Stephany D, Spriunger TA, Young HA, Shaw S (1988) Human memory T lymphocytes express increased levels of three cell adhesion molecules (LFA-3, CD2, and LFA-1) and three other molecules (UCHL-1, CDw29, Pgp-1) and have enhanced IFN g production. J Immunol 140: 1401

Scharer K (1971) Incidence and causes of chronic renal failure in childhood. In: Cameron JS, Fries D, Ogg CS (eds) Dialysis and renal transplantation. Pitman Medical Books, Berlin, pp 211–217

Schmidt MA, O'Hanley P, Schoolnik GK (1984) Gal-Gal pyelonephritis Escherichia coli pili: linear, immunogenic, and antigenic epitopes. J Exp Med 161: 705–717

Schrier RW, Harris DCH, Chan L, Shapiro JI, Caramelo C (1988) Tubular hypermetabolism as a factor in the progression of chronic renal failure. Am J Kidney Dis 12: 243–249

Skoog SJ, Belman AB, Majd M (1987) Nonsurgical approach to the management of primary vesicoureteral reflux. J Urol 138: 941–946

Slotki IN, Asscher AW (1982) Prevention of scarring in experimental pyelonephritis in the rat by early antibiotic therapy. Nephron 30: 262–268

Smellie JM, Normand ICS (1975) Bacteriuria, reflux and renal scarring. Arch Dis Child 50: 548–585

Smellie JM, Edwards D, Hunter N, Normann ICS, Prescod N (1975) Vesicoureteric reflux and renal scarring. Kidney Int 8: S65–S72

Smellie JM, Ransley PG, Normand ICS, Prescod N, Edwards D (1985) Development of new renal scars: a collaborative study. Br Med J 290: 1957–1960

Smith TW jr, Roberts JA (1978) Chronic pyelonephritis. II. Persistence of variant bacterial forms. Invest Urol 16: 154–162

Starnes HF jr, Pearce MK, Tewari A, Yim HJ, Zou J-C, Abrams JS (1990) Anti-IL-6 monoclonal antibodies protect against lethal *Escherichia coli* infection and lethal tumor necrosis factor α challenge in mice. J Immunol 145: 4185

Steele BT, Robitaile P, DeMaria J, Grignon A (1989) Follow-up evaluation of prenatally recognised vesicoureteric reflux. J Pediatr 115: 95–96

Sullivan MJ, Harvey RA, Shimamura T (1977) The effects of cobra venom factor, an inhibitor of the complement system, on the sequence of morphological events in the rat kidney in experimental pyelonephritis. Yale J Biol Med 50: 267–273

Svanborg-Edén C, Hanson LÅ, Jodal U, Lindberg U (1976) Variable adherence to normal human urinary-tract epithelial cells of *Escherichia coli* strains associated with various forms of urinary-tract infection. Lancet 2: 490–492

Svenson S, Hultberg H, Källenius G, Korhonen TK, Möllby R, Winberg J (1983) P-fimbriae of pyelonephritogenic *E. coli*: identification and chemical characterization of receptors. Infection 11: 61–67

Väisänen V, Elo J Tallgren LG, Siitonen A, Makela PH, Svanborg Edén C, Källenius G, Svenson SB, Hultberg H, Korhonen TK (1981) Mannose-resistant haemagglutination and P-antigen recognition characteristic of *E. coli* causing primary pyelonephritis. Lancet 2: 1366–1369

Van Deventer SJH, Büller HR, Ten Cate JW, Aarden LA, Hack CE, Struck A (1990) Experimental endotoxaemia in humans: analysis of cytokine release and coagulation, fibrinolytic, and complement pathway. Blood 76: 2520

Van Gool JD (1979) Bladder infection and pressure. In: Hodson J, Kincaid-Smith P (eds) Reflux nephropathy. Masson, New York, pp 181–189

Waage A, Brandtzaeg P, Halstensen A, Kierulf P, Espevik T (1989) The complex pattern of cytokines in serum from patients with meningococcal septic shock. Association between interleukin 6, interleukin 1, and fatal outcome, J Exp Med 169: 333

Walker RD (1994) Vesicoureteral reflux update: effect of prospective studies on current management. Urology 43: 279–283

Ward PA, Cochrane GC, Müller-Eberhard HJ (1965) The role of serum complement in chemotaxis of leukocytes in vitro. J Exp Med 122: 327–346

Winberg J, Andersen HJ, Berstrom T, Jacobsson B, Larson H, Lincoln K (1974) Epidemiology of symptomatic urinary tract infection in childhood. Acta Pathol Scand [Suppl 252: 1–20

Winberg J, Bollgren I, Källenius G, Möllby R, Svenson SB (1982) Clinical pyelonephritis and focal renal scarring. A selected review of pathogenesis, prevention, and prognosis. Pediatr Clin N Amer 29: 801–813

Winrow VR, Winyard PG, Morris CJ, Blake DR (1993) Free radicals in inflammation: second messengers and mediators of tissue destruction. Br Med Bull 49: 506–522

Winter AL, Hardy BE, Alton DJ, Arubs GS, Churchill BM (1983) Acquired renal scars in children. J Urol 129: 1190–1194

Wiswell TE, Smith FR, Bass JW (1985) Decreased incidence of urinary tract infections in circumcised male infants. Pediatrics 75: 901–903

Ziegler EJ, Fisher CJ jr, Sprung CL, Straube RC, Sadoff JC, Foulke GE, Wortel CH, Fink MP, Dellinger RP, Teng NNH, Allen IE, Berger HJ, Knatterud SL, LoBuglio AF, Smith CR, and the HA-1A Sepsis Study Group (1991) Treatment of gram-negative bacteremia and septic shock with HA-1A human monoclonal antibody against endotoxin. A randomized, double-blind, placebo-controlled trial. N Engl J Med 324: 429

Subject Index

Index of Volumes 86, 87 and 89 Current Topics in Pathology

Springer-Verlag
and the Environment

We at Springer-Verlag firmly believe that an international science publisher has a special obligation to the environment, and our corporate policies consistently reflect this conviction.

We also expect our business partners – paper mills, printers, packaging manufacturers, etc. – to commit themselves to using environmentally friendly materials and production processes.

The paper in this book is made from low- or no-chlorine pulp and is acid free, in conformance with international standards for paper permanency.